Changing the Global Approach to Medicine

Volume 3

Changing the Global Approach to Medicine

Volume 3

CELLULAR COMMAND AND CONTROL

Lane B. Scheiber II, MD

and

Lane B. Scheiber, ScD

iUniverse, Inc.
Bloomington

Changing the Global Approach to Medicine, Volume 3
Cellular Command and Control

This text is intended for educational and entertainment purposes. This text is not intended to take the place of a physician's evaluation or a physician's advice regarding any medical condition. It is recommended the reader consult their physician before starting any medication for any medical condition. All medications have potential side effects. Healthcare providers should review current prescribing information before prescribing medications; patients should review the latest prescribing information and side effects before taking any medication.

At the time of copyright the authors believed the concepts to be unique and different from prior art. All figures are meant to be illustrative concepts of otherwise sometimes very complex structures.

iUniverse books may be ordered through booksellers or by contacting:

iUniverse
1663 Liberty Drive
Bloomington, IN 47403
www.iuniverse.com
1-800-Authors (1-800-288-4677)

Because of the dynamic nature of the Internet, any web addresses or links contained in this book may have changed since publication and may no longer be valid. The views expressed in this work are solely those of the author and do not necessarily reflect the views of the publisher, and the publisher hereby disclaims any responsibility for them.

ISBN: 978-1-4759-2220-2 (sc)
ISBN: 978-1-4759-2221-9 (ebk)

Printed in the United States of America

iUniverse rev. date: 06/06/2012

Suggested Additional Reading:

CHANGING THE GLOBAL APPROACH TO MEDICINE, Volume 1
New Perspectives on Treating AIDS, Diabetes, Obesity, Aging,
Heart Attacks, Stroke, and Cancer
by Lane B. Scheiber II, MD and Lane B. Scheiber, ScD

CHANGING THE GLOBAL APPROACH TO MEDICINE, Volume 2
Medical Vector Therapy
Also introducing the Quantum Gene and the Quadsistor
by Lane B. Scheiber II, MD and Lane B. Scheiber, ScD

IMMORTALITY: QUATERNARY MEDICINE CODE
by Anthony Scheiber

THE HUMAN COMPUTER
by Anthony Scheiber

CURSE OF THE SNOW DRAGON
by Anthony Scheiber

EARTH PRO: The Rings of Sol
by Anthony Scheiber

Dedication

Thanks to our wives, Karin and Mary Jane,
for all of their love and support without which this
effort could never have been accomplished.
Thanks to Pat for letting us hold our workshops
in her exquisite place on the beach.

OBJECTIVE:

Deciphering COMMAND & CONTROL leads to
recognition of INTELLIGENCE,

INTELLIGENCE leads to a requirement for STRUCTURE,
rather than the alternative, that of random chaos,

ARCHITECTURE is compulsory for the presence of
STRUCTURED INTELLIGENCE,

Acknowledgement of ARCHITECTURE necessitates DESIGN,

Study of DESIGN leads to understanding the intentions of the
DESIGNER.

Seeking the DESIGNER leads to discovery of . . .
ORIGIN.

THE ASTRONOMICAL DILEMMA

Charles Darwin is globally well-recognized as a genus, especially in light of the academic standards of the eighteen hundreds. Darwin's Theory of Evolution represented a brilliant masterpiece in the amalgamation of the prevailing science and the art of scientific observation for the year 1859, when Darwin's book *On the Origin of Species* was published.

One hundred and fifty three years later, today's scientist has the advantage of a larger, more expansive data base and a more advanced understanding of science and technology with which to work with, than what was available to Charles Darwin in his time. For a Theory of Evolution based on the modus operandi that a series of random events were solely responsible for the appearance of life on Earth to be practical, such a theory would have to account for all of the following critical biophysiology:

- 3.5 billion years ago, with no cellular means or strategy or design in existence, a spherical membrane would have had to have spontaneously formed.
- A pool of twenty different nitrogen containing amino acid molecules would have had to randomly collected inside the boundaries of the spherical cell membrane.
- Amino acids can be right-handed or left-handed. Biologically active amino acid molecules are all left-handed. Therefore, all twenty different amino acids would all have to have spontaneously appeared as left-handed amino acids.
- Amongst this pool of twenty exclusively left-handed amino acids, the 327 amino acid chain necessary to generate one of the four molecules comprising the *nitrogenase molecule* would have had to have formed, lined up in the proper order, and spontaneously attached themselves together.

- Given the nitrogenase enzyme complex is a tetramer molecule consisting of two pairs of identical chains, the process of creating the nitrogenase molecules requires two different lengthy amino acid chains to have spontaneously formed with each chain occurring in the identical form twice.
- In the same primitive cell the 'reductase enzyme' would have also had to have been spontaneously generated. Nitrate reductase can be 743 amino acids in length. Reductase works with the nitrogenase enzyme to fix nitrogen.
- At this point nitrogen can be readily fixed by the primitive cell into organic molecules.
- In order to pass the blueprints of how to construct the nitrogenase molecule on to the next generation of daughter cells, spontaneously and independently four different nucleotides would have had to have appeared. These four different types of nucleotides would need to link in proper sequence of 981 nucleotides to form a DNA molecule.
- Spontaneously the machinery to transcribe the DNA, the forty proteins that comprise the transcription complex, would have had to have formed.
- Spontaneously a fifth nucleotide, Uracil, would have had to have formed and be available in a sufficient amount to be utilized by the transcription complex to form RNA.
- Spontaneously the ribosomal proteins and ribosomal RNAs would have had to have formed in order to translate the nitrogenous enzyme's RNA to produce the nitrogenase enzyme. Now there exists in this primitive cell the chance to actively replicate the nitrogenous enzyme. At this point there is only one gene. This one gene is the gene to create the nitrogenase enzyme, which is essential to life.
- Now the DNA for all of the proteins necessary for life must randomly and spontaneously form. To create the human form at least 32,000 individual segments of DNA had to have randomly and spontaneously formed all in their proper order of nucleotide sequencing.
- After the DNA forms, for genetic material to be copied such that it can be passed on to daughter cells the DNA

polymerase molecule consisting of 900-1000 amino acids needs to spontaneously appear.
- Then to generate a gene to account for the DNA polymerase molecule, a string of 2700 to 3000 nucleotides need to spontaneously line up in proper sequence and link together so that the means to replicate the DNA polymerase molecule can be passed on to future generations of daughter cells.

For all practical purposes the above is all beyond astronomical probability.

Further, if evolution was random one would see the reverse happening, i.e., animals becoming fish and going back into the sea, and that doesn't happen. Evolution may move horizontally, but generally evolution appears only to move forward.

The Astronomical Dilemma is that it is beyond astronomical calculations that organic life's critical dependency upon nitrogen as a building block to generate 'the organic molecules needed to create life' occurred by random chance or that more importantly the far more complex 'segments of genetic instructions' required to pass the information regarding the processes to generate these organic molecules on to future generations occurred by random chance.

As a result of the above observations it is obvious, an updated Theory of Evolution is needed. The new theory needs to be based on the current understanding of cell biology and genetics merged with engineering and computer science principles. In this book we begin to establish the foundation for a revolutionary new theory of how life evolved on Earth.

FOREWORD

Science has developed a nomenclature for just about everything that is known to exist, except for one very basic and fundamental set of processes . . . . the command, control, communication and intelligence functions present in a cell. The eukaryote cell represents the most reliable, most durable, the most complex piece of biologic machinery, the longest known nucleus driven inorganic system in existence and yet, how the eukaryote cell functions has remained a mystery.

This book discusses the critical concept of command and control in the cell, which is a vital concept to cell growth, maturation, operation, survival and reproduction.

In order for processes to occur in an orderly fashion, a labeling system that uniquely identifies each gene, each messenger RNA and each protein must exist. Labels can be thought of in terms of names or numbers or a combination of a name and a number. Whether the labels of this unique identification system are assigned names, numbers, or some combination, these functional labels are derived from a base-four code and are comprised of a segment of nucleotides or physical structures such as protein molecules that mimic a segment of nucleotides.

By incorporating a labeling system of unique identifiers, the eukaryote cell is able to utilize control RNAs to influence the transcriptions of specific genes, utilize ribosomal RNAs to translate specific messenger RNAs, utilize command RNAs to build specific complex proteins and utilize control proteins to provide feedback to regulate the cell's nuclear functions. Cells are able to utilize the labeling nomenclature to generate hormones in order to facilitate communication between cells in order to be able to coordinate the efforts of the nucleus of cells for the benefit of a multi-cellular organism. From these crucial concepts we develop a working nomenclature to effectively describe cellular command, control, and communications between cells and finally the intelligence of a cell.

The existence of the cell can be explained in surprising detail by simplistically surmising 'All protein production is a dynamic process created by static intelligence stored in the DNA, facilitated by command and control RNAs influencing the production of messenger RNAs which are used as templates to generate proteins, the rate of production being controlled by signaling proteins and control RNAs'.

The presence of a labeling system indicates that intelligence is structured into the DNA.

The time has come to unshackle the community from the antiquated pillars of philosophy that 'randomness' and 'chance mutation' represent the driving force that has led to evolution of life on our planet. We have arrived at the point of intellectual and scientific curiosity where the existence and actions of a Prime DNA Genome, responsible for the appearance of all organic life that has inhabited the Earth, needs to be brought to the forefront of our attention and the content of this Prime Genome defined and the knowledge carried by such a design fully explored.

This third book in this series discusses command and control aspects of the cell with the ultimate goal being to develop innovative cures for today's challenging diseases that plague the human body. Understanding the role of computer programming inherent in the DNA and the command and control instructions by which the cell operates will lead to deciphering means to adjust the programming when cells are failing or when cells are in crisis.

One such intention is to use bioprogramming repair techniques to regrow the cartilage of the knee. Osteoarthritis is a musculoskeletal joint condition where cartilage wears off the surface of joints and this afflicts pain and disability in a majority of the population as people age. At the present time there is no medical means of intervention to stop or retard this process of degeneration of cartilage. The chondrocytes that originally grew the cartilage of the knee certainly have the knowledge of how to grow the cartilage inherent in their genetic programming. Medically stimulating the chondrocytes in the proper way in order to reactivate the bioprogramming instructions to regrow the cartilage would seem a much more palatable choice than surgically removing bone and replacing it with metal and plastic as is currently the approach to the osteoarthritic knee.

This third volume opens with a brief discussion of basic cell design. The text then moves to defining the organizational principles of the programming aspects of the DNA and cell function. The concepts of command and control are brought into perspective. The organization of the DNA is defined primarily as an instruction code, the variation in the organization of the instruction coding being responsible for the differing life forms that have inhabited the Earth over the last three and an half billion years. Innovative new opportunities for medical therapies, based on a better understanding of bioprogramming and command and control, are discussed toward the end of the text. Finally, an attempt to explain magnetism and gravity is embarked upon, which the solution neatly ties the macro and micro universe together into one simple theme. Lastly, the explanation of life and evolution leads to a scientific plan to search for origin.

TABLE OF CONTENTS

Introduction...xxiii

Part 1 Cellular Basics..1

Chapter 1:   Chloroplast: The Key to Life....................................3
Chapter 2:   Basic Cell and Virus Design....................................8
Chapter 3:   Construct of the DNA...13
Chapter 4:   Construct of the Gene..16
Chapter 5:   Translation: Decoding of mRNA Produces Proteins...24
Chapter 6:   Updating the Central Dogma of Microbiology.........29

Part 2 Unique Identification..31

Chapter 7:   Concept of Unique Identification.............................33
Chapter 8:   Quantum Gene...42
Chapter 9:   Gene versus Quantum Gene...................................52
Chapter 10:   Quantum mRNA...54
Chapter 11:   Quantum rRNA..57

Part 3 Elements of Cellular Command and Control...............59

Chapter 12:   Origin of Cellular Command and Control................61
Chapter 13:   Concept of Communication...................................69
Chapter 14:   Concept of Intelligence.......................................72

Part 4 Command and Control Operations of the Cell...........79

Chapter 15:   Nuclear Signaling Proteins...................................81
Chapter 16:   Hormone: Cell-to-Cell Communication...................86

Chapter 17: Control RNA...89
Chapter 18: Command RNA: Complex Protein Manufacturing.....94
Chapter 19: Distributed Processing in the DNA........................98
Chapter 20: Mapping Out the DNA...103
Chapter 21: Genetic Reference Tables....................................107
Chapter 22: Command, Control, Communication
            and Intelligence...125
Chapter 23: Universal Dogma of Microbiology 128

Part 5 Viral Influences in Cell Command and Control.........131

Chapter 24: Viral DNA Present in Human Genome...................133
Chapter 25: Viral Influences on Cell Command and Control....135
Chapter 26: Viral Influences on DNA by Adding New DNA.......136
Chapter 27: Viral Influences on DNA by Switching Gene
            Expression On and Off.......................................138
Chapter 28: HIV: Nature's Teaching Tool...............................141

Part 6 Origin of the Atmosphere, Water, Life 145

Chapter 29: The Crux of the Nitrogen Cycle...........................147

Part 7 Ecometabolous...165

Chapter 30: Prime Genome...167
Chapter 31: Ecometabolous versus Evolution.........................171
Chapter 32: Ecometabolous and the Brain.............................180
Chapter 33: Evidence of the Prime Genome...........................184

Part 8 Opportunities 189

Chapter 34: Opportunities for Medical Therapies 191

Part 9 Summary 201

Chapter 35: Summary of Concepts 203

Post Script One..**207**

One: Bio Programming Means to Cure
             Degenerative Arthritis 207
Two: Building Hydrocarbons To Fuel The World's
             Energy Needs 211
Three: Musical Key Codes 215
Four: The Text Files Yet to be Discovered......................220
Five: The Fabric of Space: Sub^2 Atomic Particle
             Physics Theory 228
Six: The Enigma of the Magnet Solved 238
Seven: Principles of Gravity: From the Atom
             to the Black Hole..244
Eight: The Great Albatross of Physics: 'LIGHT' 273
Nine: Polymyalgia Rheumatica Explained 280
Ten: A Systems Engineer's Approach to a Cure for HIV 284
Eleven: Mars Proof-of-Origin Project 288

Glossary & Abbreviations...**307**

PATENT APPLICATIONS BOOK III **313**

No. 1: QUANTUM UNIT OF INHERITANCE VECTOR THERAPY 314
No. 2: QUANTUM UNIT OF INHERITANCE VECTOR THERAPY
        METHOD 367
No. 3: CONFIGURABLE MICROSCOPIC MEDICAL PAYLOAD
        DELIVERY DEVICE TO DELIVER NUCLEAR SIGNALING
        PROTEINS TO SPECIFIC CELLS TO MANAGE DIABETES
        MELLITUS AND GENETIC DEFICIENCY DISORDERS 420
No. 4: CONFIGURABLE MICROSCOPIC MEDICAL PAYLOAD
        DELIVERY DEVICE TO DELIVER CONTROL RNAS TO
        SPECIFIC CELLS TO MANAGE DIABETES MELLITUS
        AND GENETIC DEFICIENCY DISORDERS........................... 454
No. 5: CONFIGURABLE MICROSCOPIC MEDICAL PAYLOAD
        DELIVERY DEVICE TO DELIVER COMMAND RNAS TO
        SPECIFIC CELLS TO MANAGE DIABETES MELLITUS
        AND GENETIC DEFICIENCY DISORDERS........................... 484

INTRODUCTION

This book takes what has been a black box of genetics and cell biology and strives to create a framework with which to move forward in an effort to better define and understand the human genome and cell functions. Much of the subject matter in this text has been contrived by extrapolating information from human technologies and by seeking answers to explain intricate organic life-sustaining processes that have been ongoing for hundreds of millions of years prior to man ever setting foot on the planet. Proving some of the concepts presented in this book involves parallel data analysis of the genome of numerous species, which is achievable, but beyond the scope of this text at this time. This text is meant to act as scaffolding, from which a concrete foundation of knowledge pertaining to the biologic computer programming coded in the DNA and the biologic programming acting to control cell functions can be assimilated and defined.

This volume, of the series *Changing the Global Approach to Medicine,* is subtitled *Cellular Command and Control* because we believe this is will be the objective of the future of medical research. As one delves into the subject of command and control in the cell, clear similarities begin to emerge that parallel human computer programming strategies. To understand the importance of command and control to the health of our bodies we start with the central dogma of molecular biology. This dogma states that the genes present in the DNA are transcribed into mRNAs, which are then translated to generate proteins. The human genome contains a complete set of hereditary information which is functionally divided into genes. Each gene is a sequence of nucleotides, which will produce an RNA; in the case of a messenger RNA this is to be translated to generate a particular protein molecule. The human genome is thought to contain at least 32,000 genes.

To maintain order within a cell at least two control systems are required for the production of each protein. One control system is required at the RNA production level, while a second control system must be present at the protein production level. The cell must be capable of governing the timing of producing a specific protein as well as producing the quantity of the protein that the cell needs.

Command and control processes are intimately involved in our daily lives. Simple command and control mechanisms continuously monitor and adjust the air conditioning units that heat and cool our homes and businesses we visit. More elaborate command and control systems assist in the launch and guidance of the missiles used to place satellites in orbit around the earth. In this book we examine cellular command and control at the DNA/RNA/protein level along with the communications and intelligence necessary to generate RNA and proteins. To understand the magnitude of the problem a house generally has a few command and control systems, the heater/air conditioner being the most notable. Cars have dozens and factories have hundreds, while human cells, which we cannot ever see with the naked eye, have thousands,

In order to better understand the impact command and control has on our bodies, it is necessary to have an understanding of what a command and control system is capable of doing in the world around us. We describe the basics of command and control systems in the following using examples derived from ordinary life. Elements of this discussion can be related to the operation of a cell, e.g., the protein production processes in a cell.

Figure 1 provides a basic overview of the command and control process utilized by engineers to govern technology. The objective of the command and control system in the figure is to maintain the density of a specific protein at a specified level. This level is generally referred to as the command. The control function compares the commanded level against what its sensors sense the actual density to be. Using the result of this comparison, the control function then adjusts its input to the protein production process to bring the sensed density in line with the commanded density. In dynamic systems, where the environment is capable of changing, environmental sensors are utilized to adjust the command function such that the system meets the overall objective in face of changing requirements brought about by changes in the environment.

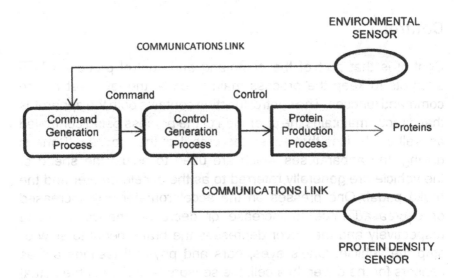

Figure 1
Overview of Cellular Command and Control

An introduction to the elements of Command and Control

Command

Command is the objective in the command and control process. For example, when driving your car you have a certain speed to maintain whether it is the posted speed limit or just keeping up with the traffic surrounding the vehicle. Cells also have command objectives. An objective in a pancreatic cell might be maintaining an adequate quantity of insulin at a specific amount stored in vacuoles within the cell to be released into circulation as required by the prevailing serum glucose level. If the level of insulin falls below the objective level the blood glucose level may not be adequately regulated. On the other hand, an oversupply of insulin could take up excessive volume within the pancreas cell and either interfere with cell function or damage the cell. Thus, Command expresses an objective like the desired density of a specific protein in the cytoplasm.

Control

Control is that part of the command and control process which attempts to keep the process maintained at the level set by the command function. The control function contains both the apparatus that directly maintains the operation of the process being controlled as well as devices that sense the output of the process. If one is driving, the apparatuses which are used to adjust the speed of the vehicle are generally referred to as the accelerometer and the brake pedal. One presses on the accelerometer with increased or decreased force to increase or decrease the car's speed respectively and the driver depresses the brake pedal to slow or stop the vehicle. One's eyes, ears and physical feelings act as sensors for the driver. In a cell, the sensors take note of the actual density of a specific protein in the cytoplasm. Thus, control is the apparatus which attempts to drive the production process such that the density of the protein being produced reaches, but does not exceed, the level dictated by the command function.

Communications

Communication is the means to send and receive data. Internal to a cell, communication is carried out via command proteins and command and control RNA molecules.

Intelligence

Intelligence interprets available data, makes decisions, and dictates to the command function that an adjustment must be made in the parameters being used in the command and control process. In the case of driving a car, if a storm is encountered the speed of the vehicle may be reduced for purposes of safe handling of the vehicle even though the posted speed limit may remain the same.

Command, Control, Communication and Intelligence as Related to Health

The human body contains numerous command and control processes, most of which regulate the health of the body at the subconscious level. In a healthy individual, the action of production of the thyroid hormone by the thyroid gland is a clear example of a command and control process.

There are numerous intracellular and extracellular communications elements present throughout the body. Hormones are obvious extracellular communications devices. These RNA molecules act as one of many intracellular communications devices. Intelligence can be appreciated at the conscious level as well as at the subconscious level of brain function. Consciously we observe and react to our environment. Subconsciously our body makes calculations and analyzes features regarding the environment that surrounds us and attempts to adjust to them.

As the features of command, control, communication and intelligence come to the forefront of awareness, it is easy to draw parallels to current computer technologies. Much of the command, control, and communications that we interact with in our daily lives are currently being aided by some form of computer technology. Present day computers rely on elaborate computer programs. The computer programs housed inside the memory devices of computers are responsible for running both the essential functions of the computer system as well as being responsible for the many applications that a computer may run for its user.

The appearance of the cell phone in the market place which is a device that provides communication from one user to another is an illustration of a one dimensional device; on the other hand, a smart phone that provides the user with not only communications but also offers computer program applications to facilitate accomplishing additional tasks, offers an entirely new dimension in mobile phone capability.

Much of the advanced technologies available to humans are dependent upon some form of computer: the computer being dependent upon one or more computer programs for its operation. If human technologies are dependent upon computer programming, it is likely that biologic cells, which are much more complex than any human-made computer, are dependent upon some form of biologic computer programming.

Early human made computers were hardwired. The program stored in the computer was build into the memory portion of the machine and could not be altered. Later, computers were provided with the capability of having a disc inserted prior to the computer being turned on. While the computer was initiating its internal systems it would read the program off the disc and temporarily store the program in its memory; this was referred to as 'booting up the computer'. Once the computer memory had transferred the operating system software from the disc to the internal memory, the original disc could be swapped out for a disc that contained data and a computer operator could run a program to accomplish a computational task. Today computer memories are dynamic, allowing computer programs and computer data to be added to a computer's memory, stored in the computer's memory and deleted from memory at the whim of the computer user.

The most obvious likeness of a cell to a computer is the cell's genetic code. The DNA present in the nucleus of eukaryote cells is thought to act as the basis for growth, maintenance, and function of the cell. Transcription complexes act as mobile central processing units that decode the DNA to produce RNA molecules. In multi-cellular organisms, this same genome exists as an identical entity in each cell of a particular species, except for the sex cells, and contains the design, organization, function and replication protocols of the multi-cellular organism. The survivability of any multi-cellular species given the environment that the species exists in, testifies that the design, organization, function and reproduction protocols operate almost to the point of perfection. Survivability of any species, given the complexity of the internal and external chemical and protein processes that are required to sustain life in a hostile environment, strongly suggest that a biological computer program, comprised of numerous subprograms, has been at work to create life, possibly from the beginning of time that life has been recognized to have existed on planet Earth.

Further, to investigate the existence of a computer program, the concepts of the quantum gene and the language of the DNA have been proposed. All computer programs are comprised of a set of instructions. Some computer programs contain data. Instructions tell the computer the processes that it is to perform for the benefit of the user of the computer. Data is generally dynamic, meaning that it is often added to, modified, and/or deleted from memory to satisfy the computer's user. Data is generally only present in a computer program if the computer program is meant to stand alone and not have access to dynamic memory or have limited use of dynamic data located outside the computer program. A movie stored on DVD might be representative of a computer program that contains all of its data, such that when the program stored on the DVD is run the user is provided the same series of images on a video screen no matter how many times the computer program is run. On the other hand, a game program played on the internet with other gamers will contain some static data to produce the general video images of the game for the user, but the computer program running the game will also actively utilize dynamic data to show the user the changing positions and actions of the user himself or herself as well as the other players participating in the game.

Concepts that are presented and discussed in this book include:

1. A unique identification numbering system exists in the cell to direct protein manufacturing.
2. Genes are associated with a unique identification which gives rise to the term 'Quantum Gene'.
3. The unique identification associated with a gene is utilized to control transcription of the gene.
4. Messenger RNA (mRNA) molecules are associated with unique identification in the 5' region.
5. Unique identification associated with messenger RNA is used to control translation of the messenger RNA.
6. Command and Control functions are necessary features of cell growth and survival.

7. Communication occurs inside the boundaries of a cell and between cells in order to orchestrate coordinated functions necessary for growth, maintenance, survival and reproduction of the life form.

8. Ribosomal RNA (rRNA) molecules are associated with a unique identification coded to engage mRNA.

9. Control RNA (cnRNA) molecules possess a unique identification that directs the RNA to a specific gene and once contact is made the RNA's tail activates a transcription complex.

10. Nuclear Signaling Proteins, by means of their three dimensional structure which mimics the unique identification of a gene, are capable of locating a specific gene and activating a transcription complex to transcribe that gene and generate positive or negative feedback to the nucleus.

11. Command RNA molecules provide the instructions and interact with fixed ribosomes in smooth endoplasmic reticulum to facilitate modifications to proteins, including folding of proteins, cleaving proteins and linking of separate proteins to build complex proteins.

12. The DNA is comprised of static intelligence made up of: (a) reference tables, (b) bundled instructions, and (c) data files.

13. In addition to protein production, functional aspects of the DNA are contained in a programming language coded into the DNA.

14. A significant portion of the 95% of human genome considered to be redundant genetic material, is in fact, comprised of the instructions needed to construct the architectural features of the cell, the organs, and the body as a whole and to operate them individually and collectively.

15. Nuclear DNA contains information that has acted as the means to change organic life in a manner that has been recognized as evolution.

16. A Prime Genome existed on Earth prior to the first appearance of life and from this Prime Genome has sprung all of the species of organic life that have ever existed on the planet.

Ecometabolous is an emerging working hypothesis which refers to morphing that has occurred to the ecosystem that existed on the planet. Examined over its timeline, organic life has undergone complete metamorphosis: all designed and intended to take advantage of the hostile features of the planet, utilize the raw chemistry and physics initially present on the planet to create an ecosystem that could support higher order life such as the human form. The basis of ecometabolous is the Prime Genome. Such a genome carried all the instruction code needed to make the existence of all the species of organic life possible.

The Prime Genome provided the basic instructions needed to generate organic life, and by varying the emphasis of these preset instructions, created each and every species in a manner that best suited survival of the species given the prevailing conditions of the environment and location where the species existed. The main objective of the Prime Genome was to establish and populate the earth with layers of an ecosystem that would be sufficient to support a species that would understand the existence of this original genome and be capable of reproducing the Prime Genome. The final objective being to extend the survival of the Prime Genome and perpetrate the influence of the Prime Genome further into the surrounding galaxy.

Part 1

Cellular Basics

CHAPTER 1

CHLOROPLAST: THE KEY TO LIFE

The chloroplast is an organelle generally present in plant cells. The chloroplast is comprised of an outer and inner membrane. Contained inside the inner membrane is a fluid medium termed the stroma. Items suspended in the stroma include thylakoids, lamella, a number of identical molecules of DNA which carries the chloroplast gene, and ribosomes. A membrane surrounds the thylakoids and the lamella. The lamella refers to a system of vesicles that may be interconnected.

Thylakoids contain four types of protein assemblies. The four systems include Photosystem I, Photosystem II, Cytochromes b and f, and ATP synthase. These four systems comprise the light reactions of photosynthesis.

Photosynthesis refers to the process of synthesizing organic molecules, such as glucose, which utilize the energy of light as the power source.

Photosynthesis can be summarized as:

$$CO_2 + 2 H_2O \xrightarrow[\text{GREEN PLANTS}]{\text{LIGHT}} (CH_2O) + O_2 + H_2O$$

(CH_2O) represents general formula for carbohydrates.

Which says that by using the chemical processes inside the chloroplast, carbon is fixed to synthesize glucose molecules. The processes of photosynthesis are conducted in two reactions. The first reaction is referred to as the light reaction of photosynthesis and the second process is referred to as the dark reaction of photosynthesis. The dark reaction of photosynthesis does not mean there is a requirement that the processes are conducted in the dark, the name simply refers to the fact that light is not necessary for the reactions to proceed.

The dark reaction of photosynthesis can be summarized as:

$$ATP + NADPH + H^+ + CO_2 = ADP + P_i + NADP^+ + carbohydrate$$

Which says that . . . . . The dark reactions of photosynthesis occur in the stroma. The RUBISCO enzymes carry out the dark reactions to convert carbon dioxide into organic molecules such as glucose. The glucose molecule is a storable currency of energy being capable of being broken down in the mitochondria of animals to create adenosine triphosphate (ATP) molecules. ATP molecules are used as energy molecules by animal cells to drive energy-requiring chemical reactions.

The segments of DNA present in the stroma of the chloroplast represents copies of the chloroplast's genome. The genes in the chloroplast contain the genetic code to generate most of the molecules required for the chloroplast to function. Other enzymes required for chloroplast operations are transcribed from the cell's nuclear DNA, then translated in the cell's cytoplasm, to be transported into the chloroplast.

The key to the means of life is locked in the efforts of the chloroplast. The capacity for the chloroplast to absorb solar energy and utilize the natural power of the sun to fix carbon atoms together to form organic molecules is the necessary step required to create life.

The wavelengths of sunlight reaching the Earth spread across a spectrum of light. Shorter wavelengths are referred to as ultraviolet. The longer wavelengths are known as infrared. Light visible to humans exists between the ultraviolet and infrared wavelengths. The human eye detects colors between the wavelengths of 400-700 nm.

The shorter the wavelength of light the more energy the light carries. Color is the result of the differential absorption of visible light by various objects. An object appears of a certain color because it reflects that color and absorbs the light of the other colors. Objects that appear white reflect all colors of light. Objects that appear black absorb all colors.

To utilize the energy in light, light must be absorbed. Pigments, light absorbing molecules, capture light's energy. Plants that contain the pigment chlorophyll appear green, because green light is reflected while other wavelengths of light are absorbed. Bands of red and blue light tend to support photosynthesis most effectively. In addition to chlorophyll, chloroplasts may have accessory pigments that absorb light of wavelengths that 'chlorophyll a' cannot absorb and may transfer this trapped energy to 'chlorophyll a'.

Red algae and blue-green bacteria contain accessory pigments of a group referred to phycobilins. Phycobilins are composed of four pyrrole groups in linear arrangement rather than the ring structured molecules found in chlorophyll. Red algae reflect the visible light in the red portion of spectrum; blue-green algae reflect the visible light in the blue-green portion of the visible spectrum.

Carotenoids represent long hydrocarbon chains with ring structures at each end. Under high light intensities, the many double bonds in the chain of a carotenoid can break and bind with oxygen. The resulting molecules are thought to protect chlorophyll molecules against damage from high intensity light. All green plants contain some carotenoids. Carotenoids are generally yellow, orange and brown in color and are responsible for the color of ripe fruits and the hues of autumn leaves.

The capability of the chloroplast to take the radiant energy of the sun and produce adenosine triphosphate (ATP) molecules, then store the energy of the ATP molecules in organic molecules such as glucose is the defining feature that has acted as the foundation of the existence of life on the surface of this planet. Other forms of life such as thermophilic archaebacteria have utilized thermal energy from volcanoes and sulfur for their metabolism. But photosynthesis has taken advantage of the abundance of radiant energy being conveyed to the earth by the sun and has provided the primary source of energy molecules for utilization by organic life.

Plants are able to utilize the process of carbon fixation of the dark reaction of photosynthesis to generate monosaccharide molecules such as glucose and fructose. Monosaccharides are simple sugars that are used to generate complex carbohydrate molecules. Carbohydrate is a general term used to refer to simple sugars or complex sugar molecules. Monosaccharides are classified by the number of carbon atoms in the molecule; triose contains three carbons, tetroses contain four carbons, pentoses contain five carbons, hexoses contain six carbons, heptose contains seven. Most monosaccharides contain five or six carbons. An important pentose sugar is 'ribose', a component of ribonucleic acids (RNA). Certain species of plants are able to combine monosaccharide molecules to produce larger disaccharide molecules and polysaccharides molecules.

Disaccharides refer to a molecule comprised of two monosaccharides linked together. Maltose refers to a molecule comprised of two glucose molecules. Sucrose refers to a disaccharide comprised of one glucose molecule and one fructose molecule.

Polysaccharides refer to a molecule comprised of multiple monosaccharides linked together which is therefore considered to be a complex sugar molecule. Polysaccharides are generally comprised of monosaccharide molecules arranged in a linear fashion or comprised of monosaccharide molecules constructed in branches. Linear polysaccharides such a cellulose can be compacted tightly to form rigid structures. Branched polysaccharides are water soluble and tend to form pastes.

Life represents the organized use of energy. The chloroplast is an essential organelle that helps to accomplish the task of organizing energy. The light reaction of photosynthesis absorbs the energy of radiant light and traps it in ATP molecules, then utilizes the chemical energy stored in ATP molecules to fix carbon into organic molecules, again trapping energy to be used at a later time as a resource for the plant or as an energy source for animals. Fixing carbon to produce complex molecules such as polysaccharides creates the capacity to generate the necessary molecules required for life such as cellulose, starches, fats, and alcohols.

Undeniably, the chloroplast is the one organelle that supports the existence of all higher orders life. Without the pigments contained in the chloroplast trapping the radiant energy of the sun, and the dark reaction of photosynthesis fixing carbon into organic molecules, animal life would not have had the necessary energy source to exist and flourish on the planet's surface.

The chloroplast is the key to life. In addition to providing an abundant source of energy molecules to animals, the chloroplast converted a hostile atmosphere to an atmosphere rich in oxygen which could support higher animal life through an aerobic respiratory process at the cell level that includes oxidative phosphorylation. The chloroplast is an intricate, double walled organelle comprised of a sophisticated orchestration of biochemical processes, the fundamentals of which still challenge the wisdom of science.

When the intricacies of the chloroplast are examined, it is difficult to fathom that the chloroplast, the essential constituent of organic life, just randomly appeared in nature near the beginning of life's timeline with no intellectual input to guide its construction. It is hard to accept that 'randomness' generated such a highly evolved energy producing factory, that by its design, still today surpasses the best that human technology can offer.

7

CHAPTER 2

BASIC CELL AND VIRUS DESIGN

The Cell

A prokaryote refers to a nonnucleated cell, such as bacteria, which has no compartment, such as a nucleus, where the genome of the organism is consolidated. Eukaryote refers to a nucleated cell. Eukaryotes comprise nearly all animal and plant cells. Fungi and Protista (protozoa and certain algae) are also considered to be eukaryote cells.

A human eukaryote cell is comprised of an exterior lipid bilayer plasma membrane, cytoplasm, a nucleus, and organelles. The exterior plasma membrane defines the perimeter of the cell. It regulates the flow of nutrients, water, and regulating molecules into and out of the cell, and has embedded into its structure receptors that the cell uses to detect properties of the environment surrounding the cell membrane. The cytoplasm acts as a filling medium inside the boundaries of the plasma cell membrane and is comprised mainly of water and nutrients such as amino acids, oxygen, and glucose.

The nucleus contains the majority of the cell's genetic information in the form of double stranded deoxyribonucleic acid (DNA). The nucleus, organelles, and ribosomes are suspended in the cytoplasm. Organelles, which carry out specialized functions of the cell, include the Golgi apparatus, mitochondria, smooth endoplasmic reticulum, and vacuoles. See Figure 2. The Golgi apparatus constructs molecules and packages these molecules in a vacuole. Vacuoles act as storage medium for chemicals, hormones and hybrid molecules. The smooth endoplasmic reticulum constructs complex protein molecules. The mitochondria act as the powerhouse of the cell converting glucose into usable chemical energy.

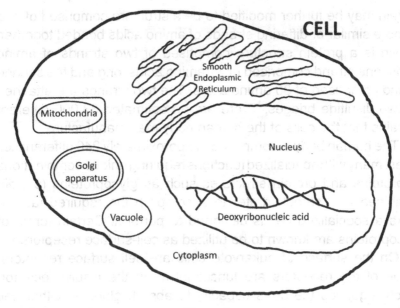

CELL

Smooth Endoplasmic Reticulum

Mitochondria

Golgi apparatus

Vacuole

Nucleus

Deoxyribonucleic acid

Cytoplasm

Figure 2
Basic Cell Structure

Floating freely in the cellular cytoplasm, but also located inside the endoplasmic reticulum and mitochondria are ribosomes. Ribosomes are complex macromolecule structures comprised of ribosomal ribonucleic acid (rRNA) molecules and ribosomal proteins. Ribosomes decode messenger RNA to produce proteins.

Messenger RNAs (mRNA) are created by 'transcription' of nuclear DNA. Messenger RNA may also be generated in the mitochondria. Messenger RNA created by transcription in the nucleus of the cell generally migrate to other locations inside the cell and are utilized by ribosomes as protein manufacturing templates. The rRNAs and the ribosomal proteins congregate to form a macromolecule structure that surrounds a mRNA molecule. Ribosomes decode genetic information in a mRNA molecule in a process termed 'translation' and manufacture proteins to the specifications of the instruction code physically present in the mRNA molecule. More than one ribosome may be attached to a single mRNA at a time.

Proteins are comprised of a series of amino acids bonded together in a linear strand, sometimes referred to as a chain. A protein may be further modified to be a structure comprised of one or more similar or differing strands of amino acids bonded together. Insulin is a protein structure comprised of two strands of amino acids; one strand comprised of 21 amino acids long and the second strand comprised of 30 amino acids. The two strands are attached by two disulfide bridges. There are an estimated 33,000 different proteins that the cells of the human body may manufacture.

The human body is comprised of approximately 240 different cell types, many with specialized functions requiring unique combinations of proteins and protein structures such as glycoproteins (protein combined with carbohydrate) to accomplish the required task or tasks a specialized cell is designed to perform. Certain forms of glycoproteins are known to be utilized as cell-surface receptors.

On the surface of eukaryote cells are cell surface receptors. Some of the receptors are functional as in the insulin receptor, which regulates the cell's capacity to absorb glucose. Other cell surface receptors act as a means of communications. Differing cells possess various combinations of cell surface receptors and markers which are used to identify cells. The immune system of a multi-celled organism needs to know which cells are suppose to be present in the body of the organism and which cells may be foreign invaders of the body. The immune system uses cell-surface receptors to identify bacteria, viruses and parasites so as to be able to mount a response against such a threat. Some cell surface receptors are utilized as means to open pathways through the cell membrane.

Viruses

A virus represents a biologic entity that is generally comprised of an outer shell and an inner core which contains the virus's genome. See Figure 3. The outer shell may be one or more layers thick. The outer most layer supports the presence of cell surface probes and receptors. Viruses tend to wish to avoid detection by an immune system, so the cell surface receptors either mimic receptors found on the surface of the host's cells or the surface receptors are the antithesis of the virus's target cell.

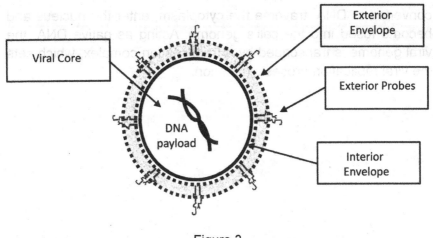

Figure 3
Basic virion structure

Viruses have no internal organelles and are unable to generate energy, thus a virus is unable to replicate itself. Viruses require the internal machinery and the chemical energy of a target host cell in order to successfully replicate. Generally a virus targets a particular type of cell as its host cell. In the case of the Human Immunodeficiency Virus (HIV) the HIV virion possess gp120 and gp41 probes on its surface which the virion uses to detect the presence of its host cell, a T-Helper cell in the human body. The HIV virion's gp120 probe engages the T-Helper cell's CD4 cell surface receptor. Once the CD4 receptor has been engaged the HIV's gp41 probe engages the T-Helper cell's CXCR4 or CCR5 cell surface receptor. Once both types of probes have successfully engaged a corresponding cell surface receptor the T-Helper cell's cell membrane is breached and the HIV virion inserts its genome into the T-Helper cell.

Viruses are classified regarding the type of genome they carry as their payload. A virus carrying a DNA genome is a DNA virus. A virus carrying one or more strands of RNA is considered an RNA virus. Once the genome has entered the host cell retroviridae RNA viruses may convert their positive single stranded RNA to DNA by means of an enzyme termed reverse transcriptase. Negative strand viral RNA genome may remain in its RNA form and act as a template for protein production. DNA genomes and RNA genomes that are converted to DNA, traverse the cytoplasm, enter the nucleus and become fused into the cell's genome. Acting as native DNA, the viral genome is transcribed by a transcription complex, which sets the viral replication process in motion.

CHAPTER 3

CONSTRUCT OF THE DNA

A 'ribose' is a five carbon or pentose sugar ($C_5H_{10}O_5$) present in the structural components of ribonucleic acid, riboflavin, and other nucleotides and nucleosides. A 'deoxyribose' is a deoxypentose ($C_5H_{10}O_4$) found in deoxyribonucleic acid.

A 'nucleoside' is a compound of a sugar, usually ribose or deoxyribose, with a nitrogenous base by way of an N-glycosyl link. A 'nucleotide' is a single unit of a nucleic acid, composed of a five carbon sugar (either a ribose or a deoxyribose), a nitrogenous base and a phosphate group. There are two families of 'nitrogenous bases', pyrimidine and purine.

A 'pyrimidine' is a six member ring made up of carbon and nitrogen atoms; the members of the pyrimidine family include: cytosine (C), thymine (T) and uracil (U). A 'purine' is a five-member ring fused to a pyrimidine type ring. The members of the purine family include: adenine (A) and guanine (G). See Figure 4. A 'nucleic acid' is a polynucleotide which is a biologic molecule such as ribonucleic acid or deoxyribonucleic acid that allow organisms to reproduce.

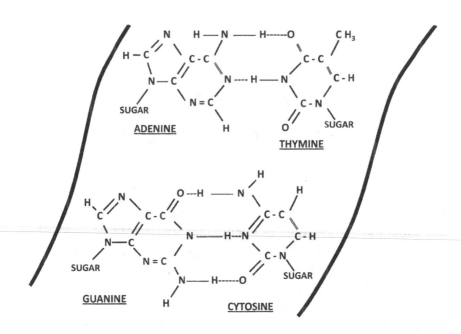

Figure 4
Chemical structures of the four nucleotides
as they exist in the DNA

A 'ribonucleic acid' (RNA) is a linear polymer of nucleotides formed by repeated riboses linked by phosphodiester bonds between the 3-hydroxyl group of one and the 5-hydroxyl group of the next. RNAs are a single strand macromolecule comprised of a sequence of nucleotides; these nucleotides are generally referred to by their nitrogenous bases, which include: adenine, cytosine, guanine and uracil. The term macromolecule refers to any very large molecule. RNAs are subset into different types which include messenger RNA (mRNA), transport RNA (tRNA), ribosomal RNA (rRNA) and a variety of small RNAs. Messenger RNAs act as templates to produce proteins.

A ribosome is a complex comprised of rRNAs and proteins and is responsible for the correct positioning of mRNA and charged tRNAs to facilitate the proper alignment and bonding of amino acids into a strand to produce a protein. A 'charged' tRNA is a tRNA that is carrying an amino acid. Ribosomal RNA (rRNA) represents a subset of RNAs that form part of the physical structure of a ribosome. Small RNAs include snoRNA, U snRNA, and miRNA. The snoRNAs modify precursor rRNA molecules. U snRNAs modify precursor mRNA molecules. The miRNA molecules modify the function of mRNA molecules.

A 'deoxyribose' is a deoxypentose ($C_5H_{10}O_4$) sugar. Deoxyribonucleic acid (DNA) is comprised of three basic elements: a deoxyribose sugar, a phosphate group and nitrogen containing bases. DNA is a macromolecule made up of two chains of repeating deoxyribose sugars linked by phosphodiester bonds between the 3-hydroxyl group of one and the 5-hydroxyl group of the next; the two chains are held antiparallel to each other by weak hydrogen bonds. DNA strands contain a sequence of nucleotides, which include: adenine, cytosine, guanine and thymine. See Figure 4. Adenine is always paired with thymine of the opposite strand, and guanine is always paired with cytosine of the opposite strand; one side or strand of a DNA macromolecule is the mirror image of the opposite strand. Nuclear DNA is regarded as the medium for storing the master plan of hereditary information.

Genes are considered segments of the DNA that represent units of inheritance.

Chromosomes exists in the nucleus of a cell and consists of a DNA double helix bearing a linear sequence of genes, coiled and recoiled around aggregated proteins, called histones. The number of chromosomes varies from species to species. Most Human cells carries twenty two pairs of chromosomes plus two sex chromosomes; two 'x' chromosomes in women and one 'x' and one 'y' chromosome in men. In a human cell, the entire nuclear genome, forty six chromosomes, is comprised of 3 billion base pairs of nucleotides.

CHAPTER 4

CONSTRUCT OF THE GENE

Current gene theory is derived from Gregor Mendel (1822-1884), who discovered the basic principles of heredity by breeding garden peas at the abbey where he resided, while teaching at Brunn Modern School. Gregor Mendel built and documented a model of inheritance, often referred to as Mendelian genetics, that has acted as the foundation of modern genetics. Gregor Mendel documented changes in characteristics of the plants he grew and described the physical traits as being related to 'heritable factors'. Over time Mendel's term 'heritable factor' has been replaced by the terms 'gene' and 'allele'. Much of what the current term of a 'gene' describes remains related to and distinctly linked to the physical traits of the live organisms they describe.

Per J. K. Pal, S.S. Ghaskabi, *Fundamentals of Molecular Biology*, 2009: 'The central dogma of molecular biology . . . states that the genes present in the genome (DNA) are transcribed into mRNAs, which are then translated into polypeptides or proteins, which are phenotypes.' 'Genome, thus, contains the complete set of hereditary information for any organism and is functionally divided into small parts referred to as genes. Each gene is a sequence of nucleotides representing a single protein or RNA. Genome of a living organism may contain as few as 500 genes as in case of Mycoplasma, or as many as 32,000 genes as in the case of human beings.'

Current computer technology utilizes the binary numeric language. Every task a computer performs is related to the language of 'ones' and 'zeros'. Transistors that comprise the inside of computer chips are either turned 'on' representing a 'one' or turned 'off' representing a 'zero'. At the core of all computer programs is the machine language of 'ones' and 'zeros'. The most sophisticated central processing unit (CPU) in the world only reads and processes the language of 'ones' and 'zeros'. All text, all pictures, all video, all sound and music is diluted down to the form of 'ones' and 'zeros', and consequently all of the computing and storage power of a computer is performed by the computer language of 'ones' and 'zeros'.

The nucleus of a biologically active cell arguably possesses the most sophisticated and well organized processing power in the world. To run such a powerful processing unit, a form of biologic computer language would seem to be a necessary foundation by which to transfer stored information from the DNA to the remainder of the biologically active portions of a cell as needed. Given that the DNA comprising the chromosomes and the mitochondrial DNA are both comprised of four different nucleotides including adenosine, cytosine, guanine and thymine, and RNA is comprised of four nucleotides including adenosine, cytosine, guanine and uracil (uracil in place of thymine), it appears evident the biologic computer language used by a cell's genome is an information language derived from base-four mathematics. Instead of current computer technology utilizing binary computer code comprised of 'ones' and 'zeros', the DNA and RNA in a biologically active cell utilize an information language comprised of 'zeros', 'ones', twos' and 'threes' to store and transfer information, which in effect represents a base-four language or quaternary language.

The above definitions of a 'gene' refer to genes residing in a specific place or locus on a chromosome. Identifying that a gene is present in a particular location is obvious to the human observer, but from a functional standpoint for cell biology this does not necessarily help a cell find or use the information stored in the nucleotide sequence of a particular gene. To rely on location alone, as a means of identifying a gene, would put the function of the entire genome at peril of failure if even a single base pair of nucleotides were added or deleted from the genome. Thus far no discussion pertaining to genes being organized utilizing a coding system of any form, other than the mention of physical location within a chromosome, has been brought forth in the medical literature.

The current understanding of the actual biologic structure of a gene is far more elaborate than the standard definition of a gene leads a casual reader to believe. Knowledge regarding structure and function of genes has evolved greatly since Gregor Mendel's work in the 19th century. A gene appears to be comprised of a number of segments loosely strung together along a particular section of DNA. In general there are at least three global segments associated with a gene which include: (1) the Upstream 5' flanking region, (2) the transcriptional unit and (3) the Downstream 3' flanking region. See Figure 5.

NUCLEAR DNA QUANTUM GENE

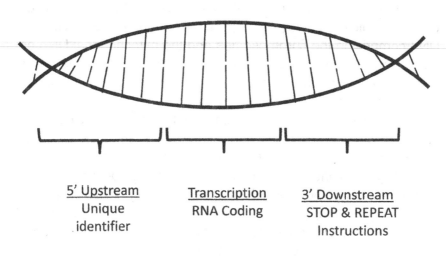

5' Upstream	Transcription	3' Downstream
Unique	RNA Coding	STOP & REPEAT
identifier		Instructions

Figure 5
Basic structure of a quantum gene

The Upstream 5' flanking region is comprised of the 'enhancer region', the 'promoter-proximal region', and 'promoter region'.

The 'transcriptional unit' begins at a location designated 'transcription start site' (TSS), which is located in a site called the 'initiator region' (inR), which may be described in a general form as Py_2CAPy_5. The transcription unit is comprised of the combination of segments of DNA nucleotides referred to as 'exons' to be transcribed into RNA and spacing units known as 'introns'. The transcription unit contains the genetic coding for a mRNA molecule, including all three elements of the mRNA that will appear in the final form of the molecule: (1) the 5' noncoding region, (2) the translational region and (3) the 3' noncoding region.

The coding region is comprised of exons, introns and segments that are not transcribed. Introns are sequences of nucleotides that are transcribed with the exons that form the precursor mRNA, but are later removed post transcription by the process of RNA splicing. Introns do not appear in the final RNA molecule. The exact role of introns remains under investigation. Introns may be rather large in size and have been reported to number up to 50 in a single gene. It is likely that the presence of introns facilitates the production of different RNA molecules. By varying which exons are retained, the end result RNA molecules can be varied. Varying the composition of a messenger RNA molecule will vary the resultant protein that is produced when the messenger RNA molecule is translated in the cytoplasm.

Removal of introns is referred to as 'RNA splicing'. Small nuclear ribonucleoprotein particles (snRNP) contain RNA segments that represent the junction between introns and the precursor RNA. The snRNPs create loops out of the introns and then facilitate removal of the introns loops and splicing together of the precursor RNA segments.

The Downstream 3' flanking region contains DNA nucleotides that are not transcribed. This region is thought to cause the transcription process to terminate and direct the transcription mechanism to disassemble. The Downstream 3' region may contain what has been termed an 'enhancer region'. An enhancer region in the Downstream 3' flanking region may promote the gene previously transcribed, to be transcribed again.

On either side of the DNA sequencing comprising a gene and its flanking regions, may be inactive DNA which act as boundaries which have been termed 'insulator elements'. The term 'upstream' refers to DNA sequencing that occurs prior to the TSS if viewed from the 5' end to the 3' end of the DNA. The term 'downstream' refers to DNA sequencing located after the TSS. In general regarding molecular biology, 'upstream' refers to the direction toward the 5' end of the molecule and 'downstream' refers to direction of the 3' end of the molecule.

The 'enhancer region' may or may not be present in the Upstream 5' flanking region. If present in the Upstream 5' flanking region, the enhancer region helps facilitate the reading of the gene by encouraging formation of the transcription mechanism. An enhancer may be 50 to 1500 base pairs in length occupying a position upstream from the transcription starting site.

The 'transcription mechanism', also referred to as 'the transcription machinery' or the 'transcription complex' (TC), in humans is reported to be comprised of over forty separate proteins that assemble together to ultimately function in a concerted effort to transcribe the nucleotide sequence of the DNA into RNA. The transcription mechanism includes elements such as 'general transcription factor Sp1', 'general transcription factor NF1', 'general transcription factor TATA-binding protein', 'TFIID', 'basal transcription complex', and a 'RNA polymerase protein' to name only a few of the forty or so elements that are used. The elements of the transcription mechanism function (1) as a means to recognize the location of the start of a gene, (2) as proteins to bind the transcription mechanism to the DNA such that transcription may occur or (3) as means of transcribing the DNA nucleotide coding to produce an RNA molecule or a precursor RNA molecule.

The process of translation where messenger RNA molecules act as the template for ribosomes to generate proteins is very much dependent upon the presence of rRNA molecules and tRNA molecules. As previously mentioned rRNAs combine with ribosomal proteins to generate ribosomes. The tRNA molecules transport individual amino acids to the ribosomes to generate the amino acid chains that comprise protein molecules. The mRNA, rRNA and tRNA molecules are transcribed using different transcription complexes. The transcription complexes vary in relation to the RNA polymerase molecule that forms an integral piece of the transcription complex.

There are at least three RNA polymerase proteins which include: RNA polymerase I, RNA polymerase II, and RNA polymerase III. RNA polymerase I tends to be dedicated to transcribing genetic information that will result in the formation of rRNA molecules. RNA polymerase II tends to be dedicated to transcribing genetic information that will result in the formation of mRNA molecules as discussed above. RNA polymerase III appears to be dedicated to transcribing genetic information that results in the formation of tRNAs, small cellular RNAs and viral RNAs.

The 'promoter proximal region' is located upstream from the TSS and upstream from the core promoter region. See Figure 6. The 'promoter proximal region' includes two sub-regions termed the GC box and the CAAT box. The 'GC box' appears to be a segment rich in guanine-cytosine nucleotide sequences. The GC box binds to the 'general transcription factor Sp1' of the transcription mechanism. The 'CAAT box' is a segment which contains the nucleotide sequence 'GGCCAATCT' located approximately 75 base pairs (bps) upstream from the transcription start site (TSS). The CAAT box binds to the 'general transcription factor NF1' of the transcription mechanism.

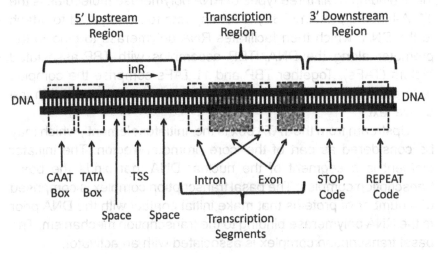

Figure 6
Detailed structure of a quantum gene

The 'core promoter' region is considered the shortest sequence within which RNA polymerase II can initiate transcription of a gene The core promoter may include the inR and either a TATA box or a 'downstream promoter element' (DPE). The inR is the region designated Py_2CAPy_5 that surrounds the transcription start site (TSS). The TATA box is located 25 base pairs (bps) upstream from the TSS. The TATA box acts as a site of attachment of the TFIID, which is a promoter for binding of the RNA polymerase II molecule. The DPE may appear 28 bps to 32 bps downstream from the TSS. The DPE acts as an alternative site of attachment for the TFIID when the TATA box is not present.

The transcription complex is comprised of different elements depending upon whether rRNA is being transcribed versus mRNA or tRNA or small cellular RNA or viral RNA. The proteins that assemble to assist RNA Polymerase I with transcribing the DNA to produce rRNA appear different from the proteins that assemble to assist RNA polymerase II with transcribing the DNA to produce mRNA and from the proteins that assemble to assist RNA polymerase III with transcribing the DNA to produce tRNA, small cellular RNA or viral RNA. A common protein that appears to be present at the initial binding of all three types of RNA polymerase molecules is the TATA-binding protein (TBP). TBP appears to be required to attach to the DNA, which then facilitates RNA polymerase to bind to the promoter along the DNA. TBP assembles with TBP-associated factors (TAFs). Together TBP and 11 TAFs comprise the complex referred to as TFIID, which has been previously mentioned in the above text.

Upstream from the TATA box is the 'initiator element', which may be considered as part of the 'core promoter' region. The initiator element is a segment of the nuclear DNA that binds the basal transcription complex. The basal transcription complex is comprised of a number of proteins that make initial contact with the DNA prior to the RNA polymerase binding to the transcription mechanism. The basal transcription complex is associated with an activator.

An activator is a protein comprised of three components: (1) DNA binding domain, (2) Connecting domain, and (3) Activating domain. When the activator's DNA binding domain attaches to the DNA at a specific point along the DNA, the activator's activating domain then causes the other elements of the transcription mechanism to assemble at this location. Generally the assembly of the other proteins occurs downstream from where the activator's DNA binding domain attached to the DNA. There is evidence that the activator is associated with the activity of small RNAs.

The design of the cell is so complex, and all of its functions so diverse and intricate, that some form of practical order is necessitated. The genes must be ordered in some fashion, especially in a human, where there are at least 32,000 different genes used by the cells. Some estimates put the total number of genes present in the human nuclear DNA genome to be closer to 100,000. If no means of order existed as to how the genes could be identified, then 'random circumstance' would dictate a cell locating a particular portion of genetic information that it requires, at any given time. Randomness tends to favor the occurrence of random events rather than a purposeful order. A 'random circumstance' approach to any living cell would tend to favor failure of the cell rather than survival of the cell. Hence, the necessity for gene IDs, referred to as quantum genes, and command and control in the cells.

23

CHAPTER 5

TRANSLATION: DECODING OF mRNA PRODUCES PROTEINS

A protein is comprised of a series of amino acids bonded together in a linear strand, sometimes referred to as a chain. A protein may be further modified to be a structure comprised of one or more similar or differing strands of amino acids bonded together. A protein comprised of more than one strand of amino acids (referred to as subunits) may be referred to as a protein complex. Insulin is a protein structure comprised of two strands of amino acids, one strand comprised of 21 amino acids long and the second strand comprised of 30 amino acids; the two strands attached by two disulfide bridges. There are an estimated 33,000 different proteins the cells of the human body may manufacture. The human body is comprised of a wide variety of cells, many with specialized functions requiring unique combinations of proteins and protein structures such as glycoproteins (protein combined with carbohydrate) to accomplish the required task or tasks a specialized cell is designed to perform. Forms of glycoproteins are known to be utilized as cell-surface receptors.

Messenger RNAs (mRNA) are created by transcription of DNA. See Figure 7. Messenger RNA generated by transcription of nuclear DNA, migrate out of the nucleus of the cell, and are utilized as protein manufacturing templates by ribosomes. Different mRNAs code for different proteins. As previously mentioned, there are at least 32,000 human genes, therefore there are at least 32,000 different mRNA molecules.

A ribosome is a protein complex that manufactures proteins by deciphering the instruction code located inherent in a mRNA molecule. When a specific protein is needed, pieces of the

24

ribosome complex bind around the strand of mRNA that carries the specific instruction code that will generate the required protein. The ribosome traverses the mRNA strand and deciphers the genetic information coded into the sequence of nucleotides that comprise the mRNA molecule.

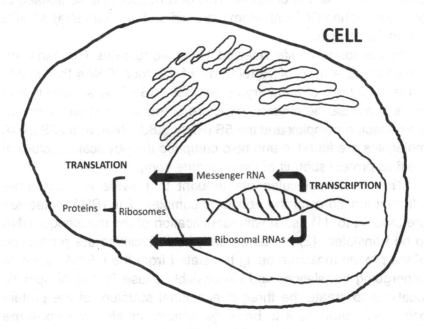

Figure 7
Process of transcription to translation

A ribosome is complex macromolecule comprised of ribosomal RNA (rRNA) molecules and ribosomal proteins. Ribosomal RNAs and ribosomal proteins are often designated with a number measured in Svedberg (S) units, which represents the sediment coefficient. The sediment coefficient is influenced by both molecular weight of the molecule and surface area of the molecule. In humans there are generally recognized at this time two mitochondrial rRNAs identified as 12S rRNA and 16S rRNA, and there are generally recognized four rRNAs that reside in the cytoplasm of a cell identified as 5S rRNA, 5.8S rRNA, 18S rRNA and 28S rRNA. There may be other rRNAs, as of yet unidentified, that reside in some of the other structures in the cell that engage in manufacturing of macromolecules, such as the smooth endoplasmic reticulum, the rough endoplasmic reticulum and the Golgi complex.

In eukaryotes, in the cytoplasm, the ribosome complex is referred to as an 80S ribosome. Generally two ribosomal proteins comprise a ribosome complex. This 80S ribosome is comprised of one 'dome-shape' 60S ribosomal protein and one 'cap-shaped' 40S ribosomal protein.

In the forms of life referred to as vertebrates (Humans are classified as a form of vertebrate), of the four rRNAs that reside in the cytoplasm of a eukaryote cell, the 18S rRNA is found in and helps comprise the physical structure of the 40S protein subunit of the ribosome complex and the 5S rRNA, 5.8S rRNA, and 28S rRNA molecules are found in and help comprise the physical structure of the 60S protein subunit of the ribosome complex.

The rRNA molecules are thought to provide at least three different functions for the ribosome complex. The rRNA molecules are thought to: (1) assist with identification of the messenger RNA to be translated, (2) act as an enzyme to facilitate the production of the protein molecule being translated from the mRNA molecule undergoing translation, and (3) possibly cause folding at specific locations to create the three dimensional structure of the protein being generated as it is being generated, or after the ribosome complex has decoded the mRNA molecule.

Ribosomal RNAs (rRNA) are generated by 'RNA Polymerase I' molecules deciphering the instruction code present in the DNA. The rRNAs generally migrate to locations where mRNAs are to be utilized as templates. The rRNA molecules connect to their respective ribosome proteins and this macromolecule complex, referred to as a ribosome or ribosome complex, surrounds the beginning 5' segment of a mRNA molecule.

Utilizing inherent coding, the rRNA molecules direct the ribosome pieces to build the ribosome complex around a particular strand of mRNA or particular type of mRNA. Given there are four unique types of nucleotides that make up the physical linear strand of any RNA molecule, these four unique types of nucleotides may in some circumstances represent a base-four numbering system. As an analogy, at the core of the current digital computer technology, binary coding or base-two coding, which is comprised of 'ones' and 'zeros', is utilized in certain formats to code for names and numbers. The inherent coding the rRNA molecules harbor is a sequence of nucleotides which represent a unique 'name' (coded in the base-four numbering system), unique 'base-four number' or unique 'combination of a name and base-four number' that corresponds to a particular mRNA or particular type of mRNA. In this manner, rRNAs act to control which mRNA molecule will undergo translation to produce proteins, rather than a ribosome complex randomly engaging any mRNA template that happens to be available. With the DNA producing rRNA molecules that cause a ribosome to attach to a particular mRNA molecule or particular type of mRNA molecule, the DNA is able to exert control over the manufacturing capacity of the cell and produce proteins as needed, rather than producing proteins in a random fashion. Producing proteins as needed by the cell, rather than in a random fashion, conserves valuable resources and conserves energy inside the cell.

RNAs are generally degraded by enzymes known as ribonucleases or RNAases. Ribonucleases act to split RNA molecules, which tends to inactive the RNA molecules; preventing RNA molecules from performing their duties. Different RNAs have different half-lives. A 'service life' refers to the amount of time an RNA molecule may participate in the biologic functions it was originally created to participate in within a cell. A 'half-life' or 'service half-life' is the amount of time it takes for half of a given amount of RNA molecules to degrade to a form to which the RNA molecules are unable to participate in the biologic processes they were created to participate in within a cell. The 'life' or 'service life' or 'time span of participation in biologic processes' of biologic macromolecules is generally measured and reported in the science community in terms of the macromolecule's half-life. The nucleotide sequencing of the rRNA molecule could be altered from that of the naturally occurring molecule to lengthen or shorten the service half-life of the native rRNA. Lengthening the service life of rRNA molecules such that the rRNAs could combine with ribosomal proteins to participate in ribosomes over a longer than the naturally occurring period of

27

time would be especially useful in diabetic patients to facilitate a greater production of insulin molecules in the Beta cells.

The rate of degradation of rRNA molecules by ribonucleases could be varied by changing the nucleotide sequence of the rRNA molecule or by altering the folding characteristics of the rRNA molecule or by altering both the nucleotide sequence and the folding characteristics of the rRNA molecule. By making changes to the nucleotide sequence and/or the folding characteristics of the rRNA molecules, the rate of degradation of the rRNA molecules by ribonucleases could be caused to vary in length of time from seconds to minutes to hours to days to weeks to months to years.

Transport RNAs (tRNA) are constructed in the nucleus and in the mitochondria, and are coded for one of the 20 amino acids the cells of the human body use to construct proteins. Once a tRNA is created by transcription of the DNA, the tRNA seeks out the type of amino acid it has been coded for and attaches to one of that specific type of amino acid. The tRNA then delivers the amino acid it carries to a ribosome that is waiting for that specific amino acid. Proteins are manufactured by the ribosomes binding together sequences of amino acids. The order by which the amino acids are bonded together is dictated by the way the mRNA is constructed and how the ribosome interprets the information encoded in the string of nucleotides present in the mRNA strand.

A sequence of three nucleotides present in a mRNA molecule represents a unit of information referred to as a codon. Codons code for all of the 20 amino acids used to construct protein molecules and also for START and STOP commands. In the process known as translation, the ribosome decodes the codons present in the mRNA, initiating the protein manufacturing process at a START codon, then interfacing with tRNAs carrying the amino acids that match the sequence of codons in the mRNA as the ribosome traverses the length of the mRNA molecule. The ribosome functions as a protein factory by taking amino acids delivered by tRNAs and binding the amino acids together in the order dictated by the sequence of codon instructions coded into the mRNA template as directed by the manner of the nucleic acid arrangement in the mRNA molecule. Protein synthesis ceases when a ribosome encounters a STOP code. Once complete, the protein molecule is released by the ribosome.

CHAPTER 6

UPDATING THE CENTRAL DOGMA
OF MICROBIOLOGY

The central dogma of molecular biology serves as the central concept in Molecular Biology. The central dogma of molecular biology refers to the detailed flow of genetic information from the DNA to the construction of a polypeptide molecule. A peptide being a molecule comprised of two or more amino acids linked by a peptide bond. A peptide bond joins two amino acids together. A peptide bond in a polypeptide molecule, such as a protein, is formed by a condensation (water-loss) reaction between the carboxyl group of one amino acid and the amino group of the next amino acid. Therefore, proteins are formed by the linear arrangement of amino acids in a particular order.

The central dogma of microbiology in essence states that 'coded genetic information is hard-wired into the DNA genome, that a portion of this genetic information is transcribable to produce messenger RNA and once the messenger RNA has migrated to the cytoplasm of the cell, the messenger RNA acts as a template for ribosomes to translate the messenger RNA to generate proteins'.

The central dogma falls short of describing how a particular gene is selected for transcription, and further falls short of describing how a particular gene is located amongst the 32,000 genes thought to exist amongst the 46 chromosomes that comprise the human genome. The central dogma does not address how complex proteins, comprised of more than one protein molecule, are constructed. The central dogma fails to discuss the intracellular feed-back mechanism whereby proteins which are required to be regularly manufactured to meet chronic supply needs of the cell are generated by the cell such that the quantity manufactured is exactly proportionate to the needs of the cell.

The central dogma also falls short in adequately explaining what orchestrates the construction of complex molecules whereby proteins are fused to other organic molecules. Glycoproteins represent complex molecules comprised of at least one protein fused to at least one lipid. The central dogma offers an explanation for the production of the protein portion of the molecule, but what of the production of the lipid. Chemical reactions and chains of chemical reactions that run in the presence of adequate energy and enzymes are thought to be responsible for the inherent construction and disassembly of various molecules. Still, there needs to be some intelligent mechanism responsible for fusing the right protein to the right lipid.

Part 2

Unique Identification

CHAPTER 7

CONCEPT OF UNIQUE IDENTIFICATION

What is a Gene?

The gene is the recognized unit of heredity for organic life. The central dogma of microbiology dictates that within the boundaries of the nucleus of a biologically active cell, genes are transcribed to produce messenger ribonucleic acid molecules (mRNAs); these mRNAs migrate to the cytoplasm where they are translated by cellular machinery to produce proteins. One of the great unknowns that has challenged the study of microbiology is the subject of understanding of how the genes, comprising the genome of a species, are organized such that the nuclear transcription machinery can efficiently locate specific transcribable genetic information and instructions that the cell requires to maintain itself, grow and conduct cell replication.

Decoding the means as to how the genetic information contained in the nuclear deoxyribonucleic acid (DNA) of a cell is 'organized' contributes to furthering the efforts to produce an effective gene therapy treatment strategy. Understanding the basis of nature has labeled and cataloged the genetic information comprising the human genome, makes inserting biologic instruction into the DNA of cells a practical and effective means of treating a wide variety of challenging medical conditions. It would seem the biologic instructions necessary to build and maintain the human body are individually labeled with some form of unique identification code to assist the nuclear machinery in locating and utilizing the genes when needed.

The human genome is comprised of 3 billion base pairs (bp) of nucleotides. Each nucleotide represents one bit of information.

33

These three billion bits of deoxyribonucleic acid (DNA) are separated into 46 chromosomes. A chromosome consists of a DNA double helix bearing a linear sequence of genes, coiled and recoiled around aggregated proteins, termed histones. The number of chromosomes varies from species to species. Most human cells carries twenty two pairs of chromosomes plus two sex chromosomes; two 'x' chromosomes in women and one 'x' and one 'y' chromosome in men. The number of nucleotide base pairs per chromosome is presented in Table 1.

Chromosome	Number of base pairs	Chromosome	Number of base pairs
1	247,199,719	13	114,127,980
2	242,751149	14	106,360,585
3	199,446,827	15	100,338,915
4	191,263,063	16	88,822,254
5	180,837,866	17	78,654,742
6	170,896,993	18	76,117,153
7	158,821,424	19	63,806,651
8	146,274,826	20	62,435,965
9	140,442,298	21	46,944,323
10	135,374,737	22	49,528,953
11	134,452,384	X	154,913,754
12	132,289,534	Y	57,741,652

Table 1
The number of base pairs of nucleotides associated
with each chromosome.

The chromosomes are subdivided into genes. Genes represent units of transcribable DNA. A little over 32,000 genes are listed in Table 2. The number of genes per chromosome varies with the least number of genes being 379 on chromosome 11 and the most being 4220 genes on chromosome 2. Transcription of the DNA refers to generating one RNA molecule or a variety of RNA molecules by decoding the genes. Regarding the human genome, currently it is estimated that 5% of the total nuclear DNA is thought to represent genes and 95% is thought to represent redundant non-gene genetic material.

Chromosome	Number of Genes	Chromosome	Number of Genes
1	4,220	13	924
2	1,491	14	1,347
3	1,550	15	921
4	446	16	909
5	609	17	1,672
6	2,281	18	519
7	2,135	19	1,555
8	1,106	20	1,008
9	1,920	21	578
10	1,793	22	1,092
11	379	X	1,846
12	1,430	Y	454

Table 2
The number of genes associated with each human chromosome.

The DNA genome in a cell is comprised of transcribable genetic information and nontranscribable genetic information. Transcribable genetic information represent the segments of DNA that when transcribed by transcription machinery yield RNA molecules, usually (in the case of RNAs destined to become mRNAs) in a precursor form that require modification before the RNA molecules are capable of being functional. The nontranscribable genetic information represent segments that act as either points of attachment for the transcription machinery or act as commands to direct the transcription machinery or act as spacers between transcribable segments of genetic information or have no known function at this time. A segment of nontranslatable DNA that is coded as a STOP command, under the proper circumstances, will cause the transcription machinery to cease transcribing the DNA at that point.

A segment of DNA coded to signal a REPEAT command, will cause the transcription machinery to repeat its transcription of a segment of genetic information.

Locating the proper gene in a timely fashion enables a cell to properly operate, survive, grow and replicate.

Various standard definitions of a gene exist:

Per *Stedman's Medical Dictionary*, 24th edition, copyright 1982: 'The functional unit of heredity. Each gene occupies a specific place or locus on a chromosome, is capable of reproducing itself exactly at cell division, and is capable of directing the formation of an enzyme or other protein. The gene as a functional unit probably consists of a discrete segment of purine (adenine and guanine) and pyrimidine (cytosine and thymine) bases in the correct sequence to code the sequence of amino acids needed to form a specific peptide. Protein synthesis is mediated by molecules of messenger RNA formed on the chromosome with the gene unit of DNA acting as a template, which then pass into the cytoplasm and become oriented on the ribosomes where they in turn act as templates to organize a chain of amino acids to form a peptide. Genes normally occur in pairs in all cells except gametes as a consequence of the fact that all chromosomes are paired except the sex chromosomes (x and y) of the male.'

Per *Dorland's Pocket Medical Dictionary*, 23rd edition, copyright 1982 the definition of 'gene' is 'the biologic unit of heredity, self-producing, and located at a definite position (locus) on a particular chromosome.'

Per the text *Understanding Biology*, Second Edition, Peter Raven, George Johnson, Mosby, copyright 1991: 'Gene: The basic unit of heredity. A sequence of DNA nucleotides on a chromosome that encodes a polypeptide or RNA molecule and so determines the nature of an individual's inherited traits.'

Per *The New Oxford American Dictionary*, Second Edition, copyright 2005: 'Gene: A unit of heredity that is transferred from a parent to offspring and is held to determine some characteristic of the offspring: proteins coded directly by genes. In technical use: a distinct sequence of nucleotides forming part of a chromosome, the order of which determines the order of monomers in a polypeptide or nucleic acid molecule which a cell (or virus) may synthesize.'

Per MedicineNet.com. (*Current as of the time of this publication*): According to the official Guidelines for Human Gene Nomenclature, a 'gene' is defined as "a DNA segment that contributes to phenotype/ function. In the absence of demonstrated function a gene may be characterized by sequence, transcription or homology." DNA: Genes are composed of DNA, a molecule in the memorable shape of a double helix, a spiral ladder. Each rung of the spiral ladder consists of two paired chemicals called bases. There are four types of bases. They are adenine (A), thymine (T), cytosine (C), and guanine (G). As indicated, each base is symbolized by the first letter of its name: A, T, C, and G. Certain bases always pair together (AT and GC). Different sequences of base pairs form coded messages. The gene: A gene is a sequence (a string) of bases. It is made up of combinations of A, T, C, and G. These unique combinations determine the gene's function, much as letters join together to form words. Each person has thousands of genes—billions of base pairs of DNA or bits of information repeated in the nuclei of human cells—which determine individual characteristics (genetic traits).'

Per Wikipedia.com, referenced to: Group of the Sequence Ontology consortium, coordinated by K. Eilbeck, cited in H. Pearson. (2006). Genetics: what is a gene? *Nature*, 441, 398-401 (*Current as of the time of this publication*): A modern working definition of a gene is '*a locatable region of genomic sequence, corresponding to a unit of inheritance, which is associated with regulatory regions, transcribed regions, and or other functional sequence regions.*'

The above definitions of a 'gene' are fairly detailed and at present time generally universally accepted in the science and medical communities as representing the definition of a gene. There is a distinct lack of any previous reference in the medical science literature to a unique identifier associated with genetic material.

Human computer programs, commonly utilized in desk top computers, laptop computers, and mainframe computers, are comprised of a series of software instructions and data likened to genetic information in a specie's genome. In order for a computer program to run its digital programming in an orderly fashion, each software instruction and each element of data is assigned or associated with a 'unique identifier', such that the software instructions can be carried out in an orderly fashion and each element of data can be efficiently located when there is a need to process that data element. Similarly, each gene or unit of genetic information comprising the nuclear DNA of a specie's genome must have a unique identifier assigned to it such that the genetic information can be readily located by the transcription machinery and utilized when needed by a cell.

Current computer technology utilizes the binary numeric language. Every task a computer performs is related to the language of 'ones' and 'zeros'. Transistors that comprise the inside of computer chips are either turned 'on' representing a 'one' or turned 'off' representing a 'zero'. At the core of all computer programs is the machine language of 'ones' and 'zeros'. The central processing unit (CPU) is the heart of any computer. The most sophisticated CPU in the world only reads and processes the language of 'ones' and 'zeros'. All text, all pictures, all video, all sound and music is diluted down to the form of 'ones' and 'zeros', and consequently all of the computing and storage power of a computer is performed by the computer language of 'ones' and 'zeros'.

In order to keep the computing power of a CPU and associated memory storage devices in synch, all computer instructions and data elements are labeled with unique identifiers. In early generations of computers every line of a computer program was identified with a sequential number. As technology progressed, the distinct sequential numbering system evolved into utilizing names or numbers to label segments of computer code. Instructions and data elements retain unique identification in order to be located and processed by the CPU in an orderly fashion.

If a computer's CPU processing loses tract of computer instructions or data elements, the CPU becomes dysfunctional. Older generations of computers frequently experienced disparity in the sequencing of instructions and data. Once a computer's CPU lost tract of which instruction to process next or lost tract of the data it was to process, the computer would shut down; in older computers this often occurred and is referred to as a computer 'crash'. In the event a computer's CPU shut down, the computer screen generally freezes and the input and output devices became disabled. Often the only remedy to bring a frozen computer back to life is to turn off the power to the computer. Once a computer is restarted, the CPU automatically reboots itself at a known point of instruction code and is able to carry on deciphering further instruction code in an orderly fashion. Although today's computers are less likely to exhibit such behavior, they are not completely immune to the problems.

The nucleus of a biologically active cell arguably possesses the most sophisticated and well organized processing power in the world. To run such a powerful processing unit, a form of biologic computer language would be a necessary foundation with which to transfer and process stored information located in the DNA. Given that the DNA comprising the chromosomes and mitochondrial DNA are both comprised of four different nucleotides (adenosine, cytosine, guanine and thymine), and RNA is also comprised of four nucleotides with uracil in place of thymine, it appears evident the biologic computer language used by a cell's genome is an information language consistent with base-four mathematics. Instead of current computer technology utilizing binary computer code comprised of 'ones' and 'zeros', the DNA and RNA in a biologically active cell utilize an information language comprised of 'zeros', 'ones', twos' and 'threes' to store and transfer information, which in effect represents a base-four language or quaternary language.

The set of genes acting as the template dedicated to the construct of eukaryote cells is conserved in nature and utilized across those species utilizing eukaryote cells as their platform to generate the body tissues for a particular species.

The sharing of genetic information between differing species requires a global numbering system to be present in the genome. Within each species the physical location of genes would most likely change, since the size of the genome will be different per species. Physical location of the genetic information becomes irrelevant if the position of a gene changes with different species. Since it is known that Nature has shared genetic information between species, some form of a unique identification labeling segments of genes becomes imperative for the proper utilization of such genetic information as needed by each species.

Introducing the Unique Identifier

To allow a cell to utilize the biologic information stored in a gene, a 'unique identifier' must be associated with or attached to each gene's specific nucleotide sequence. In the human genome, the cell's transcription mechanism require an organized means to locate and transcribe any given gene's nucleotide sequence amongst the 3 billion nucleotides that reside in the 46 chromosomes that comprise human DNA. Given how the transcription mechanism assembles upstream from the portion of the gene to be transcribed, the nucleotide sequence acting as a unique identifier associated with a specific gene would be positioned upstream from the transcription start site.

The transcription complex (TC) engages the DNA upstream from the genetic information segment the TC transcribes. The unique identifier may be attached directly to the RNA coding segment of genetic material, or there may exist one or more base pairs physically separating the unique identifier and the RNA coding portion of genetic material. Regarding some genes, there may be numerous base pairs separating the unique identifier from the transcribable region of the gene.

A unique identification may exist as (1) a single contiguous segment or (2) two or more segments, with unrelated base pairs of nucleotides present between the segments. In the case where a unique identification exits as two or more segments, combined, these segments represent the unique identification of the associated quantum gene.

Naturally occurring unique identifiers in the nuclear genome may occur in numerous forms. Since humans share 47% of their DNA with bananas and 95% of their DNA with monkeys, a portion of the unique identifiers associated with genes in the human nuclear DNA may not be specific to a human. Unique identifiers most likely have a global utility, with a portion of the genome of any organism being shared amongst numerous species. The rational would be that once Nature developed an adequate fundamental design for a particular facet of biologic organisms, this information may be shared amongst numerous species that would benefit from the design. An example might be the basic design of a eukaryote cell;

this information would be shared amongst all life that utilized the basic eukaryote cell design rather than each successive multi-celled species having to repeatedly re-invent the design of a eukaryote cell. Some unique identifiers may be specific to and help define a particular Phylum, Class, Family, Genus or Species. One outcome of this is its aid in helping to understand evolution.

To support the theory of evolution, genes need to be present in the DNA and these genes need to be turned on or activated and turned off or deactivated when it is to the advantage to the survival of the organism. When a gene is activated, the gene must be able to be identified so that it can be located and used by the organism. Activated genes, either in combination or by themselves, often express some form of phenotypical feature that acts as a means of recognizing a particular species from another species. When genes are activated and linked to other genes and provide enough genetic information to produce a unique species, activated genes need to be able to be easily identified and located by the processing units in the cell's nucleus so that the genetic information can be easily utilized by the biologic machinery of a cell.

In order for the knowledge base of cellular genetics to progress forward, the definition of a gene must be expanded to include the presence of a 'unique identifier' associated with each gene present within the DNA. The basis for the presence of the unique identifier associated with each active gene is such that the cell can locate the biologic information stored in the DNA nucleotide sequence of the gene. An active gene refers to those genes present in the genome that are utilized by a particular species to support conception, development, maintenance and reproduction of the species.

CHAPTER 8

QUANTUM GENE

Introducing the Quantum Gene

Upon adding the concept of a unique identifier to the definition of a gene, the current term 'gene' is thus expanded to the term 'quantum gene'. The term 'quantal' in biology generally refers to an 'all or nothing' state or response. The term 'quantal' is a derivative of the word quantum. The term 'quantum' means a quantity or amount, a discrete quantity of energy, a discrete bundle of energy, or a discrete quantity of electromagnetic radiation.

A 'quantum gene' is comprised of a sequence of nucleotides that represents a 'unique identifier' physically linked to a sequence of nucleotides that represent a discrete quantity of genetic information; these sequences of nucleotides being comprised of some combination of the nucleotides being referred to by their nitrogenous base as adenine (A), thymine (T), cytosine (C), and guanine (G). The genetic information associated with the unique identifier may be comprised of a portion of transcribable genetic information and a portion of nontranscribable genetic information which together comprise a specific gene.

Similar to how a gene is described, with regards to a quantum gene, the term 'upstream' refers to DNA sequencing that occurs prior to the transcription start site (TSS) if viewed from the 5' end to the 3' end of the DNA; where the term 'downstream' refers to DNA sequencing located after the TSS.

Similar to the previously described organization of a standard gene found in nuclear DNA, a quantum gene is structured with at least three global segments which include: (1) the Upstream 5' flanking region, (2) the transcriptional unit and possibly instructional units and (3) the Downstream 3' flanking region. The 'unique identifier' is located in the Upstream 5' flanking region. See Figure 8. The current standard definition of a gene strictly encompasses the concept that a gene is comprised of a segment of nuclear DNA that when transcribed produces RNA. Therefore, the differences between the current standard definition of a 'gene' and the definition of a 'quantum gene' is that a quantum gene includes both a unique identifier and a segment of nuclear DNA that when transcribed produces RNA. The segment of nuclear DNA that when transcribed produces RNA is comprised of one or more segments of transcribable genetic information that may be accompanied by one or more segments of nontranscribable genetic information. Nontranscribable segments of genetic information include segments that are removed or ignored during the transcription process or segments that act as commands which includes START code, STOP code, and REPEAT code.

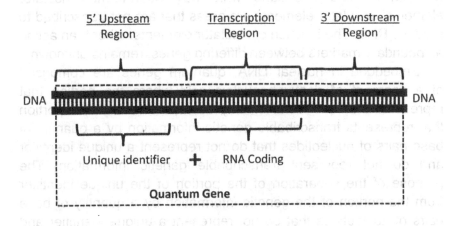

Figure 8
Quantum Gene

Analogous to the standard description of a 'gene', a quantum gene's Upstream 5' flanking region is comprised of the 'enhancer region', the 'promoter-proximal region', and 'promoter region'.

Similar to the standard description of a 'gene', a quantum gene's 'transcriptional unit' begins at a location designated TSS, which is located in a site called the 'initiator region' (inR), which may be described in a general form as Py_2CAPy_5. The transcription unit is comprised of the combination of segments of DNA nucleotides to be transcribed into RNA. In the cases where the RNA is to become mRNA spacing units known as 'introns' that are transcribed, but removed post transcription, such that they do not appear in the final mRNA molecule. That is, in the case of a gene coding for a mRNA molecule, the final transcription unit will contain all three elements of the mRNA, which includes: (1) the 5' noncoding region, (2) the translational region and (3) the 3' noncoding region.

Comparable to the standard description of a gene, with regards to the quantum gene, the Downstream 3' flanking region contains DNA nucleotides that are not transcribed and may contain what has been termed an 'enhancer region'.

On either side of the DNA sequencing comprising a gene and a quantum gene are flanking regions which represent inactive DNA, which act as boundaries which have been termed 'insulator elements'. Insulator elements are areas that are not transcribed to produce RNA. The function of insulator elements, other than acting as boundary markers between differing genes, remains unknown.

Embedded in nuclear DNA, quantum genes are comprised of a segment of deoxyribonucleic acid where the portion that represents a unique identifier may be separated from the portion that represents transcribable genetic information by a quantity of base pairs of nucleotides that do not represent a unique identifier and do not represent transcribable genetic information. The purpose of the separation of the portion of the unique identifier from the portion of the genetic information by a quantity of base pairs of nucleotides that do not represent a unique identifier and does not represent genetic information may be to act to facilitate a transcription complex attaching to the quantum gene upstream from the portion of the quantum gene that represents genetic information so that transcription of the biologic information associated with the quantum gene may occur at the designated starting point.

In a base four language, a string of nine nucleotides is needed to code for 256,144 individual genes. If there were over a million quantum genes, then a string of ten nucleotides could be used since ten nucleotides could represent 1,024,576 unique numbers in a base-four number system.

Utilizing a base four number system a string of twenty-five nucleotides would represent the number 1,125,899,906,842,624, which could account for 200,000 different quantum genes in 5 billion different species. (By contrast, to show how powerful a base-four system is compared to a binary number system, the digital technology that acts as the platform for all current computer services, can only represent approximately 17 million different numbers utilizing a string of 25 bits.) By current estimates, 200,000 different quantum genes represents more than enough genetic information to produce a biped form of life.

The differing number of species of organisms is recorded to be approximately 1.8 million. There are recorded 4,000 differing bacteria, 80,0000 differing protocitists, 72,0000 differing fungi, 270,000 differing plants, 1,272,0000 differing animal invertebrates and 52,0000 animal vertebrates for a total of 1,750,000 recorded species. The recorded species have been approximated to account for only a small number of actual species that inhabit the planet. It is estimated that 5-14 million different species actually exist on the planet today.

The time the average species is thought to be in existence is estimated to be 10 million years. It is also believed that 99% of the species that have ever existed have already become extinct. Given it is generally accepted that life has existed on earth for 3.5 billion years, it has been estimated that the number of species that has ever existed on the planet is between 200 million and 1 billion. Since a grouping of twenty-five base-four bits offers 5 billion possibilities, given 200,000 possible genes per species, utilizing this base-four mathematics, the genome could account for all of the possible species that have already existed on the planet. Considering that much of the genome required to construct a particular species is potentially shared with other species, especially basic microbiology such as cell constructs, the 200,000 genes allocated to contrive a species may indeed be too excessive of a number, since the number of genes necessary to produce a particular species may be a much smaller number of genes, thus conserving the unique identifier. This suggests that a unique identifier consisting of a string of twenty-five characters offers an even larger number of possible species beyond 5 billion.

In the human genome 5% of the 3 billion base pairs are considered to represent genes by the current definition of a gene. If 5% of the human genome were to represent 100,000 quantum genes (the upper estimate of the number of human genes, the lower estimate is 32,000 genes) in the nuclear DNA, then on average 1500 nucleotides can be dedicated to each gene within this 5% of DNA nucleotides. If 25 nucleotides are dedicated to a unique address or unique identifier, then there remains 1475 nucleotides, on average, to be utilized for coding the biologic information associated with each of the 100,000 quantum genes estimated to exist in the human genome.

By recognizing that a unique identification exists, it may be determined that a portion of the 95% of the human genome not presently considered to represent genes may indeed represent genes that have been unrecognized in their role as a gene. There may be numerous 'command instruction codes' associated with quantum genes that do not have a phenotypical role, but exist as a function role in the construction and maintenance of a cell, that have yet to be identified.

In nuclear DNA, there are several places in the upstream segment of a quantum gene where a contiguous segment of twenty-five, or more, or less, base pairs could exist that acts as the unique identifying code that uniquely identifies the segment of transcribable genetic information. Though a unique identifier having a length of 25 base pairs of nucleotides would serve the purpose of the concept of a unique identifier, a unique identifier may exist as a larger or smaller string of base pairs of nucleotides. The transcription start site (TSS) is present upstream from a segment of transcribable genetic information. In many genes there exists a segment of 25 bps upstream from the TSS that occupies the space along the DNA between the TSS and the TATA box. There exists the downstream promoter element (DPE) 28 bps to 32 bps downstream from the TSS. The DPE acts as an alternative site of attachment for the TFIID when the TATA box is not present. Within the 28 bps to 32 bps of DNA separating the DPE from the TSS may also be a convenient location for a unique identifying code to reside and be associated with the genetic information located just downstream. Living cells exists with numerous inherent variability.

There exists variation in the arrangement of the elements upstream from the transcribable genetic information; therefore various sites upstream from the transcribable genetic information may function as the unique identifying code for some quantum genes.

Computer software programs are comprised of lines of code. See Table 3. Each line of code generally represents an instruction or a unit of data. Early computer programming required each line of code to be identified by a unique number. The earliest programming required these unique numbers to be in a sequential order. As computer processors became faster and more powerful, computer programming techniques became less rigid. Large computer programs often are divided into groups of lines of code. A group of lines of code is termed a 'subprogram' and subprograms are often identified by a unique name. The group of instructions comprising a subprogram could then be accessed by the main program by simply referencing the unique name of the subprogram.

Line Number	Program Instruction Statement
001	START
002	INPUT A
003	INPUT B
004	C = A + B
005	PRINT C
006	STOP

Table 3
Line numbered steps comprising a simple addition computer program.

Table 3 illustrates a computer program comprised of six lines. Each line of the program has a unique line number. The program starts at line 001. Line 002 asks for the variable A to be input. Line 003 asks for the variable B to be input. Once the two variables have been inserted Line 004 represents the command that adds the two variables together. Line 005 prints the result of adding variable A to variable B. Line 006 stops the program.

The term ASCII is an abbreviation for American Standard Code For Information Interchange. The ASCII code was originally developed for teletypewriters but eventually found wide application in personal computers. The initial standard ASCII code used seven-digit binary numbers. By utilizing numbers consisting of various sequences of 0's and 1's, the code could represent 128 different characters.

ASCII was a standard data-transmission code that was used by smaller and less-powerful computers to represent both textual data (letters, numbers, and punctuation marks) and non-input device commands (control characters). Like other coding systems, it converts information into standardized digital formats that allow computers to communicate with each other and to efficiently process and store data.

In 1981, International Business Machines Corporation (IBM) introduced an extended ASCII code, an eight-bit system, for use with its first model of personal computer. Current digital computer technology uses a binary code that is arranged in groups of eight rather than of seven bits. Each such eight-bit group is referred to as a byte. By utilizing an eight-bit system, the number of characters the code could represent increased to 256.

The first 32 characters (0-31) of the extended ASCII code are unprintable and are used to control peripheral devices. Printable characters are from binary codes 32 to 127. Numbers from 'zero' to 'nine' are characters are 48 to 57. The upper case letters 'A' to 'Z' are characters 65 to 90. The lower case letters 'a' to 'z' are characters 97 to 122. As an example, Table 4 demonstrates the decimal numbers '0' to '9' and the associated binary numbers as seen in the extended ASCII code.

ASCII Code	Number	Binary Number
48	0	00110000
49	1	00110001
50	2	00110010
51	3	00110011
52	4	00110100
53	5	00110101
54	6	00110110

55	7	00110111
56	8	00111000
57	9	00111001

Table 4
Numbers 0 to 9 represented as their ASCII binary numbers.

As far as the entire scope of digital computer technology is concerned, all numbers, letters, characters and instructions are represented as differing strings of one's and zero's. The strings of one's and zero's are linked together to produce numbers, words, text and computer commands. Individual segments of information stored in a computer are tagged with a unique address identifier to facilitate quickly locating the information amongst everything else stored in memory, when the specific information is needed by the computer's central processor.

The core concept of a 'quantum gene' is the association of a 'unique identifier' with a segment of 'translatable DNA'.

Since it is estimated that humans share 47% of their genome with that of the genome of a banana, and 95% of their genome with the genome of a monkey, more than likely genetic instructions are grouped together. This grouping of genetic instructions facilitates the design of segments of a cell not having to be re-invented by each succeeding species.

Table 5 illustrates the concept that a biologic genetic program could be organized in the DNA utilizing a unique identifier comprised of a string of 25 characters. Insulin is a protein structure constructed of two protein molecules, each comprised of a differing chain of amino acid molecules. Insulin is generated inside the Beta cells located in the Islets of Langerhans inside the organ known as the pancreas. A set of programming instructions is required to produce each of the two chains of protein. A more complex set of instructions would be required to construct a Beta cell. Further, an even more complex set of instructions would be necessary to construct the organ referred to as the pancreas. Any organism sophisticated enough to require a pancreas may carry and utilize the universal set of genes that are utilized to construct the pancreas, the Islets of Langerhans, the Beta cells and the insulin protein.

49

Number	Unique Identifier 25-characters (base 4)	Transcript Region	Transcription Instructions
1	3000000000000000001000000	1	Design of Pancreas
2	3000000000000000001100000	2	Design of Islet of Langerhans
3	3000000000000000001110000	3	Design of Beta Cell
4	3000000000000000001110100	4	Insulin Protein 1
5	3000000000000000001110110	5	Insulin Protein 2

Table 5

Example of how the unique identifier may be used
to organize instructions.

All of the genetic instruction code necessary to build each and every structure comprising the human body could have a unique identifier comprised of 25-characters associated with it to act as a label so that the instruction code can be located when needed. All of the data required to build the various structures of the human body would similarly be labeled and stored in an organized fashion in the DNA of the nucleus. See Figure 9. In Figure 9 a series of generic unique identifiers are illustrated along with a series of generic transcribable regions. UI 1 represents a unique identifier for transcribable region 1, while the remaining unique identifiers are associated with other unique transcribable regions.

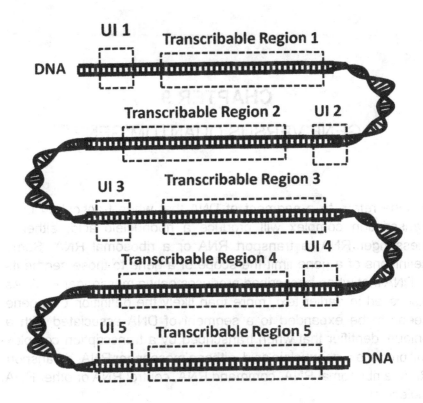

Figure 9
Unique Identifiers are associated with individual
Transcription Regions

CHAPTER 9

GENE VERSUS QUANTUM GENE

A gene refers to a segment of DNA that when transcribed by a transcription complex will produce a ribonucleic acid, either a messenger RNA, a transport RNA or a ribosomal RNA. Some definitions of a gene limit the scope of a gene to those segments of DNA that when transcribed produces only a messenger RNA. As discussed in earlier text, more than likely the definition of a gene needs to be expanded to a segment of DNA associated with a unique identifier that when transcribed by a transcription complex will produce a ribonucleic acid, either a messenger RNA, a transport RNA, a ribosomal RNA, command RNA, control RNA or other RNA molecules.

A quantum gene is a segment of DNA associated with a unique identifier that when transcribed by a transcription complex will produce a ribonucleic acid, either a messenger RNA, a transport RNA, a ribosomal RNA, command RNA, control RNA or other RNA molecules.

Quantum genes may be comprised of a segment of DNA that when transcribed produces one ribonucleic acid or a quantum gene may be comprised of multiple genes, with each gene being capable of generating a ribonucleic acid when transcribed.

Quantum genes may act as control switches. If it is necessary for a specific set of genes to be transcribed in a certain order or all at a particular time, then such genes may be bundled together and associated with one unique identification. Once the cell's transcription complex locates the unique identifier associated with the first gene in the bundled series, all of the genes in the series will be transcribed in the order they appear in the series. Therefore, not all genes need to have a unique identification.

The existence of quantum genes is associated with certain viral genomes such as HIV's DNA genome. There is a unique identification associated with HIV's DNA genome located in the 5' region. Following this unique identifier all of HIV's genes are bundled downstream in the transcription region.

Recognized switch genes have been referred to as Hox genes in the literature. Hox genes that have a unique identifier would represent a subset of quantum genes. Quantum genes represent a wide scope of functional genes including any gene labeled with a unique identifier.

CHAPTER 10

QUANTUM mRNA

Messenger RNA molecules are comprised of three regions (or segments). These three regions include: (1) a 5' untranslatable region, (2) a coding region and (3) a 3' untranslatable region. The '5' untranslatable region' acts as the initiation point for a ribosome to attach to the mRNA. The 'coding region' acts as the template from which a protein is constructed.

An 'untranslatable region' represents a segment of a messenger RNA molecule that does not code for a protein, is not used to yield a protein, and therefore 'translation' does not occur in such a region. The 3' untranslatable region is associated with the degradation of the usefulness of the mRNA. Different mRNAs have different service life expectancies. The half-life of the naturally occurring mRNA that acts as the template responsible for the production of the protein 'glucokinase' is two hours. The half-life of the naturally occurring mRNA that acts as the template that produces the protein 'alcohol dehydrogenase' is ten hours. The half-life of the naturally occurring mRNA that acts as the template to produce the protein 'glucuronidase' is thirty hours. By modifying the nucleotides that comprise the 3' untranslatable unit of an mRNA the service half-life of the mRNA may be lengthened or shortened depending upon the need for the quantity of protein and timeframe over which the mRNA is required to produce the protein coded in the protein template of the mRNA's coding region.

Research has demonstrated that natural proteins can be altered to produce medically beneficial effects. The parathyroid hormone (PTH) is one example. Intact PTH is produced by cells in the parathyroid glands. There are four parathyroid glands present in the neck, generally in the vicinity of the thyroid gland. The term 'para' means 'next to', so early anatomists identified the four glands 'parathyroid glands' because they were generally found 'next to' the thyroid gland in the neck. Parathyroid hormone is released in response to the cells of the parathyroid gland sensing a decline in the level of serum calcium.

Parathyroid hormone, in its natural state, acts to stimulate osteoclast cells present in bone to release calcium from bone, thereby returning the serum calcium level to the normal range. On the other hand, it has been well demonstrated that if (1) the amino acid chain of the parathyroid hormone is shortened and (2) the shorter parathyroid hormone molecule is pulsed, by injecting it into the body once a day, the action of this modified parathyroid hormone molecule is opposite of the intact parathyroid hormone. One such form of a shorter length parathyroid hormone molecule is termed 'teriparatide'. Teriparatide (1-34) has the identical sequence from 1 to the 34th N-terminal amino acids of the 84-amino acid endogenous human parathyroid hormone. The skeletal effects of the modified protein molecule act on bone cells to preferentially cause osteoblastic activity over osteoclastic activity, which results in storage of calcium into bone, rather than a release of calcium from bone if the teriparatide is administered once a day. Teriparatide has been a recognized and widely used treatment of osteoporosis, dating to its introduction to the medical community at least as far back as the year 2000.

Modifying the 'coding region' of a messenger RNA will modify the protein the messenger RNA will produce when the ribosomes decode such a modified messenger RNA. As demonstrated by the case of modifying the naturally occurring parathyroid hormone by administering a molecule that is comprised of fewer amino acids than the original PTH molecule, modifying proteins the messenger RNAs produce may provide health care providers with an entirely new and widely spanning armamentarium of medically beneficial therapies.

Messenger RNAs (mRNA) are created by 'transcription' of nuclear DNA. Messenger RNA may also be generated in the mitochondria. Messenger RNA created by transcription in the nucleus of the cell generally migrate to other locations inside the cell and are utilized by ribosomes as protein manufacturing templates. The rRNAs and the ribosomal proteins congregate to form a macromolecule structure that surrounds a mRNA molecule. Ribosomes decode genetic information in a mRNA molecule in a process termed 'translation' and manufacture proteins to the specifications of the instruction code physically present in the mRNA molecule. More than one ribosome may be attached to a single mRNA at a time.

The 5' untranslatable region of a messenger RNA molecule is used to identify the messenger RNA. It is also utilized as a point of attachment by ribosomes to the messenger RNA molecule.

Modifying the 5' untranslatable region by altering the nucleotide sequence in the 5' untranslatable region may make it easier to identify a modified messenger ribonucleic acid molecules in a fashion that the modified ribonucleic acid molecules can be engaged by ribosomes. Altering the nucleotide sequence of the 5' untranslatable region of a modified messenger ribonucleic acid molecule to create a unique identifier would facilitate ribosomes to preferentially engage the modified messenger ribonucleic acid molecule to preferentially produce the protein for which the modified messenger ribonucleic acid molecule is acting as a template. Supplying cells with exogenous rRNA molecules and exogenous mRNA molecules coded with a similar unique identifier such that the rRNA molecules will engage the mRNA molecules, facilitates the production of a desired protein.

CHAPTER 11

QUANTUM rRNA

Within eukaryotes, in their cytoplasm, the ribosome complex is referred to as an 80S ribosome. Generally two ribosomal proteins comprise a ribosome complex. This 80S ribosome is comprised of one 'dome-shape' 60S ribosomal protein and one 'cap-shaped' 40S ribosomal protein. Ribosomal proteins are associated with rRNA molecules.

Eukaryote cells have given rise to multi-cellular life forms including vertebrates (multi-cellular animal organisms with spines). Humans are classified as a form of vertebrate. Of the four rRNAs that reside in the cytoplasm of a eukaryote cell, the 18S rRNA is found in and helps comprise the physical structure of the 40S protein subunit of the ribosome complex and the 5S rRNA, 5.8S rRNA, and 28S rRNA molecules are found in and help comprise the physical structure of the 60S protein subunit of the ribosome complex.

The rRNA molecules are thought to provide at least three different functions for the ribosome complex. The rRNA molecules are thought to: (1) assist with identification of the messenger RNA to be translated, (2) act as an enzyme to facilitate the production of the protein molecule being translated from the mRNA molecule undergoing translation, and (3) possibly cause folding at specific locations to make the three dimensional structure of the protein being generated as the ribosome complex decodes the mRNA molecule.

Ribosomal RNAs (rRNA) are generated by RNA Polymerase I molecules that transcribe the instruction code present in the DNA. The rRNAs generally migrate to locations where mRNAs are to be utilized as templates. The rRNA molecules connect to their respective ribosome proteins and this macromolecule complex, referred to as a ribosome or ribosome complex, surrounds the beginning 5' segment of a mRNA molecule. Utilizing inherent coding, the rRNA molecules direct the ribosome pieces to build the ribosome complex around a particular strand of mRNA or particular type of mRNA.

Given there are four unique types of nucleotides that make up the physical linear strand of any RNA molecule, they may in some circumstances represent a base-four numbering system. As an analogy, at the core of the current digital computer technology, binary coding or base-two coding, which is comprised of 'ones' and 'zeros', is utilized in certain formats to code for names and numbers. The inherent coding the rRNA molecules harbor is a sequence of nucleotides which represent a unique 'name' (coded in the base-four numbering system), unique 'base-four number' or unique 'combination of a name and base-four number' that corresponds to a particular mRNA or particular type of mRNA. In this manner, rRNAs act to control which mRNA molecule will undergo translation to produce proteins, rather than a ribosome complex randomly engaging any mRNA template that happens to be available. With the DNA producing rRNA molecules that cause a ribosome to attach to a particular mRNA molecule or particular type of mRNA molecule, the Command and Control which is embedded in the DNA is able to exert control over the manufacturing capacity of the cell and produce proteins as needed, rather than producing proteins in a random fashion. By controlling the number of rRNA molecules produced, the genetic based Command and Control processes can control the number of a specific protein that is generated by the translation of a specific mRNA molecule. Producing proteins as needed by the cell, rather than in a random fashion, conserves valuable resources and conserves energy inside the cell.

Part 3

Elements of Cellular Command and Control

CHAPTER 12

ORIGIN OF CELLULAR COMMAND
AND CONTROL

Nature and the random expression of energy

Energy exits in various different microscopic and macroscopic forms in the environment. The physical nature of the earth is etched in the crust of the planet by the continuous battle waged between the trapping of energy and the release of energy. The release of energy creates force, motion and heat. The trapping of energy creates a source of energy in one location as related to a relative void of energy in a different location. The environment is in constant flux. Radiation from the sun continuously adds energy into the planet's environment, stimulating the build up and release of energy. Left to its own, nature creates dramatic, wondrous artistic displays of what unbridled energy is capable of accomplishing. The Hubble telescope has revealed colossal cosmic artwork. For the most part, energy behaves according to the known laws of physics. As our knowledge of the universe expands, mankind's written laws of physics are in continuous need of refinement especially as we discover more about the concept of energy and the power it can exhibit.

Nature represents the expression of energy that often appears to be random outbursts of thermal, radiant, electrical or exertional forces, but all are under the auspice of the laws of physics. In nature, the construct of command and control need not be present. There is only one rule of law energy needs to abide by in nature, which is the law of 'equilibrium'. Energy must exist in balance or must be progressing toward a state of balance between opposing forces. Energy flows from one form to another form in order to serve its master, the state of equilibrium.

Planet earth is always in an imbalance regarding energy. The sun continuously feeds the earth energy. The planet rotates on its axis. The Moon revolves around the Earth in a slightly eccentric orbit at a mean distance of 238,600 miles and exerts a dynamic gravitational pull on the Earth's surface as seen by the rhythmic control over the tides. As the sun exposed surface of the planet absorbs solar radiation and heats up, then cools as the planet rotates, energy transcends through energy absorbing mediums present in the atmosphere, on the surface and immediately below the surface of the planet. Energy transcends mediums in an attempt to establish equilibrium. Movements of wind, water, surface debris is related to transfer of energy. Other forces acting on the planet include gravitational forces exerted by passing comets, extraterrestrial bodies such as meteorites striking the earth and forces generated by movement of the molten core located at the center of the planet.

Life: The Purposeful Use of Energy

In contrast to nature's indiscriminate utilization of energy's power, life represents the purposeful use of energy. Life bridles energy and puts energy to constructive use.

The existence of a cell is the defining line between energy with no purpose and energy that is capable of creating useful things. The chloroplast inside a plant cell is capable of taking the sun's radiant energy and converting it to chemical energy that can be stored in adenosine triphosphate (ATP) molecules. The energy stored in ATP molecules is then capable of combining carbon dioxide (CO_2) molecules with water molecules (H_2O) and producing glucose ($C_6H_{12}O_6$) molecules. Glucose is the elemental form of sugar. Glucose is a relatively stable form of energy storage that can be used by the plant that created the sugar at a later time, or can be transferred to other forms of life to be utilized as an energy source.

Animal cells lack chloroplasts, thus animal cells are unable to directly harness the energy of the sun to generate chemical energy. Animal cells, like all cells, require energy in order to promote and sustain the chemical processes that support the existence of the cell. Animals must consume sugars or consume fats or starches and break these more complex molecules down into simple sugar. Animal cells must absorb glucose and derive their energy from metabolizing glucose molecules.

Animal cells utilize an organelle called the mitochondria to metabolize glucose molecules to obtain the ATP molecules they require to conduct biochemical reactions. In the presence of oxygen, the cell utilizes three processes termed (1) glycolysis, (2) tricarboxylic acid cycle (also referred to as the Kreb's cycle) and (3) oxidative phosphorylation, in an effort to gain 38 ATP molecules from the metabolism of one glucose molecule. The ATP molecules are then utilized throughout the cell as the energy source to perform tasks such as energy requiring biochemical reactions and to construct proteins to build intracellular and extracellular molecules and structures.

Mitochondria are found in nearly all eukaryote cells. The number of mitochondria present in a cell varies depending upon the energy requirements of a cell. The number of mitochondria in a cell may range from one large mitochondria to thousands. For example, human liver cells contain up to 2,200 mitochondria.

If an insufficient amount of oxygen is present to a cell, a cell is still able to harvest ATP from glucose molecules, but in a much less efficient manner. Utilizing the enzyme lactate dehydrogenase, a cell is able to convert pyruvate to lactic acid. The anaerobic respiration process is capable of yielding two ATP molecules for each glucose molecule. In certain cells with high needs of ATP molecules, this may be inadequate and cell damage or cell death might occur.

Enzymes are a subset of proteins that represent a means to circumvent energy requirements and facilitate chemical reactions. Enzymes both lower the activation energy necessary for chemical reactions and dramatically speed up the rate of chemical reactions. Human cells are capable of producing potentially 33,000 differing proteins. Human cells function to harness energy to create, operate and maintain physical structures to accomplish tasks.

In order for any process to be successfully carried out there needs to exist ingredients or substrates, an energy source, a means of direction for the processes to produce the necessary products and a means of removing waste. Cells successfully accomplish innumerable processes in an effort to support life.

Introduction to Cellular Command & Control

Command addresses the means of constructing and maintaining a living system. Control represents the means to successfully utilize available resources to maintain, and when possible, expand the existence of life in the face of a hostile environment.

Cellular command and control is a fractal concept. Fractal refers to a rough or fragmented geometric shape that can be split into parts. Coined by Benoit Mandebrout in 1975, the term fractal was derived from the Latin fractus meaning broken or fractured. Fractal is a term often used to describe a concept that is connected to a very complex process comprised of seemingly innumerable parts. Cell metabolism is an extremely complex array of biochemical processes requiring a very high level of orchestration for the cell to exist.

Command and control is the purposeful influence that facilitates the production and utilization of energy in an organized fashion to insure that the necessary cellular processes occur in a resolute manner.

Command and control is predicated on the existence of feedback loops. A feedback loop is a process where an action occurs, the occurrence of the action produces a product, the existence of the product acts to suppress the activity level of the process when a certain level of need has been reached.

Life in general, even at the cellular level, exists with a definitive amount of energy and resources required with survival being the primary objective beyond all other concerns. Inside the external membrane of a cell, thousands of differing processes occur. Command and control functions provide means to conduct a necessary process at a necessary rate, which includes reducing or increasing the rate as necessary or to shut the process off if the process is no longer needed. By being able to control processes, resources are conserved and products of processes are produced in adequate supplies not just to insure survivability of a cell, but to ensure correct operation of the cell as well.

In the human body, the existence of feedback loops act to conserve resources and to facilitate the production of cellular products in an efficient, organized, and balanced manner. Feedback loops control the rate of processes. Feedback loops are essential for the existence of cell operations occurring in an organized manner and rate.

Chemical production in a cell is accomplished by reactions driven by enzymes which occur to balance energy in a cell. Chemical reactions occur in relation to the amount of energy present in a cell and the availability of the necessary chemicals needed to facilitate the chemical process. Enzymatic chemical processes require no form of intelligence: just energy, one or more enzymes and raw materials.

The production of proteins, molecules existing as complex three dimensional structures comprised of one or more chains, is a process that requires a certain level of intelligence. Producing a single chained protein requires a template, referred to as a messenger RNA, from which to construct the protein. Generation of a multi-chained protein often requires more than one type of template and requires the proper linkage of the differing sub-protein chains to produce the required multi-chained macromolecule.

Hemoglobin is a macromolecule present in red blood cells. The function of hemoglobin is to act as a transport mechanism to carry oxygen from the lungs to the various tissues in the body. In the case of the hemoglobin, four protein sub-chains are joined together along with an iron atom to create the necessary macromolecule. Without hemoglobin, human life would not be possible as we know it.

The biologic effort required to create a macromolecule such as hemoglobin is defined by the command function of a cell. The instructions present in the DNA that lead to the cellular actions which create such a molecule are referred to as the command function of the cell. Both of these efforts are expressions of static intelligence present in a cell.

Both command and control are necessary for every intercellular processes, as well as intracellular processes, to exist.

An example of an extracellular feedback loop is seen in the function of the thyroid gland. The pituitary gland, located in the brain, produces the thyroid stimulating hormone (TSH). TSH is released into the blood when circulating thyroid levels are determined to be low. Presence of the TSH in the blood results in the thyroid gland being stimulated to produce and release thyroid hormone into the blood stream. The thyroid hormone circulates through the blood and eventually is detected by the pituitary. Receptors located on the surface of the pituitary cells monitor the level of the thyroid hormone circulating in the blood. When there is excess circulating thyroid hormone, the production of TSH is suppressed. When there is too little thyroid hormone circulating in the blood stream, under normal circumstances, the production and release of TSH is increased. TSH stimulates the thyroid gland to produce thyroid hormone, the resultant thyroid hormone acts in a dual manner as a master hormone in the body and also acts in a negative feedback function to down-regulate the production of TSH when there is an adequate supply of thyroid hormone.

An example of an intracellular feedback loop can be seen in diabetes mellitus. Beta cells in the islets of Langerhans in the pancreas produce insulin to be released into circulation to regulate blood sugar. Beta cells generate insulin and store the insulin in vacuoles inside the cell. Surface receptors located on the exterior of Beta cells are sensitive to fluctuations in blood sugar. When the amount of glucose circulating in the blood rises above the appropriate physiologic level, Beta cells release insulin into the blood stream. Insulin circulating in the blood engages receptors located on cell surfaces. Once engaged by an insulin molecule, an insulin receptor will facilitate the transfer of glucose from the blood, through the cell's outer membrane and into the cytoplasm of the cell. Insulin, circulating in the blood assists the cells in the body with absorption of glucose to provide cells with the energy they require to conduct chemical reactions. A physiologic normal level glucose circulating in the blood acts as a negative signal to reduce the release of insulin. Higher than physiologic levels of glucose circulating in the blood stream acts as a positive signal to stimulate the release of insulin into the blood stream.

Without the presence of command and control, cellular processes would be conducted in a random and haphazard manner. With regards to a Beta cell's production of insulin, if there existed no feedback loop, insulin molecules would be generated solely according to the amount of amino acids that could be strung together to construct insulin molecules or the amount of energy a Beta cell could generate and direct toward the cellular protein building processes utilized to generate insulin. If the insulin generating process was not contained by features of command and control, Beta cells might fill up with excess amounts of insulin beyond their normal capacity and rupture their outer membrane, damaging or destroying the cell.

Command and control is essential to the existence and survival of every single-cell or multi-cellular living organism.

Tyrosine Kinases

Tyrosine kinase refers to a number of molecules that cells use to convey instructions inside cells. Tyrosine kinases are a subclass of protein kinases which are enzymes that can transfer a phosphate group from adenosine triphosphate (ATP) molecule to a protein. The function of transferral of a phosphate group acts as an 'on' or 'off' switch in a cell. Phosphorylation of proteins regulates many cellular activities.

Tyrosine kinase molecules are often components of cell receptors. Often, once a cell surface receptor is activated, tyrosine kinase molecules either participate by propagating the signal to other molecules through phosphorylation or undergo molecular transformation to act itself as an intracellular signal. In addition to transmembrane signaling, tyrosine kinases participate in signal transduction to the nucleus, cell-cycle control, and a means of regulating the properties of transcription factors.

Mutations of tyrosine kinases and their associated receptors are thought to contribute to various forms of cancer and autoimmune diseases by causing certain cell functions, such as cycle-control, to become misregulated. Oncologists are actively working on strategies to block or down regulate tyrosine kinases in cancer cells. Rheumatologists and immunologists are researching means to regulate tyrosine kinase activity to treat inflammatory conditions. There are at least 90 tyrosine kinase genes in the human genome. The subject of tyrosine kinases is expansive enough, that to do the subject justice is beyond the scope of this text; the subject of tyrosine kinases is a more mechanical signaling, where the subjects of this text are more related to programming signals. Certainly, as the research into the cellular role of tyrosine kinases is further detailed, a large segment of cellular command and control will continue to be attributed to the activity of tyrosine kinases; this subject deserves its own textbook.

CHAPTER 13

CONCEPT OF COMMUNICATION

Communication is necessary for coordinated efforts to occur inside a cell and between cells. Multi-cellular organisms require communications to coordinate the efforts of numerous cells to facilitate growth, maintenance, survival and reproduction of the organism. Communication occurs at numerous levels in the body including signals generated between organs, signals generated within an organ to regulate organ function, cell-to-cell communication and intracellular communication; where intracellular communication includes signal transduction occurring in the cytoplasm of a cell, signal transduction from the cytoplasm to the nucleus, signal transduction occurring inside the nucleus of the cell, as well as numerous signals originating in the nucleus to be conducted to the cytoplasm.

Communication between neighboring cells in an organism occurs in two fashions including surface markers and proteins. A multi-cellular organism such as the human body contains as many as 240 different types of cells. Cells have surface markers that identify the type of cell it is to neighboring cells. Proteins are passed between cells to act as update mechanisms to coordinate the efforts of a cell with its neighbors.

Multi-cellular organisms, such as the human body, require communication between cells in one organ to other organs.

The nervous system is comprised of a network of nerve cells. Electrical activity stimulates chemical activity amongst nerve cells and sensors.

The human body's nerve center is comprised of (a) the brain and spinal cord, referred to as the central nervous system, and (b) nerves that connect the organs, muscles and skin to the spinal cord, referred to as the peripheral nervous system. The system of nerves communicates the intentions of the brain to the organs and individual muscles of the body. A variety of sensors connected to the peripheral nerves communicate the status of the body's organs to the brain, so that the brain can be apprised of injury, illness, failure and performance readiness of the organs of the body.

Outside the central and peripheral nervous system, communications between organs is facilitated by proteins. These proteins are generated by organs referred to as glands and are generally referred to as hormones. Hormones travel through the blood stream and are capable of inducing effects at one or more locations throughout the body. Hormones can be created to affect only one cell type, though numerous hormones produce a response in multiple organs simultaneously.

The responses produced by a hormone vary depending upon the construct of the cell surface receptor the hormone encounters. The same hormone might up-regulate cell activity in one type of cell, while it down-regulates activity in other types of cells.

Adrenaline is a hormone. Most people consider adrenaline to be the 'fight or flight' hormone. When a person is suddenly threatened with bodily harm, the tendency is to either fight the threat or flee the danger. When a threat is recognized 'adrenaline' is released into the blood stream. Most people equate the release of adrenaline with a burst in energy. Rightfully such a boost of energy might be necessary to either do battle with a harmful threat or to run to escape danger.

As adrenaline is released, there is a sudden burst of energy in the muscles, but other actions also occur. Adrenaline affects to heart cells in the SA node causing an increase in heart rate, an action that facilitates the pumping of oxygenated blood to the muscles. At the same time, adrenaline slows down the peristalsis activity of the intestinal tract since the act of processing food is not needed at the time of fighting or fleeing a threat.

Intracellular communication takes a variety of forms. There are numerous means of signal transduction occurring in the cytoplasm of a cell, signal transduction from the cytoplasm to the nucleus, signal transduction occurring inside the nucleus of the cell, as well as numerous signals originating in the nucleus to be conducted to the cytoplasm. Tyrosine kinases and ribonucleic acids are responsible for many of the intracellular signals which are generated in the cytoplasm and nucleus of the cell.

Communication in various forms is necessary for the coordinated actions of a single cell as well as a multi-celled organism to occur successfully to insure survivability of the organism.

CHAPTER 14

CONCEPT OF INTELLIGENCE

Intelligence is a word that is often taken for granted. The textbook definition of the word intelligence refers to the ability to acquire and apply knowledge and skill. Most individuals know what the general concept of 'intelligence' 'is', by means of knowing what intelligence 'is not'. A person driving their car in reverse down a busy road during rush hour would generally be considered not-intelligent.

The concept of intelligence is often measured by scholastic prowess. But it is well recognized that some people who are 'book smart' are not necessarily 'street smart'.

But what is really meant by intelligence and how does one come by it? To neurologists the brain remains a mysterious black box. Much of what is known about the function of the brain has been learned by what happens when one or more parts of the brain has failed or has been injured or has been invaded by a cancer. If a stroke occurs in a certain portion of the brain and the stroke leads to a recognizable deficit in function of either the brain or body, then such a loss has been noted. The assimilation of data regarding failure of the brain has lead to the medical discipline referred to as neurology.

How a person's brain generates 'intelligence' is often thought to be related to how well a person strives to learn what they are taught in the school system. Still, there are those high achievers that seem to know more than what the general body of students is taught and appear to expend little effort in attaining their academic prowess. Academic intelligence is often thought to be the product of either (1) a natural talent to absorb information or (2) a meticulous effort by an individual to learn what is taught in the school system. The detailed reasons as to why some individuals have a recognized innate tendency toward intelligence or that some individuals are able to generate intelligence by working at learning, while others are not, remains a mystery to medical science and is beyond the scope of this book and medical science in general, at this time.

The concept of intelligence can be thought of in two manners (1) dynamic intelligence and (2) static intelligence.

Dynamic Adaptable Intelligence

Dynamic adaptable intelligence is what we generally recognize as being functionally intelligent. Dynamic intelligence refers to the capability to sense the environment, learn and analyze the environment, then problem solve to facilitate maintenance, survival and reproduction of the organism. Some would include 'retaining memory of details regarding the environment' and the capacity to 'actively utilize such memories' as necessary components of a dynamic intelligence. Many would require that to be classified as 'intelligent' an organism, such as a human, needs to exhibit 'a high level of awareness and appreciation of the environment that surrounds the organism' and in some cases, be able to express this appreciation in either a verbal or written format.

Naming things is a part of our general communication using words and language; it is an aspect of every day taxonomy as we distinguish the objects of our experience, together with their similarities and differences, which we identify and classify. The use of names, as the many different kinds of nouns embedded in different languages, connects nomenclature to theoretical linguistics, while the way we mentally structure the world in relation to word meanings and experiences relates to philosophy of language.

Humans tend to learn in terms of data files organized from experiences learned by our five senses. The most abundant learned filing system is in terms of pictures, rather than numbers. Many of us 'learn' in terms of pictures because the human brain is equipped with a means to stores memories in multi-dimensional data files.

Computers utilize a core system of ones and zeros to store and process computer programs and data. Certain business software is able to organize data in two or three dimensional spread sheets.

Users of a computer are able to view and manipulate the data displayed in such spread sheet software.

Humans utilize a more powerful data storage system termed multi-dimensional data files (MD^2F). Humans are equipped to learn what one or more of the five senses is telling them of their environment and attach numerous data elements to that file including name, picture, texture, odor, color scheme, fragility or volatility, value, threat level to personal safety, ownership, etc.

The human brain is built and functions much like a network of computer processors. The brain's network of computer processors is controlled by a complex computer program referred to as the Brain Operating System Software (BOSS). The brain's operating system is written in a base-four software language and it accesses the memory data stored in complex data files.

A reflection of dynamic intelligence exhibited by the human brain is comprised of (a) how much information is stored in the multi-dimensional data files, (b) the proficiency of the pathways connecting the network of computer processors, (c) the response time regarding data retrieval and (d) capacity to analyze data and make appropriate decisions based on a combination of data being actively streamed into the brain per the body's array of sensory equipment and data or decision algorithms stored in the memory files of the brain.

An individual with academic prowess generally possesses in their brain a library of data files filled with facts or opinions thought to be academically important. Often a learned person has passed some academic test that testifies that the individual has stored enough textbook information in the data files of their brain to have answered an appropriate number of questions on a test to deem the individual as adequately smart. A person with street smarts is generally equipped with a library of data files related to experience the person has encountered. Often street smarts are generated by making numerous bad decisions and learning from the negative outcomes of those experiences.

Static Nonadaptable Intelligence

Static nonadaptive intelligence is a more fundamental form of intelligence. Static intelligence surrounds us, is a necessary part of our lives, and often controls our behavior, but is often not recognized with regards to its importance. The concept of static intelligence refers to a set of algorithms that form decision trees that generate cause and effect relationships in the physical world functioning with regards to how it is programmed, but not adapting to its environment.

The idea of a static intelligence is possibly best thought of as a computer program. Computer software is comprised of a series of instructions that are arranged to produce one or more actions inside a computer. An example of a very basic computer program would be a set of software instructions that would take two numbers and add these numbers together to achieve a sum. A slightly more complex program would send this 'sum' to a video screen to be viewed or send the 'sum' to a printer to be printed on a medium such as paper. Loop programs may add two arrays of numbers to produce an array of sums; these sums might be viewed on a video screen, printed or stored in the computer's memory for later use.

Computer programs often make comparisons of values and then generate actions based on the results of comparisons. The static intelligence of a thermostat in a house may regularly compare the air temperature in a room to a selected temperature. A thermostat may trigger the furnace to be turned on when the air temperature in the room falls below the selected temperature.

Static intelligence might be likened to a city's computerized traffic network. A computerized traffic network changes the traffic light signals at intersections, varying the 'timing' of the lights as related to the time of day and expected traffic flows utilizing the streets under control of each traffic light. The static intelligence takes the place of human traffic officers standing in intersection and directing traffic. The static intelligence of a traffic network is derived from a set of instructions that produce an algorithm that results in a decision tree that controls the traffic lights. The traffic network acting in the role of static intelligence operates to facilitate a smooth flow of traffic. A static intelligence system such as a traffic system tends to operate despite the event of a drastic change in traffic flow, such as the occurrence of an accident at the intersection. It is generally recognized that if an accident were to occur in an intersection, the traffic lights would continue to switch seemingly incognizant of the abrupt stoppage of traffic flow. Static intelligence systems do not generally operate outside the guidelines of a preset algorithm.

The average desktop computer is filled with numerous static intelligence software programs. When the power button is properly depressed numerous functions automatically begin to occur that make it possible for the user to operate the computer. Software present in the computer performs a multitude of tasks which include initializing the operating system, activating the graphics card and turning on the computer screen, seeking out hardware connected to the computer, and turning on the internal fan to keep the central processing unit cool. Software programs internal to the computer, that require no human input, automatically ready the computer for service by the human user. Static intelligence software programs have become a necessity to daily life and save humans a considerable amount of time and effort every waking moment of the day.

The concept of static intelligence can be extrapolated to include how an organism conducts certain functions in a precise format to properly achieve growth, maintenance, survival and/or reproduction. The intelligence of many animals is often referred to as 'instinct' because humans recognize that animals grow, seek food, defend themselves and mate without consulting a guidebook or attending a class or accessing the Internet for their information. We concede that animals must possess a form of intelligence; however, we generally will not concede that animals possess enough intelligence to generate truly creative thoughts or actually have the capacity to understand and appreciate the environment that they live in.

The concept of static intelligence may be best applied to the activities of the genome of a species. In sexual mating, two cells, each containing half the required genetic material for the organism, unite and form one cell. The one cell, referred to as a zygote, contains all the genetic information required to construct the life form. In the case of a complex multi-celled human, it generally takes nine months for the zygote to grow, divide, multiply, and differentiate enough to generate the fetal form of a human that has a high probability of surviving outside the womb. The very technical processes of cell growth, cell division, and cell differentiation proceed millions of times in the developing fetus, in a very regimented manner, in an automatic fashion, to eventually produce a human infant capable of transiting from the womb to an air environment.

The genome of a species exerts intelligence in the manner of being able to reliably produce copies of the organism in a predictable manner. The intelligence in this case refers to the processes stored in the DNA of a species that facilitate growth, maintenance, survival and reproduction of a cell, which in a coordinated effort leads to growth, maintenance, survival and reproduction of the organism. Information is stored in all DNA in a base-four language as a series of nucleotide bases known as adenine (A), cytosine (C), guanine (G), and thymine (T). Information is also stored in RNA in a base-four language of as a series of nucleotide bases, but these are known as adenine (A), cytosine (C), guanine (G), and uracil (U).

Part 4

Command and Control Operations of the Cell

CHAPTER 15

NUCLEAR SIGNALING PROTEINS

A 'nuclear signaling protein' (NSP) molecule is a protein molecule intended to attach to nuclear deoxyribonucleic acid (DNA), by means of zinc fingers, for the purpose of initiating or inhibiting the process of transcription of a segment of the deoxyribonucleic acid. See Figure 10. Nuclear signaling protein molecules include nuclear binding proteins (NBP), artificial transcription factors (ATF), and nuclear receptors (NR).

Nuclear signaling proteins provide a means of feedback to the nucleus from the organelles in the cell's cytoplasm. When another messenger RNA is needed to produce a specific protein, a nuclear signaling protein is generated by an organelle. The nuclear signaling protein migrates from the cytoplasm into the nucleus. Once in the nucleus, the nuclear signaling protein binds to the DNA at the site of unique identifier that the nuclear protein has been constructed to physically interface with when it reaches the proper segment of DNA. Once bound to the unique identifier of a quantum gene, the nuclear signaling protein acts in a manner similar to a control RNA in that the binding action stimulates or inhibits the assembly of a transcription complex in order to facilitate or discourage transcription of the transcribable region of the quantum gene.

Nuclear signaling proteins, when bound to the unique identifier of a quantum gene, can act in a positive manner to activate the assembly of a transcription complex to facilitate transcription of the transcribable region of a quantum gene. Nuclear signaling proteins can also exhibit the opposite effect. The reversible binding of certain nuclear signaling proteins to the unique identifier of a quantum gene may block the assembly of a transcription complex at that site. The feature of reversible blocking of a quantum gene allows for negative feedback to occur. If a particular protein is being made in excess inside a cell, a nuclear signaling protein can be generated that reversibly binds to the quantum gene responsible for transcribing the messenger RNA that codes for the protein, which will act to shut off the manufacture of the messenger RNA, in turn terminates the production of the protein. After a certain period of time lapses, the nuclear signaling protein will degrade and become disengaged from the DNA. Once the nuclear signaling protein is degraded and disengaged from the nuclear DNA, the quantum gene is available again to be transcribed to produce messenger RNA.

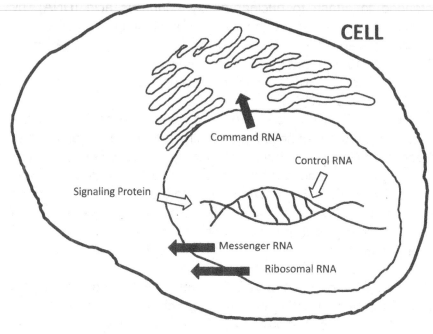

Figure 10
Intracellular signals

Proteins are comprised of one or more linear strings of amino acids. Particular segments of a protein may be termed a 'domain'. Zinc fingers refer to small protein domains that are folded, with these folds stabilized by one or more zinc ions. The three dimensional physical structure that is the result of the folding of the zinc finger

DNA binding domain facilitates the protein molecule's ability to attach to deoxyribonucleic acid (DNA), ribonucleic acid (RNA), other proteins or small molecules.

In the case whereby a zinc finger DNA binding domain facilitates a nuclear binding protein molecule to bind to nuclear DNA, the physical structure of the folding of the zinc finger DNA binding domain engages and makes contact with a specific sequence of DNA bases. A particular zinc finger DNA binding domain therefore attaches to a specific sequence of DNA bases. Once a zinc finger DNA binding domain binds to the DNA, this facilitates or represses the possible transcription of a specific segment of the DNA located near the site where the zinc finger DNA binding domain caused the nuclear binding protein molecule to bind to the DNA.

Nuclear binding proteins (NBP), also referred to as 'DNA binding proteins', are subset into at least two categories, which include: (1) immediately active nuclear binding proteins (iaNBP) and (2) delayed activity nuclear binding proteins (daNBP). Nuclear binding proteins do not require to be attached to a ligand prior to attaching to the DNA; but a nuclear binding protein may be influenced by a ligand once the NBP has attached to the DNA.

A ligand is a molecule that acts to convey a signal by binding to one or more other molecules to form a molecular complex. The presence of a ligand causes the resultant molecular complex to perform an intended function; the absence of the ligand prevents the molecular complex from performing the intended function. In the case of a daNBP, the daNBP does not require an atom or molecule to attach to it to form a complex molecule in order for the daNBP to exert an effect on the DNA.

Immediately active nuclear binding proteins (iaNBP) at a minimum are comprised of a zinc finger DNA binding domain, a transactivation domain, a C-terminal region and a N-terminal region. There may exist more than one transactivation domain. There may exist a hinge domain. There may exist more than one zinc finger DNA binding domain. The zinc finger DNA binding domain attaches its nuclear receptor to the DNA at a specific site along the DNA. The transactivation domain interacts with transcription proteins that ultimately assemble to form a transcription complex. The iaNBP attaches to a specific segment of the DNA as dictated by the zinc finger DNA binding domain present within the iaNBP. Once the iaNBP has bound to the DNA, the iaNBP activates transcription proteins to assemble into a transcription complex. The transcription complex then transcribes a segment of the DNA.

Delayed activity nuclear binding proteins (daNBP), at a minimum, are comprised of a ligand binding domain, a zinc finger DNA binding domain, a transactivation domain, a C-terminal region and a N-terminal region. There may exist more than one transactivation domain. There may exist a hinge domain. There may exist more than one zinc finger DNA binding domain. The zinc finger DNA binding domain attaches the nuclear receptor to the DNA at a specific site along the DNA. The transactivation domain interacts with transcription proteins that ultimately assemble to form a transcription complex. The ligand binding domain acts as a receptor for a ligand to bind to. The daNBP binds to the DNA per attachment of the zinc finger DNA binding domain to the DNA. The daNBP may sit attached to the DNA without activating transcription proteins, until a ligand becomes attached to the daNBP's ligand binding domain. Once a ligand binds to the ligand binding domain of the daNBP, a conformation change occurs in the daNBP molecule. The conformation change in the daNBP activates transcription proteins. Activated transcription proteins assemble into a transcription complex. The transcription complex then transcribes a segment of the DNA.

Artificial transcription factors (ATF) have been created that utilize zinc finger DNA binding domains to attach to DNA. Artificial transcription factors are comprised of a zinc finger DNA binding domain and either a domain that activates transcription or a domain that represses transcription. Artificial transcription factors attach to the DNA at a specific binding site as dictated by the construction of the zinc finger DNA binding domain. Once an artificial transcription factor binds to the DNA, if the zinc finger DNA binding domain is physically attached to an activating domain, then transcription proteins become activated and a transcription complex is assembled. If an artificial transcription factor binds to the DNA and the zinc finger DNA binding domain is physically attached to a repressor domain, then this form of artificial transcription factor prevents the assembly of a transcription complex, which results in the adjacent DNA not being able to be transcribed. Zinc finger DNA binding domains can be readily designed to attach to specific sequences of the DNA. Artificial transcription factors may be comprised of protein domains exclusively, or a combination of one or more protein domains and one or more non-protein elements. Artificial transcription factors may have a ligand binding domain as part of the molecule.

Nuclear receptors are proteins that sense the presence of ligands such as steroids, thyroid hormones, and certain other proteins. In general, nuclear receptors exist in a nonactive form until a ligand binds to the ligand binding domain. When a ligand binds to a nuclear receptor, the now activated nuclear receptor migrates to the DNA and attaches to the DNA at a specific binding site as dictated by the zinc finger DNA binding domain present within the nuclear receptor.

CHAPTER 16

HORMONE: CELL-TO-CELL COMMUNICATION

Hormones represent a group of organic substances that are produced in a cluster of cells referred to as a gland which exerts a predictable effect on one or more tissues that are adapted to respond to the presence of the hormone. A hormone is generally thought of as a substance released into the blood stream with the intent to cause one or more cellular actions to occur. The role of hormones is to regulate physiologic activities and promote homeostasis. Hormones are also generated and released by neurosecretory cells, in some instances intended to affect other nerve cells. Some hormones known as pheromones are released external to the body and act as a form of sexual attractant. Often the release of hormones is controlled by tightly regulated feedback control loops.

Thyroid Stimulating Hormone (TSH), a glycoprotein (protein and carbohydrate combination) is generated and stored in pituitary cells located in the human brain. When the pituitary gland senses the level of thyroid hormone circulating in the blood is lower than the acceptable range, the pituitary secretes TSH into the blood stream. The TSH circulates the body until it reaches the thyroid tissues present in the neck. The TSH acts to stimulate thyroid tissues to produce and release thyroid hormone into the blood. Once the thyroid gland has successfully raised the amount of thyroid hormone circulating in the blood stream, the pituitary gland ceases the release of TSH.

Nuclear receptors are proteins that sense the presence of ligands such as steroids, thyroid hormones, and certain other proteins. The description of a nuclear receptor is varied in the literature. For purposes of this text, nuclear receptors are commonly comprised of a N-terminal domain, one or more zinc finger DNA binding domains, one or more transactivation domains, a hinge region, a ligand binding domain and a C-terminal domain. In general, nuclear receptors exist in a nonactive form until a ligand binds to the ligand binding domain. Prior to a ligand binding to the nuclear receptor, the nuclear receptor may be prevented from attaching to DNA by the presence of neutralizing proteins. A ligand binding to the ligand binding domain causes: (1) a conformational change in the nuclear receptor which activates the nuclear receptor and (2) removal of the presence of any neutralizing proteins.

Separating neutralizing proteins from a nuclear receptor frees the nuclear receptor to traverse to a specific site along the deoxyribonucleic acid. The zinc finger DNA binding domain attaches the nuclear receptor to the DNA at a specific site along the DNA. The transactivation domain interacts with other transcription proteins that ultimately assemble to form a transcription complex. The transcription complex transcribes genetic information in the nuclear DNA. The hinge region is thought to facilitate changes in the three-dimensional shape of the nuclear protein.

Nuclear receptors are subset into at least four categories. The four categories include: (1) Nuclear receptors that originally reside in the cytoplasm and sense the presence of extrinsic ligands, (2) Nuclear receptors that reside in the cytoplasm and sense intrinsic ligands, (3) Nuclear receptors that reside in the nucleus and sense the presence of extrinsic ligands, and (4) Nuclear receptors that reside in the nucleus and sense the presence of intrinsic ligands. Nuclear receptors that sense 'intrinsic' ligands are often referred to as 'orphan' nuclear receptors.

When an extrinsic ligand or an intrinsic ligand binds to a nuclear receptor that resides in the cytoplasm, the now activated nuclear receptor traverses the cytoplasm, enters the nucleus, traverses the nucleus and attaches to the DNA at a specific binding site as dictated by the zinc finger DNA binding domain present within the nuclear receptor.

When an extrinsic ligand or an intrinsic ligand binds to a nuclear receptor that resides in nucleus, the now activated nuclear receptor traverses the nucleus and attaches to the DNA at a specific binding site as dictated by the zinc finger DNA binding domain present within the nuclear receptor.

Examples of extrinsic ligands are steroids and thyroid hormones, which enter the cell from the external environment surrounding the cell. Once an extrinsic ligand enters the cell it attaches to the ligand binding domain of a nuclear receptor residing in the cytoplasm or it attaches to the ligand binding domain of a nuclear receptor residing in the nucleus.

CHAPTER 17

CONTROL RNA

The concept of a unique identifier is only feasible if there is a means of utilizing the segment of DNA that comprises the unique identifier. The antithesis of the unique identifier would be either in the form of a nuclear signaling protein or a Control RNA (cnRNA).

A cell that is at rest, has a moderate number of proteins to generate for the purposes of maintenance of the cell. A cell preparing for cell division is generating numerous proteins to construct numerous parts of itself to divide amongst the resultant daughter cells. Likewise, the cells of the adult stage of a life form are generally attending to general maintenance needs, where in the embryonic stage of a life form where cells are growing and dividing at an accelerated rate, they require numerous proteins to be generated.

If nuclear signaling proteins, specifically nuclear binding proteins, were the only mechanism to identify quantum genes and activate transcription to produce proteins, that would mean that for every differing type of protein to be produced the DNA would first have to be transcribed to produce the messenger RNA for the nuclear signaling protein (mRNA-NSP) that would be used to transcribe the specific quantum gene. This mRNA-NSP would have to migrate to the cytoplasm and be translated by a ribosome to produce the intended nuclear signaling protein. This nuclear signaling protein would then have to migrate back to the nucleus and locate the specific quantum gene that it is configured to bind with in order to effect transcription of the proper messenger RNA to generate the protein that is required. Though plausible, this seems to be a labor intensive effort on the part of the cell.

There is known to exist numerous types of small nuclear RNA molecules. These short chain RNA molecules are thought to perform several duties inside the nucleus of the cell including RNA splicing. Once a gene has been transcribed, introns are excised from the original transcription product and the exons are spliced together by small nuclear RNA molecules to produce the final messenger RNA.

It would seem that a more efficient manner to transcribed specific quantum genes would be to transcribe small nuclear RNA (snRNA) molecules. Once transcribed, a snRNA would seek out and bind to the specific unique identifier of quantum gene that the snRNA is coded for and activate the construction of a transcription complex to effect the transcription of the quantum gene. The nucleotide sequence of such an RNA is already the antithesis of the unique identifier of the quantum gene and would be an effective promoter of transcription.

A control RNA (cnRNA) refers to a form of RNA small in size that exerts its effects inside the nucleus of the cell. A cnRNA may not be much larger than 25 nucleotides in length. A cnRNA is coded to attach to a particular segment of nuclear DNA that represents a specific unique identifier. See Figure 11. By the action of the control RNA attaching to the DNA at the unique identifier, this assists in the assembly of a transcription complex in the 5' Upstream region of the quantum gene so that the translatable region of the quantum gene can be decoded. See Figure 12.

Control RNA molecules represent a subset of small nuclear RNA molecules. Control RNA molecules are comprised of a portion that attaches to the unique identifier on the nuclear DNA and a segment that acts as a tail, which attracts one or more molecules that assemble into a transcription complex. The control RNA generally attaches to the nuclear DNA between the TATA box and the TSS.

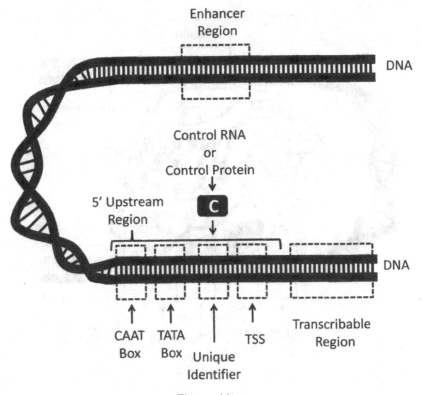

Figure 11
Control RNA or Nuclear Signaling Protein binding
to the Unique Identifier

Control RNA molecules are derived from transcribing the DNA. In order for a stepwise process to occur in an efficient manner, one gene would need to be able to point to a subsequent gene to continue certain processes of building or maintaining biologic structures. While a gene is being transcribed, a portion of the transcription process produces one or more control RNAs. These control RNAs, generated when a quantum gene is transcribed, cause other subsequent quantum genes to be transcribed by the nucleus. Control RNAs may even cause the gene that produced the control RNA to be reread, in order to form a looping action, where certain RNAs are required to be continuously produced to maintain either the cell's health or the body's health.

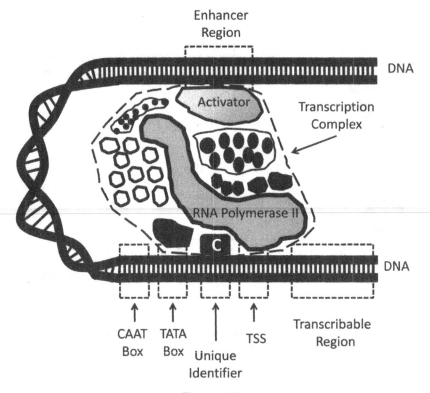

Figure 12
Presence of Control RNA or Nuclear Signaling Protein
activates assembly of a Transcription Complex

By their construction, a control RNA or a nuclear signaling protein can act to block the transcription complex from forming at the site of a specific gene. See Figure 13.

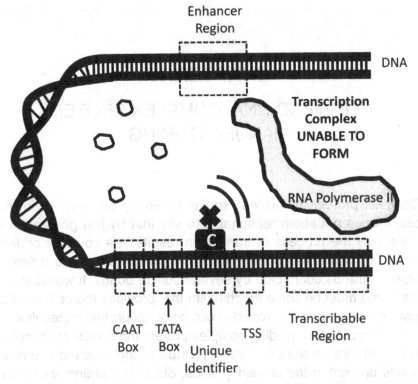

Figure 13
Control RNAs are capable of blocking transcription

A control RNA or a nuclear signaling protein, depending upon its configuration, may act to initiate the transcription of a quantum gene by stimulating the assembly of a transcription complex or inhibit the transcription of a quantum gene by acting to block the assembly of a transcription complex at the site of the quantum gene.

CHAPTER 18

COMMAND RNA: COMPLEX PROTEIN MANUFACTURING

Complex protein molecules require assembly somewhere in the cell. It does not seem reasonable to say that by just generating a protein by the process of translation results in a complex protein such as insulin. The protein insulin is comprised of two different protein strands connected by several sulfide bonds. It would seem that there must be some mechanism that provides the cell with the instructions on how to properly build complex protein molecules.

The process of building complex protein molecules could occur in one of three manners. First, by virtue of the inherent chemical bonds present in the protein strands, differing proteins are drawn together in the cytoplasm and combine to form a complex protein molecule. The problem posed by the construct of the insulin molecule is 'how do the known sulfide bonds become attached between the two protein strands?' This might occur naturally or there is some process that actively attaches such bonds at their proper locations.

Second, in a structure like the smooth endoplasmic reticulum, an extensively convoluted membrane structure present in the cytoplasm, complex proteins and lipids are constructed in an organized manner. The endoplasmic reticulum appears to be functioning as a protein manufacturing and enhancement facility. Large proteins and complex protein molecules may be formed preferentially inside such a structure. Bonding of multiple chains of proteins and bonding of proteins to other molecules such as lipids and carbohydrates may also occur in the endoplasmic reticulum.

The endoplasmic reticulum is comprised of a rough endoplasmic reticulum (RER) and the smooth endoplasmic reticulum (SER).

The rough endoplasmic reticulum is named due to the many ribosomes that appear attached to the outer surface of the structure. Ribosomes produce proteins by translating the genetic information from messenger RNA. The smooth endoplasmic reticulum is comprised of a fine meshwork of tubular membrane vesicles. Smooth endoplasmic reticulum generates phospholipids and cholesterol molecules. In specialized cells such as the liver, the SER engages in detoxification of various compounds produced by metabolic processes.

The endoplasmic reticulum packages up various molecules into vesicles and transfers these products to the Golgi apparatus. The Golgi apparatus is comprised of five to eight flat disc-shaped membrane defined cisternae (flattened vesicle) arranged in a stack. The Golgi apparatus appears to provide services essential in the maturation of certain molecules such as secretory proteins, plasma membrane proteins, lysosomal proteins, glycoproteins, and glycolipids.

Instructions on how to produce complex molecules such as combining differing proteins together or combining a protein with a fatty acid, or a protein with a lipid or a protein with a carbohydrate may be inherent in the endoplasmic reticulum or the Golgi apparatus. Similar to an automobile manufacturing plant that produces one model of car, raw materials enter the plant and due to the manner by which the assembly line is constructed a series of the same type and model of a vehicle will exit the automobile factory. No variability is necessarily required. Blue cars are made if blue paint is supplied to the manufacturing plant. High performance engines are installed in the vehicles if high performance engines are delivered to the plant to be placed in the vehicles. But what if a customer wants a sunroof?

The presence of sunroofs in vehicles is extremely common in the automotive market place today. Several decades ago this was not the case. In the past, the sunroof was not present in the early version of the car. In its infancy, the sunroof was created post production by cutting a hole in the roof of an existing vehicle. The popularity of the sunroof eventually caused this option to be offered as a feature in new cars and became part of the initial design of many vehicles.

In the automotive industry, there needs to be a means of creating enough vehicles to meet the demands of those buyers who wish to purchase cars without a sunroof and those cars that are equipped with factory installed sunroofs. Consumers appreciate factory installed sunroofs due to the lower likelihood that the seals around the sunroof panel will leak when it rains. Given the variability in fashion, the sales of sunroof equipped vehicles will change from year to year. To meet the demand for vehicle sales, the owner of an automotive company can build a separate factory to construct vehicles specifically with a sunroof and a separate factory to construct vehicles that are not equipped with a sunroof. An alternative to building separate factories is that the owner of the automotive company sends a message to his one factory to direct the factory's employees to build one quantity of vehicles equipped with a sunroof and a different quantity of vehicles without sunroofs, with the total number of vehicles targeted at aligning production with demands in vehicle sales to maximize profit.

Changing the production of cars to meet an ever changing demand in sales by the marketplace is a necessity for the survival of business. Unless the amount of production of a vehicle necessitated the construction of a new manufacturing plant, a single automotive manufacturing plant would be retooled to the point to produce all options available regarding a particular model and type of a vehicle. The number of differing types of vehicles produced would be communicated to the factory employees by those managing the factory.

The cell must find itself in a similar situation regarding variations in protein production as the owner of an automobile manufacturing plant. With the cells comprising the human body being capable of producing approximately 33,000 different proteins, there exists a significant variability in the amino acids comprising proteins, size and folding of the proteins as well as variability in the types of molecules proteins may be merged with to produce the various organic molecules that are required. The cell does not have the luxury to have a separate endoplasmic reticulum or Golgi apparatus to generate each and every protein molecule that it needs. There must exist some form of communication from the nucleus delivered to the endoplasmic reticulum and Golgi apparatus in order to produce the proper complex protein molecules required by the various cell functions.

Since the nucleus generates mRNAs, rRNAs, tRNAs and a wide variety of small nuclear RNAs, it would seem practical that the transcription process whereby RNAs are produced from a transcription complex decoding the DNA would produce an RNA that would carry instructions to the endoplasmic reticulum and Golgi apparatus with regards to the design parameters detailing 'how' complex protein molecules were to be constructed. Given the endoplasmic reticulum is contiguous with the nucleus, RNA molecules could easily migrate to the endoplasmic reticulum.

Command ribonucleic acid (cmRNA) molecules refer to RNAs that provide instruction to the endoplasmic reticulum and Golgi apparatus with regards to the design parameters detailing 'how' complex protein molecules are to be constructed. CmRNAs are generated by transcribing the nuclear DNA. CmRNAs may actually be present in the collection of introns that are sequences transcribed along with messenger RNAs that to this point have no known function.

The command RNAs traverse the nucleus to the endoplasmic reticulum. A subset of cmRNAs traverse the length of the endoplasmic reticulum to the cytoplasm to eventually migrate to the Golgi apparatus. Inside the endoplasmic reticulum the cmRNAs provide the proper instructions and prompts to effect splicing and folding of proteins to produce complex multi-chain protein macro molecules.

CHAPTER 19

DISTRIBUTED PROCESSING IN THE DNA

The average desk top or laptop computer is fundamentally comprised of a single central processing unit (CPU) which may have multiple cores, a hard drive that acts as a memory, a video output such as a computer screen, a graphics card to display complex video images, USB ports and a disc drive. The desk top computer, the laptop computer, notebook computer and now the smart phone and tablets function by streaming necessary information through the single CPU. In a basic system, all intelligent functions are coordinated by the CPU. See Figure 14.

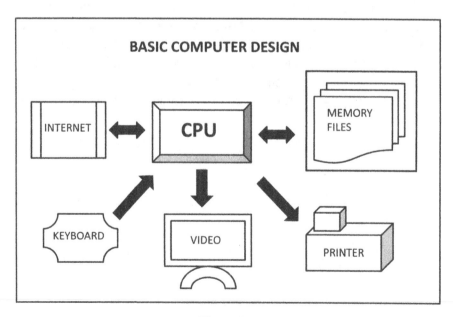

Figure 14
Components of a computer

The new age of computers have multiple core central processing units. Altering the core of the central processing unit allows the central processor to increase its efficiency by multi-tasking. Math processing units have been associated with CPUs for over a decade, whereby any math problem is shunted to the math unit for performance of the calculation while the CPU busies itself with other tasks. Most recently there has been a trend of employing two or more CPU operating units working in conjunction with each other in order increase the speed by which the computer complex can attend to tasks.

The central processing unit of the cell's nucleus is the transcription complex. See Figure 15. The transcription complex is assembled at the site of a quantum gene to be transcribed. The transcription complex is comprised of at least 40 proteins. Following assembly of the transcription complex upstream from the transcribable region of a quantum gene, the transcription complex moves downstream and generates at least one RNA molecule.

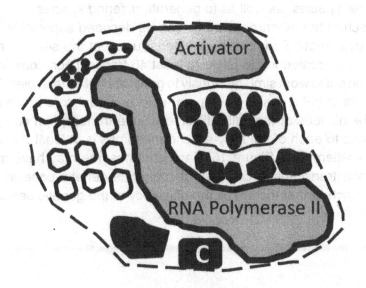

**Transcription
Complex**

Figure 15
The transcription complex

Within the human genome there are 46 individual chromosomes. Contained in the 46 chromosomes are 3 billion nucleotide base pairs, each representing a 'character', to comprise the DNA's programming language. The 3 billion characters are divided into meaningful data, which it has been estimated to be 5% of the genome, and redundant data which accounts for the remaining 95% of the genome. Associated with the 5% of the human genome that represents meaningful data, this portion of the DNA has been subdivided into at least 32,000 genes. Since a gene is a unit of heredity and codes for the production of a protein and since there are at least 33,000 proteins, this is what leads to the estimate of number of genes present in the human genome. Current understanding suggests some genes code for more than one protein due to alternative splicing. Alternative splicing refers to the same genetic segment may be transcribed but differing exons may be used to comprise the final messenger RNA molecule. Nature utilizes this process to conserve genetic information yet still generate variations amongst species, as well as to generate differing species.

Each of the 46 chromosomes can be decoded separately. The cell's transcription complexes are constructed at the site of where the data is located in the DNA. At least 46 transcription complexes could be put to work simultaneously to generate RNA molecules. This suggests that if a desktop computer utilizes a dual core processor, that the nucleus of the cell with at least one transcription complex assigned to each of the forty-six chromosomes is at least 23 times more efficient. See Figure 16. Each chromosome may have more than one transcription complex decoding its genetic code at one time, which further increases the efficiency of the genetic decoding system.

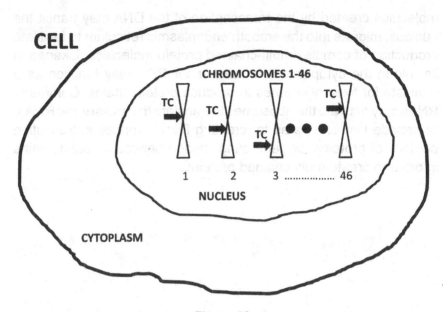

Figure 16
Each chromosome can be transcribed independently

Since there are differing RNA polymerase molecules that are used to generate the different RNAs, the processing power of the nucleus of a cell may be much more advanced than our current computer system. RNA Polymerase I is used to transcribe rRNA, RNA Polymerase II is used to transcribe mRNA and RNA Polymerase III is used to transcribe tRNA, snRNA, and other RNA molecules. When a cell is not dividing, the DNA is often stretched out, unraveled at differing locations. Multiple transcription complexes may be at work transcribing one chromosome simultaneously, again increasing the processing power of the nucleus to read and act on the data stored in the memory of the DNA.

In a desktop or laptop the data is fed to the CPU and processed. With regards to the human genome, the processor or reader goes to the data. The transcription complex forms around the DNA at the 5' end of the gene, upstream of the transcription start point.

There may be exceptions. The smooth endoplasmic reticulum attached to the nucleus of the cell may function similar to the CPU of a computer. Messenger RNA molecules and command RNA molecules created by the transcription of the DNA may transit the nucleus, migrate into the smooth endoplasmic reticulum to facilitate production of complex multi-chained protein molecules. Likened to its role in the cytoplasm, the messenger RNA may function as a template for fixed ribosomes to produce protein chains. Command RNAs may activate the ribosomes to translate the messenger RNAs, or provide instructions as to; creating folds in proteins, truncating portions of proteins, or generating linkage between protein chains in order to create multi-chained proteins.

CHAPTER 20

MAPPING OUT THE DNA

Once the concepts of unique identifiers, reference tables, bundled programming instructions, feedback mechanisms and data files have been recognized, the functions that they represent can be used as search tools to decode the human genome.

If we recognize that unique identifiers exist and would be comprised of approximately twenty-five characters in length, then the three billion base-pairs of nucleotides comprising the DNA can be searched for segments of approximately twenty-five characters that appear to be exhibiting a sequential number system.

Once a sequential numbering system has been established, one could then take existing DNA data pertinent to segments of the DNA that have been previously identified as to representing genes. Genes are either data files, if their presence dictates a physical characteristic of a specimen of a species (such as eye color, hair color, skin color, height, etc.), or they contain instructions related to the means to conduct a process. Arranging the known gene information by chromosome and location along the chromosomes will assist in mapping out the remaining DNA.

Five percent of the DNA has been identified as being related to genes. The remaining 95% of the DNA has been thought to represent redundant genetic material or genetic garbage. Within the scope of the remaining 95% of the DNA, more likely a portion is related to instructions. Instructions are more difficult to identify since they code for the means to conduct chemical or protein building processes and they code for the manner by which an organelle, a cell, an organ or overall how the body as a whole is constructed, rather than physical characteristics of an organism.

The DNA is known to contain genes that are associated with human proteins, but there is also information stored in the human genome that can be traced to similar genetic information found in plants. It has been suggested that humans share 47% of their genome with a banana. There is also a portion of the human genome that is related to viral DNA. It has been estimated that there are elements of at least 450,000 virus genomes present in human DNA. Contrasting and comparing the human genome with both the genome of other living organisms as well as viral genomes will assist in decoding and subdividing the human genome into an understandable biologic computer language. All organic life on the planet uses the same fundamental building blocks to generate their particular genome. All organic life shares a basic set of instruction code in order to create and maintain essential cellular functions.

It would be logical to consider that likened to desktop computer software, there would be basic essential programming instructions that would represent 'IF THEN', GO TO, as well as ADDITION and SUBTRACTION functions. Understanding the behavior of currently recognized genes would lead to decoding the instructions that comprise these genes.

Human programmers often place text inside their computer programming code to identify important facts about the computer program or the subprograms that comprise the program. When deciphering the computer language used to create the human genome, it is important to remember that text files could exist. The text would play no active role in how a program functions. A text file may be comprised of simply a word used to identify a subprogram or line of programming, or a text file might be represented as a string of words or symbols that discusses a portion of the program in detail.

The human genome is therefore comprised of differing sections. The 3 billion base pairs of the human genome would be divided into data files, instruction files, remnants of viral genomes and possibly text files.

Data files contain the parameters of physical features of the body. Data files are easy to understand and locate in the human genome since they generally dictate the recognizable physical features of the body such as height, skin color, eye color, and hair color. Over the years data files have been referred to as genes.

Instruction code is more difficult to identify due to the lack of direct attachment to a physical feature of the body. Understanding and locating instruction code in a biologic program necessitates at least a rudimentary understanding of the syntax use by the writer of the programming instructions. Genetic instructions may be silently present since physical error or damage involving one or more nucleotide bases comprising a genetic instruction or the deletion of one or more nucleotide bases comprising certain a genetic instruction may or may not produce a physical effect in the body that can be easily detected by a researcher.

The human genome is therefore thought to be comprised of at least the 5% of the DNA that has been recognized as genes. The remaining 95% of the human genome that currently is recognized as nonfunctional or redundant genetic information.

The 95% of the human genome is comprised of micro instructions, command and control instructions, macro instructions, remnants of viral genomes and text files. See Figure 17. The micro instructions include instruction on how to construct the cell, information regarding the chemical processes performed by the cell, instructions on how to build the various organelles present in cells and instructions on how to generate specialized cells. The macro instructions are needed as the means to generate the organs of the body and to orchestrate the overall physical design of the body.

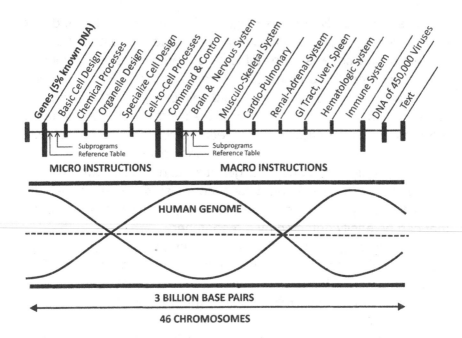

Figure 17
The Human Genome is divided into data files
and genetic instruction code, traces of viral genomes and text files

The instructions, which in the case of the genome dictate the means and manner by which the structures of the human body are generated, require far more detail due to the complexity than the details of the physical attributes of a structure. If the physical attributes such as dimensions, color, and content represent 5% of the genome of an intricate structure such as the human body, the instructions required to build the structures of the human form may require the majority of the remaining 95% of the genome.

CHAPTER 21

GENETIC REFERENCE TABLES

Reference Tables in the Genome

In addition to unique identifiers being present in the 5' Upstream segment of a quantum gene, unique identifiers may comprise an important part of reference tables. To facilitate the physical construction of a species, more than likely there are reference tables present in the chromosomes, which are comprised of an organized list of unique identifiers. Such reference tables represent a list of addresses of the locations of quantum genes. Each of the unique identifiers in the reference table would point to a specific gene necessary to be manufactured for a particular species. As each unique identifier is selected, the gene associated with the unique identifier is located and a transcription complex is formed to facilitate transcription of the gene. Such a reference table would insure the genes were transcribed in an orderly fashion to promote the successful production of a representative of a particular species.

Mathematical systems tend not to be arbitrary. Table 6 demonstrates comparison of the four nucleotides. In comparison of total bonds, total atomic number and total atomic weight the rankling of the four nitrogenous bases used to construct the four nucleotides comprising DNA from smallest to largest is Cytosine, then Thymine, then Adenine and finally Guanine. The actual numbering system present in the genome is likely related to the size or weight of the molecule. A comparison of the four nitrogenous bases is presented in Table 6. In a mathematical system the first element would represent a zero. Utilizing the ranking of the four nitrogenous bases mentioned above to designate the order, Cytosine would represent the 'zero' since it is the smallest of the four nitrogenous bases. Thymine would represent the 'one' being the next nitrogenous base. Adenine represents the 'two' being ranked third. Guanine represents the 'three' since it is the largest of the four nitrogenous bases. C=0, T=1, A=2, G=3.

Nitrogenous base	Hydrogen Atoms	Nitrogen Atoms	Carbon Atoms	Oxygen Atoms	Total Bonds	Total Atomic Number	Total Atomic Weight	Rank
Cytosine	4	3	4	1	16	57	110.0939	1
Thymine	5	2	5	2	17	65	125.1052	2
Adenine	4	5	5	0	19	69	134.1186	3
Guanine	4	5	5	1	20	77	150.118	4

Table 6

Comparison of the nitrogenous bases used in construction of DNA.

There may be a number of different reference tables written into the chromosomes to provide an organized plan to construct a wide variety of physical structures comprising the body of an organism. There would be a reference table dictating the construction sequence of the body of a species as a whole. There may be a reference table dedicated to the construct of each organ of a body. There may be a reference table regarding the construction of each of the different cell types comprising a body. There may be a reference table dedicated to the construct of a basic cell design. There may be reference tables defining the construction of each organelle found in a cell. There may also be reference tables assigned to listing a series of unique identifiers that are associated with the maintenance of the body as a whole and/or for each of the different cells comprising a body. Reference tables and the quantum genes they point to are most likely conserved between species. A generic reference table dictating basic construction of a generic cell might appear as the example presented in Table 7.

Number	Unique Identifier 25-characters	Transcript Region	Cell Components
1	0000000000000100000000000 CCCCCCCCCCCCCCTCCCCCCCCCCC	1	Genes to construct cell membrane
2	0000000000000111000000000 CCCCCCCCCCCCCCTTTCCCCCCCCC	2	Genes to construct chloroplast
3	0000000000000112 000000000 CCCCCCCCCCCCCCTTACCCCCCCCC	3	Genes to construct mitochondria
4	000000000000011 3010000000 CCCCCCCCCCCCCCTTGCTCCCCCCC	4	Genes to construct Golgi Apparatus
5	0000000000000111 111 000000 CCCCCCCCCCCCCCTTTTTTCCCCCC	5	Genes to construct rough endoplasmic reticulum
6	0000000000000111111 2 00000 CCCCCCCCCCCCCCTTTTTTACCCCC	6	Genes to construct smooth endoplasmic reticulum
7	000000000000011112 1 000000 CCCCCCCCCCCCCCTTTTATCCCCCC	7	Genes to construct flagella
8	00000000000001111 31000000 CCCCCCCCCCCCCCTTTTGTCCCCCC	8	Genes to construct micro tubular network
9	0000000000000111 221000000 CCCCCCCCCCCCCCTTTAATCCCCCC	9	Genes to construct lysosomes
10	0000000000000111 223000000 CCCCCCCCCCCCCCTTTAAGCCCCCC	10	Genes to construct vacuoles
11	0000000000000200000000000 CCCCCCCCCCCCCCACCCCCCCCCCC	11	Genes to construct nuclear membrane
12	000000000000022 1111 000000 CCCCCCCCCCCCCAA TTTTCCCCCC	12	Genes to construct chromosomes
13	000000000000022 3111 000000 CCCCCCCCCCCCCAAGTTTCCCCCC	13	Genes to construct nucleosides
14	000000000000022 32111 00000 CCCCCCCCCCCCCAAGATTTCCCCC	14	Genes to construct mitotic spindles

Table 7

Example of how unique identifiers may organize construction of a cell*.

*all numbers presented as unique identifiers are meant to be for illustration purposes only; where C=0, T=1, A=2, G=3 have been assigned based on molecular weight.

The information presented in Table 7 is only meant to act as a simplified example of what a reference table for constructing a cell might appear like in the chromosomes. Tables such as this may be widespread throughout the DNA and function to orchestrate the construction of all types of physical elements comprising the body. Reference tables may be even present at the level of providing the proper sequence of steps required to manufacture individual chemical molecules needed by the cell. In Table 7, under the heading of 'Unique Identifier 25-characters' is presented both the numerical and the nucleotide sequence for the unique identifier.

Given that there is a base-four mathematical system comprising the DNA of all organic species it is reasonable to extrapolate that quantum genes have been lumped together into four organized branches. Table 8 is an illustration of a very rudimentary level of organization.

Number	Unique Identifier 25-characters	Branch	Genes to Construct
1	0000000000000000000000000 CCCCCCCCCCCCCCCCCCCCCCCCC	1	Cell and Proteins
2	1000000000000000000000000 TCCCCCCCCCCCCCCCCCCCCCCCC	2	Prokaryotes
3	2000000000000000000000000 ACCCCCCCCCCCCCCCCCCCCCCCC	3	Viruses
4	3000000000000000000000000 GCCCCCCCCCCCCCCCCCCCCCCCC	4	Eukaryotes

Table 8
Arbitrary starting point per unique identifiers to identify
the four branches of genes*.

*all numbers presented as unique identifiers are meant to be for
illustration purposes only; where C=0, T=1, A=2, G=3 have been
assigned based on molecular weight.

In of themselves, reference tables would have no phenotypical characteristics to identify their presence in the DNA. Reference tables represent a series of commands manifested by pointing to a series of quantum genes that are arranged in an orderly fashion to act as a guide to insure the proper construction of the physical elements comprising a cell. More than likely, reference tables occupy a portion of the DNA that at this time is considered to be meaningless genetic code or as some have described 'useless genetic junk'. Much of the generic code considered to be useless at this time, because it does not exhibit the phenotypical features of the currently known genes, is comprised of the instructions necessary to utilize the known body of genes.

Genetic Reference Tables: Basis of Observed Evolution

Unique identifiers make it possible to locate quantum genes in the nuclear DNA. Reference tables provide an orderly means for transcribing a group of quantum genes. Speed of transcription becomes an important factor in cell growth and metabolism. It is also important to the survival of the entire organism. How fast the nucleus can locate a quantum gene may be just as important as locating and transcribing the gene. Since there are forty-six chromosomes comprising human genetics, knowing which chromosome harbors a particular quantum gene is vital to locating the quantum gene.

There may be one or more reference tables that identify, amongst the forty-six chromosomes, where each quantum gene resides.

Control of transcription of quantum genes may be a hybrid of (1) directions provided by a reference table, but may also be related to (2) instructions present in the end of the transcription region or in the 3' Downstream segment of a quantum gene.

After the transcribable region of a quantum gene has been transcribed, the transcription complex may proceed to transcribe one or more control RNA (cnRNA) molecules. The purpose of the control RNA molecules would be to: (1) point back to the reference table or (2) point directly to the next gene that is required to be transcribed. Once a control RNA molecule is generated, either the molecule traverses the nucleus to the location of the reference table to provide feedback that indicates that the required quantum gene was indeed transcribed and the next quantum gene in the series should be transcribed or the control RNA molecule traverses the genome and directly activates a transcription complex at the site of the next quantum gene. Control RNA molecules may be manufactured as the antithesis of the unique identifier found either in the reference table or in the 5' Upstream region of a quantum gene to facilitate the act of binding of the control RNA molecule to the unique identifier.

The changes that have occurred to the life forms that have inhabited the planet, as been documented by paleontologists and geneticists, has been referred to as evolution. Evolution has been thought to be related to alterations in the genes of species, these alterations occurring randomly, but being responsible for the development of new forms of life. Changes in the DNA that have led to evolutionary changes may actually in part be due to functional changes that have occurred within the bounds of the genetic reference tables stored in the genome. If genome reference tables direct the order by which transcription of genes occurs, then an alteration of a genome reference table would change which quantum genes were transcribed or the order of when quantum genes were transcribed.

Histones are alkaline protein molecules that exist alongside nuclear DNA. Histones are thought to be associated with the physical state of the chromatin during cell division and transcription of genetic material. The exact role of histones is not entirely clear. The assumption is that these proteins help with packing of the DNA into tightly wound units to facilitate cell division. Histones may, in part, be responsible for allowing certain quantum genes to be transcribed versus blocking the transcription of certain quantum genes. The actions of histones may in fact be a mechanism that turns on and turns off genes by physically preventing various genes from being transcribed by preventing the DNA from opening up and allowing a transcription complex to assemble in the 5' Upstream region of a quantum gene. In the case of a reference table, the position of histones along the nuclear DNA may allow certain portions of a reference table to be transcribed, while other portions of the reference table may be blocked from being transcribed.

A master genome reference table may be associated with each species. Genome reference tables represent a list of addresses of the locations of quantum genes. A generic master genome reference table may be refined to specific details associated with most species.

This generic master genome reference table may be altered by various external or internal factors that lead to the master genome reference table for each species. This would suggest that genes comprising the DNA may be transcribed or not transcribed. If a quantum gene is necessary for the construction or the maintenance of a species it is transcribable. If a quantum gene is not necessary it is dormant and is never transcribed during the lifecycle of the species.

A species generic master genome reference table would be present in some form for all organisms. Smaller, more truncated forms of the master genome reference table may be present in more primitive organisms. The concept of a generic master genome reference table would help explain why the single celled organism Red Algae possesses 60 chromosomes, while humans possess only 46 chromosomes. As life forms develop into more sophisticated and diverse organisms there may not be a need to conserve all of the genetic instructions from one species to another or from one generation to another. More sophisticated life forms could discontinue replicating genes that will never be used in succeeding generations or succeeding species, thus conserving resources and energy. Conversely, if a catastrophic disaster were to strike the earth leading to mass extinction of a majority of the species, as has been estimated to have occurred at least six times in earth's history, primitive life, if it survived, could recultivate the earth by acting as a reservoir for the DNA genome.

Universal Genome Reference Table

A universal genome reference table would be comprised of quantum genes from all four branches of genes. Similar to that seen in Table 8, the information present in Table 9 demonstrates a evidence of divisions of the last two branches to demonstrate the presence of Archaebacteria and Eubacteria and the four major taxonomy kingdoms including Fungi, Protista, Plantae and Animalae. Table 9 is a very elementary representation of what a universal genome reference table would appear like. An actual universal genome master genome reference table would be much more elaborate and far more detailed.

Number	Unique Identifier 25-characters	Branch	Genes to Construct
1	000000000000000000000000000 CCCCCCCCCCCCCCCCCCCCCCCCC	1	Cell and Proteins
2	100000000000000000000000000 TCCCCCCCCCCCCCCCCCCCCCCCC	2	Prokaryotes
3	110000000000000000000000000 TTCCCCCCCCCCCCCCCCCCCCCCC	2	Archaebacteria
4	130000000000000000000000000 TGCCCCCCCCCCCCCCCCCCCCCCC	2	Eubacteria
5	200000000000000000000000000 ACCCCCCCCCCCCCCCCCCCCCCCC	3	Viruses
6	300000000000000000000000000 GCCCCCCCCCCCCCCCCCCCCCCCC	4	Eukaryotes
7	300000000000000000000000000 GCCCCCCCCCCCCCCCCCCCCCCCC	4	Protista
8	310000000000000000000000000 GTCCCCCCCCCCCCCCCCCCCCCCC	4	Fungi
9	320000000000000000000000000 GACCCCCCCCCCCCCCCCCCCCCCC	4	Plantae
10	330000000000000000000000000 GGCCCCCCCCCCCCCCCCCCCCCCC	4	Animalae

Table 9

Arbitrary starting point per unique identifiers to identify the two branches of Prokaryote genes and four branches of Eukaryote genes*.

*all numbers presented as unique identifiers are meant to be for illustration purposes only; where C=0, T=1, A=2, G=3 have been assigned based on molecular weight.

Each of the four major taxonomy kingdoms of classification including Protista, Fungi, Plantae and Animalae would have their own generic master genome reference table comprised of the list of quantum genes that can be selected to support a viable species. Ultimately, most likely there was one original universal genome reference table that described all quantum genes. The universal genome reference table would have been modified into smaller reference tables per Kingdom, Phylum, Family and Order for ease of replication. Diversity amongst life may be related to the switching on and off of genes that are present in generic reference tables.

If the genomes of all forms of life were to be combined together and redundant segments reduced to only one copy, the universal master genome reference table could be recompiled; though some of the genes utilized exclusively by the most primitive life forms may have been lost when those forms of life became extinct.

The concept of a universal genome reference table would provide an explanation as to why fish in the oceans could over time evolve into legged creatures and birds. An overly simplified version of a universal genome reference table is present in Table 10. A universal master genome reference table coincides with the observations that the basic construct of fins lead to legs and then led to the construct of wings. The genes related to the construct of fins became untranscribable (deactivated), while the genes that led to the construct of legs and wings became transcribable (activated) as necessary. The genes that provide the instructions as to how the physical features are constructed don't necessarily change, the master generic reference tables derived from the universal master genome reference table select combinations of features that provide plant and animal species that are intended to have the optimal chance at survival given the prevailing environmental conditions at the time. Reference tables changing versus genes changing makes for both (1) an organized and adaptable evolutionary process regarding species development, as well as (2) a balanced ecosystem. The concept of reference tables provides the needed explanation of organization leading to a successful viable ecosystem, which has otherwise been explained as the result of sheer randomness.

For adaption to occur the option to adapt must already be available to the species. The concept of survival of the fittest hones the possible variations of a species to a more survivable form or selects which species will flourish and which will become extinct given the constraints of the prevailing environment, but the option to create a new species must already be present. Random mutations don't grow limbs from flat bodies, that extends three or more feet and terminate into a thumb and fingers with a dedicated nerve supply, blood supply, and microscopic sensor array when no such structure ever previously existed in the history of the planet.

Branch	Unique Identifier 25-characters	Instructions to manufacture species
1	000000000000100000000000 CCCCCCCCCCCCCTCCCCCCCCCC	Genes to construct cell membrane
1	000000000000111000000000 CCCCCCCCCCCCCTTTCCCCCCCCC	Genes to construct chloroplast
1	000000000000112000000000 CCCCCCCCCCCCCTTACCCCCCCCC	Genes to construct mitochondria
1	00000000000001 13010000000 CCCCCCCCCCCCCTTGCTCCCCCCC	Genes to construct Golgi apparatus
1	000000000000011 1121000000 CCCCCCCCCCCCCTTTTATCCCCCC	Genes to construct flagella
1	00000000000001111 31000000 CCCCCCCCCCCCCTTTTGTCCCCCC	Genes to construct micro tubular network
1	000000000000200000000000 CCCCCCCCCCCCCACCCCCCCCCCC	Genes to construct nuclear Membrane
1	000000000000221111 000000 CCCCCCCCCCCCCAATTTTCCCCCC	Genes to construct chromosomes
1	000000000000022 3211000000 CCCCCCCCCCCCCAAGATTCCCCCC	Genes to construct mitotic spindles
2	110000000000000000000000 TTCCCCCCCCCCCCCCCCCCCCCCC	Genes to construct Archaebacteria
2	130000000000000000000000 TGCCCCCCCCCCCCCCCCCCCCCCC	Genes to construct Eubacteria
3	210000000000000000000000 ATCCCCCCCCCCCCCCCCCCCCCCC	Genes to construct viruses Prokaryotes
3	210000000000000000000000 ATCCCCCCCCCCCCCCCCCCCCCCC	Genes to construct viruses Eukaryotes
3	23 123 10310000031103 021 033 AGTAGTCGTCCCCCGTTCGCATCGG	Genes to construct HIV
4	300000000000000000000000 GCCCCCCCCCCCCCCCCCCCCCCCC	Genes to construct Protista
4	310000000000000000000000 GTCCCCCCCCCCCCCCCCCCCCCCC	Genes to construct Fungi
4	320000000000000000000000 GACCCCCCCCCCCCCCCCCCCCCCC	Genes to construct Plantae
4	320000000001 1223 211000000 GACCCCCCCCCTTAAGATTCCCCCC	Genes to construct hypha
4	3200000000 111 22 3211000000 GACCCCCCCCCTTTAAGATTCCCCCC	Genes to construct spores
4	320000000001222 3 211000000 GACCCCCCCCCCTAAAGATTCCCCCC	Genes to construct seed
4	320000000001 32232 11 000000 GACCCCCCCCCCTGAAGATTĊCCCCC	Genes to construct leaves

4	330000000000000000000000000 GGCCCCCCCCCCCCCCCCCCCCCCCC	Genes to construct Animalae
4	3300000000111 22 3211 000000 GGCCCCCCCCCTTTAAGATTCCCCCC	Genes to construct skeleton
4	33000000001 22 300001000000 GGCCCCCCCCCTAAGCCCCTCCCCCC	Construct a heart
4	330000000022 22 00001000000 GGCCCCCCCCAAAACCCCTCCCCCC	Construct lungs
4	3300000000 3222 00001000000 GGCCCCCCCCGAAACCCCTCCCCCC	Construct a kidney
4	3300000000000000000 1000000 GGCCCCCCCCCCCCCCCCTCCCCCC	Genes to construct a pancreas
4	330000000033 22 00001000000 GGCCCCCCCCGGAACCCCTCCCCCC	Genes to construct a liver
4	3300000000000 22 3211000000 GGCCCCCCCCCCCCAAGATTCCCCCC	Genes to construct a fin
4	3300000000000 2232 11100000 GGCCCCCCCCCCCCAAGATTTCCCCC	Genes to construct an arm limb
4	3300000000000 223 211110000 GGCCCCCCCCCCCCAAGATTTTCCCC	Genes to construct a leg limb
4	3300000000000 223 211300000 GGCCCCCCCCCCCCAAGATTGCCCCC	Genes to construction of a tail

Table 10

Simplified version of a Universal Genome Reference Table*.

*all numbers presented as unique identifiers are meant to be for illustration purposes only; where C=0, T=1, A=2, G=3 have been assigned based on molecular weight.

There is most likely an element of randomness when it comes to appearance of species over the last 3.5 billion years that life has existed on the planet. If the generic master genome reference table produces a species specific reference table which defines certain phenotypic features that are to comprise a species, if that species is produced it is necessary that it survive to pass on its new arrangement of transcribable genes. Many variations of species specific reference tables have probably been attempted that have never survived, or survived only over the course of a few generations. All known species have appeared and become extinct, except for those in existence today; average life of a species is considered to be 10 million years. The law of survival of the fittest still empowers some species to survive while others become extinct. Species that survive most likely are the product of a species specific reference table that dictates a series of transcribable quantum genes that takes best advantage of the environmental conditions that exist on the planet at the time the species lived on the planet. At least to date, all species eventually die out and become extinct; most likely related to the ever changing environmental factors.

Another observation that generic master genome reference tables helps to explain is that if evolution occurred due purely to random chance, then we should see the development of individual species going forward into more sophisticated forms as well as backwards into less sophisticated or defined forms. That is, random chance works both ways. The number of positive steps forward should equal the number of negative steps backwards. For the most part, life appears to have evolved from more primitive forms to more sophisticated and complex forms. The utilization of generic master genome reference tables capable of being influenced by external signals such as environmental factors and producing more complex multi-cell organisms, would explain the tendency toward evolution from more primitive forms to more sophisticated life forms.

A generic master genome reference table would also help explain how, following each of the estimated six occurrences when life on the planet experienced a catastrophic event that caused the extinction of ninety percent of the species, that the ecosystem was able to rebuild itself. Evolution, based on random chance would have an extremely difficult time surviving in the face of harsh, sudden, unpredictable changes to the habitat; such as a meteorite six miles wide colliding with the earth. A generic master genome reference table would be able to offer options to rearrange the groupings of transcribable quantum genes to produce new life forms that could adapt and flourish in a changing environment.

Master Reference Table for Plants

As mentioned above, the plant kingdom would have its own master genome reference table, which would be further subdivided to provide the necessary instructions to produce all of the individual species of plants. Such a reference table, see Table 11, for each plant species would contain instructions to produce a basic cell and instructions to produce each individual component of the plant necessary to produce each specific plant species. The reference table would be stored in the seed of the plant and provide the genetic direction as to how to construct the plant in an orderly step-wise fashion. As in the life of a seed, the reference table could lay dormant for any length of time, until the proper environmental conditions exist necessary to activate the seed.

As a seed is activated, pointers systematically traverse the entries present in the master genome reference table, which in turn facilitates the transcription of transcribable quantum genes or activates other reference tables, which in turn facilitate the transcription of transcribable genes. Mutations, replication errors, selections, viruses or environmental factors may be responsible for certain quantum genes being transcribable versus untranscribable.

Higher orders of plants would not need to contain any genetic material regarding the genes required for the construction of animal species except in a rudimentary form. The genes present in plants would be mostly from branches 1, 2, and 4. Genes in a species genome would include quantum genes to construct basic cell structures and macro molecules, quantum genes from viruses that utilize plant cells as hosts and quantum genes dedicated to generating the plant species.

Branch	Unique Identifier 25-characters	Instructions to manufacture species
1	00000000000000100000000000 CCCCCCCCCCCCCCTCCCCCCCCCCC	Genes to construct cell membrane
1	00000000000000111000000000 CCCCCCCCCCCCCCTTTCCCCCCCCC	Genes to construct chloroplast
1	00000000000000112000000000 CCCCCCCCCCCCCCTTACCCCCCCCC	Genes to construct mitochondria
1	000000000000011 3010000000 CCCCCCCCCCCCCCTTGCTCCCCCCC	Genes to construct Golgi Apparatus
1	000000000000011 1131000000 CCCCCCCCCCCCCCTTTTGTCCCCCC	Genes to construct micro tubular Network
1	00000000000000200000000000 CCCCCCCCCCCCCCACCCCCCCCCCC	Genes to construct nuclear Membrane

1	00000000000002211 11000000 CCCCCCCCCCCCCCAATTTTCCCCCC	Genes to construct chromosomes
1	000000000000022 3211100000 CCCCCCCCCCCCCAAGATTTCCCCC	Genes to construct mitotic spindles
4	3200000000001 22 3211000000 GACCCCCCCCCCTAAGATTCCCCCC	Genes to construct seed
4	320000000000 2223 211000000 GACCCCCCCCCCAAAGATTCCCCCC	Genes to construct leaves
4	32 00000003000223 211000000 GACCCCCCCGCCCAAGATTCCCCCC	Genes to construct flowers
4	32000000002002 23 211000000 GACCCCCCCCACCAAGATTCCCCCC	Genes to construct roots system
4	3200000000 220223 211000000 GACCCCCCCCAACAAGATTCCCCCC	Genes to construct stem and Branches

Table 11

Simplified version of a master genome reference table for plants*.

*all numbers presented as unique identifiers are meant to be for illustration purposes only; where C=0, T=1, A=2, G=3 have been assigned based on molecular weight.

Master Reference Table for Animals

As mentioned above, the animal kingdom would have its own master genome reference table, which would be further subdivided to provide the necessary instructions to produce all of the individual species of animals. Such a reference table, see Table 12, for each animal species would contain instructions to produce a basic cell and instructions to produce each individual component of the animal necessary to produce each specific animal species. The reference table would be stored in the genome of the animal and provide the genetic direction as to how to construct the animal in an orderly step-wise fashion.

As an animal species' genome is activated, pointers systematically traverse the entries present in the master genome reference table, which in turn facilitates the transcription of transcribable genes or activates other reference tables, which in turn facilitate the transcription of transcribable genes. Mutations, replication errors, selections, viruses or environmental factors may be responsible for certain quantum genes being transcribable versus being untranscribable.

Higher orders of animals would not need to have their genome contain any genetic material regarding the genes required for the construction of plant species or fungi species or Protista species except in a rudimentary form. The genes comprising the genome of a particular animal species would be mostly from branches 1, 2, and 4. The genome of an animal would include quantum genes to construct basic cell structures and macromolecules, quantum genes from viruses that utilize animal cells as hosts and quantum genes dedicated to generating the animal species.

Branch	Unique Identifier 25-characters	Instructions to manufacture species
1	0000000000000100000000000 CCCCCCCCCCCCCTCCCCCCCCCCC	Genes to construct cell membrane
1	0000000000000112000000000 CCCCCCCCCCCCCTTACCCCCCCCC	Genes to construct mitochondria
1	0000000000000113 010000000 CCCCCCCCCCCCCTTGCTCCCCCCC	Genes to construct Golgi Apparatus
1	0000000000000111121000000 CCCCCCCCCCCCCTTTTATCCCCCC	Genes to construct flagella
1	00000000000001111 31000000 CCCCCCCCCCCCCTTTTGTCCCCCC	Genes to construct micro tubular Network
1	0000000000000200000000000 CCCCCCCCCCCCCACCCCCCCCCCC	Genes to construct nuclear Membrane
1	000000000000022 1111 000000 CCCCCCCCCCCCCAATTTTCCCCCC	Genes to construct chromosomes
1	000000000000022 32111 00000 CCCCCCCCCCCCCAAGATTTCCCCC	Genes to construct mitotic spindles
3	2300000000000000000000000 AGCCCCCCCCCCCCCCCCCCCCCCC	Genes to construct human viruses
4	330000000000022 3 211000000 GGCCCCCCCCCCCAAGATTCCCCCC	Genes to construct skeleton
4	33000000001 223 00001000000 GGCCCCCCCCCTAAGCCCCTCCCCCC	Construct a heart
4	3300000000 22220000 1000000 GGCCCCCCCCCAAAACCCCTCCCCCC	Construct lungs
4	3300000000 3222 00001000000 GGCCCCCCCCCGAAACCCCTCCCCCC	Construct a kidney
4	330000000000000000 1000000 GGCCCCCCCCCCCCCCCCCTCCCCCC	Genes to construct a pancreas

4	3300000000 33 2200001000000 GGCCCCCCCCGGAACCCCTCCCCCC	Genes to construct a liver
4	3300000000000 2232 11000000 GGCCCCCCCCCCCAAGATTCCCCCC	Genes to construct a fin
4	3300000000000 22 3211100000 GGCCCCCCCCCCCAAGATTTCCCCC	Genes to construct an arm limb
4	3300000000000 223 21111 0000 GGCCCCCCCCCCCAAGATTTTCCCC	Genes to construct a leg limb
4	3300000000000 223 211300000 GGCCCCCCCCCCCAAGATTGCCCCC	Genes to construct a tail

Table 12

Simplified version of a Universal master genome reference table for animals*.

*all numbers presented as unique identifiers are meant to be for illustration purposes only; where C=0, T=1, A=2, G=3 have been assigned based on molecular weight.

Hierarchy of Genome Reference Tables

As a genome reference table (GRT) is read by a GRT transcription complex one or more control RNA molecules are generated. These control RNA molecules traverse the nucleus and bind to the unique identifier of a specific quantum gene and activate the formation of a transcription complex to transcribe the quantum gene. In this manner, quantum genes are utilized in a precise and organized manner.

Genome reference tables (GRT) provide groups of instructions for various levels of construction of any given organism. The hierarchy of reference tables presented in Table 13 demonstrates the various GRTs from higher order to the lower order reference tables. Process specific GRT (#9) involving the least number of instructions or references to quantum genes, therefore represents the lowest order GRT.

No.	GENOME REFERENCE TABLE	*Includes list of quantum genes to—*
1	Universal Genome Reference Table	*All inclusive genome
2	Kingdom specific Master GRT	*construct a kingdom*
3	Species specific GRT	*construct a specific species*

4	Organ specific GRT	*construct an organ*
5	Physical Feature specific GRT	*generate limbs & features*
6	Cell specific GRT	*construct cells of each cell design*
7	Organelle specific GRT	*build each organelle*
8	Molecular specific GRT	*produce each molecule*
9	Process specific GRT	*conduct each necessary process*

Table 13
Hierarchy of genome reference tables.

Genome Reference Tables are capable of producing variable outcomes. Amongst the list of quantum genes present in any given reference table, not all quantum genes may be read by a GRT Transcription Complex. Influences to the GRT Transcription Complex may cause certain quantum genes to be activated versus other available quantum genes left idle. This may occur as an active process while an organism is alive; or it may be an event that occurs while sex cells are being generated by an organism. Imprinting may occur as a genome is being generated in sex cells. Imprinting may occur to activate or deactivate available instructions present in a reference table.

A GRT at any level of the hierarchy may be comprised of a number of references to quantum genes, but not all of the available references will be utilized by any given species. Imprinting designates which of the available references in a GRT will be used. In the circumstance where a limp specific GRT exists, it may be comprised of the instructions necessary to produce either an arm, a wing or a fin. Imprinting selects to activate the list of quantum genes necessary to produce an arm, while leaving the quantum genes dedicated to producing a wing or fin deactivated or in a dormant state.

Certain GRTs, such as lower order GRTs, may not exhibit much variability. The GRTs to produce organelles, molecules, and direct processes may be very well conserved. Higher order GRTs may exhibit the kind of variability that have been necessary to produce the evolutionary process as recorded by science.

The existence of a hierarchy of GRTs facilitates the fact that the earth supports a very well balanced ecosystem. Despite the variety of environmental ranges that exist on the planet, an ecosystem comprised of various life forms can be found across the globe inhabiting nearly every part of the earth. Despite severe stresses to the earth, some of which have catastrophically eradicated numerous species, the life forms comprising the ecosystems on the planet have adapted to the climate changes and rebuilt complex food chains that have been able to survive. It would appear that the master genome reference tables utilized by kingdoms and species are able to dynamically alter the list of activated quantum genes, selecting or experimenting with dormant quantum genes to select which life forms will survive the best given the prevailing environmental conditions.

CHAPTER 22

COMMAND, CONTROL, COMMUNICATION AND INTELLIGENCE

As previously noted, Command, Control, Communication and Intelligence represent four cellular functions that are intimately tied together and are necessary participants in a multi-cellular organism such as the human body.

Command is the instructions that dictate to the cell how macro molecules are constructed. Command instructions are carried in Command RNA (cmRNA) molecules.

Control is represented by instructions regarding the transcription of the next quantum gene. Control is produce by nuclear signaling proteins (NSP), also referred to as DNA binding proteins, or control RNA (cnRNA) molecules.

Communication is a necessity of multi-cellular organisms to coordinate the actions of the individual cell types in an effort to best insure survival of the overall organic life form. Cell to cell communication occurs by the actions of various hormones. Nerve cells are able to communicate by the secretion of chemicals or secretory proteins. Cell surface receptors are a passive means of communications between cells. The immune system probes cell types by physical contact with cell surface receptors to judge which cells comprise the human body versus which organic entities represent an invader posing a threat to the body.

Intelligence is divided into active intelligence and static intelligence. Active intelligence is able to utilize reason and analysis to make decisions. A static intelligence impacts decisions by means of interpreting present algorithms. The genome of a species is considered a static intelligence. The static intelligence of the genome may create a means of generating an active intelligence by causing the body to generate a brain which is capable of reason and analysis, and provides benefits from learned behavior. Both active intelligence and static intelligence are critically important to the health and survivability of the human body.

In essence, static intelligence of the human body facilitates the ability for the human brain to take the time to exercise its capacity for active intelligence. If the conscious brain had to concern itself with all of the housekeeping duties required to maintain the human body such as minute to minute temperature control, blood pressure control, heart rate, thyroid hormone excretions, and the thousands of other functions the subconscious brain attends to by means of static intelligence control dictated by the action of the DNA of specialized cells, there would never be time for any of the creative thoughts humans pride themselves as having. These thoughts and expressions in the form of our writing, our music and our art is what we hold so precious as the essence of what separates humans from the lower order organic life that we share this planet with at this time.

In a cell a nuclear signaling protein or a control RNA molecule will trigger the transcription of a command RNA molecule. See Figure 18. A command RNA may instruct the endoplasmic reticulum to produce one of various types of hybrid protein molecules. For cell to cell communication, the command RNA may instruct the endoplasmic reticulum to produce a hormone.

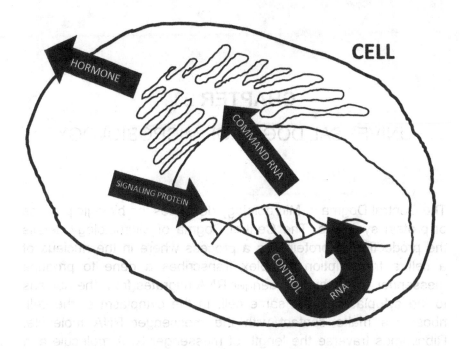

Figure 18
Nuclear signaling protein or a control RNA
generates a command RNA, which subsequently generates
a hormone to be utilized as intracellular communication
or intercellular communication

Hormones are collected together and stored in vacuoles. Homes are generally released as part of a command and control strategy to effect a cellular response in a remote portion of the body.

CHAPTER 23

UNIVERSAL DOGMA OF MICROBIOLOGY

The Central Dogma of Microbiology describes the biologic process of protein synthesis. The Central Dogma of Microbiology details the production of proteins as a process where in the nucleus of a cell a transcription complex transcribes a gene to produce messenger RNA, this messenger RNA migrates from the nucleus to the cytoplasm of the same cell. In the cytoplasm of the cell, ribosomes make contact with the messenger RNA molecule. Ribosomes traverse the length of messenger RNA molecule and as the ribosome does so, through the process of translation, each ribosome generates a single-stranded protein.

Numerous questions are left unanswered by the Central Dogma of Microbiology. Questions such as how a particular gene is identified to be transcribed, why ribosomes are constructed with ribosomal RNA molecules, and what is the feedback mechanism that regulate how much of each type of protein is to be manufactured by a cell.

The Universal Dogma of Microbiology states 'All protein production is a dynamic process created by a static intelligence stored in the DNA, facilitated by control RNAs and DNA binding proteins to produce messenger RNA which are used as templates to generate proteins, the rate of production being controlled by nuclear signaling proteins and control RNAs and the construction of complex protein molecules being directed by the collaboration of static chemical processes, production rate of enzymes and command RNA molecules'.

The Universal Dogma of Microbiology (UDM) is an expansion upon the principles detailed in the Central Dogma of Microbiology. The UDM addresses that a cell process such as the production of a protein molecule is a dynamic process requiring a means to enhance production of the protein and a competing means to slow down and even terminate production of a protein. UDM is inclusive of Command, Control, Communication and Intelligence features of a cell. See Table 14.

COMMAND	CONTROL	COMMUNICATION	INTELLIGENCE
>Messenger RNA >Command RNA	>Control RNA >Control Proteins >Hormones	>Hormones >Cell Membrane receptors >Proteins traversing cell membrane to neighboring cells	>Reference Tables >Bundled Instruction codes >Primary Programming code

Table 14
Table of independent portions
of the Universal Dogma of Microbiology.

Command and control are necessary functions required for the survival of an individual cell and are necessary for the survival of the body as a whole. The Universal Dogma of Microbiology addresses the need to include the elements of command and control in the production of proteins either for intracellular use or for extracellular functions.

Part 5

Viral Influences in Cell Command and Control

CHAPTER 24

VIRAL DNA PRESENT IN HUMAN GENOME

It has been estimated that the human genome contains physical evidence of the genome of at least 450,000 viruses. Since the human genome contains evidence of viral genomes then either the human genome has spawned these viruses or these viruses have invaded sex cells of primitive humans, along with their ancestors, and added their viral DNA to the human genome. Either way, the genetic composition of viruses and humans are intimately tied together.

The presence of viral DNA in human DNA may also be a reflection that viruses have evolved, over time, with all forms of life, including the previous stages of genomes that lead to the human genome. The genome of a virus may not represent the entire genetics of a virus, but instead just the essential DNA. DNA of viruses that infect humans may act as a primary template to trigger genes already physically present in human DNA. In this instance, this would indicate an extremely high level of conservation and organization by nature. It would also indicate a symbiotic relationship between animal cells and viruses that is far more intimate that any other symbiotic relationship described previously. Nature may have produced viruses in their most simplistic (smallest) form as a means to insure the survival of the virus as well as construct the most effect means to bypass an animal's immune system safeguards in order to insure that the virus would be capable of successfully infecting animal cells in order to modify existing species or create new species.

Viral DNA genomes present in the human genome may represent the footprints of the influence viruses have had since the beginning of life on planet earth. There are more species of virus than there are species of all organic life combined. HIV teaches us that when a viral genome accesses the inner boundaries of a cell, the virus's genome may not activate right away. There may be a significant time delay prior to the infecting viral genome becoming active and taking control of the host cell's protein producing machinery to effect the production of copies of the virus's virion. Traces or even complete copies of a viral genome may be passed from one generation of an organic life form to the next generation in certain circumstances.

In the case of a single celled organism such as protozoa, a virus targeting this organic life form may indeed infect the protozoa. The infecting virus might insert its DNA into the protozoa's DNA. The viral DNA may lay dormant for a period of time, even during replication of the protozoa. Future generations of the protozoa may contain viral DNA. At some point, the viral genome present in one of the offspring of the original protozoa activates and sets in motion the viral replication process in that particular protozoa. The remaining protozoa may continue to survive and replicate transferring the viral genome on to other future generations of protozoa.

In multi-cellular organisms, viruses would have to infect the sex cells and alter the specie's DNA in order for all or part of a viral genome to be present in the genome of future genomes of the species. The potential influences that any virus has on the sex cells of a species are a subject that may uncover secrets of a symbiotic existence that is not well understood at this time.

The presence of genetic traces of 450,000 viruses present in the human genome suggest that: (1) during the human existence human sex cells have been infected and the DNA influenced by this number of viruses, or (2) that viruses have infected lower order life forms during their life time and the traces of these infections are visible in the human genome, or (3) viral DNA has been present with the DNA of organic life since the beginning of organic life on this planet. All three concepts are deeply profound statements.

In the case of the 450,000 viral species having infected lower order organic life, it may be possible to contrive a road map, a timeline, and a lineage of how the human species developed from lower order organic life by correlating which viruses infected which species of organic life that have existed over time.

CHAPTER 25

VIRAL INFLUENCES ON CELL COMMAND AND CONTROL

A cell grows, maintains itself and replicates due to a very elaborate, yet strict set of command and control functions. Dysfunction of the command and control structure of a cell leads to failure due to under production or over production of proteins, which eventually leads to death of the cell.

A viral genome generates instructions that override the normal command and control functions of a cell. A viral genome takes over cell functions necessary to generate copies of the virus's virion. The virus's genome is generally not concerned with the overall survivability of the host cell. The virus's genome's only intention is to generate copies of the virus's virion, which are then able to escape the confines of the host cell that manufactured the copies, and are free to seek out an alternative host cell to infect and repeat the replication cycle.

In order to produce copies of the virion, the virus must exert its own agenda in a manner that overrides the cells normal cell function. The virus's genome disperses within the host cell its own series of command and control RNAs, and command and control proteins, to effect the production of viral proteins needed to generate as many copies of the virion as possible to insure survival of the virus.

Infection by a virus usually results in the breakdown of the host cell's normal cell functions, which leads to failure of essential cell metabolism, which leads to death of the infected host cell.

CHAPTER 26

VIRAL INFLUENCES ON DNA
BY ADDING NEW DNA

The cell, by itself, has no known clear identifiable means to constructively add nucleotides to the DNA. An exception may be in the chance that fragmentation occurs to a chromosome in a sex cell, which accidently finds its way to adhering to the DNA of a daughter sex cell, reducing the DNA content of DNA in one haploid daughter sex cell and increasing the DNA content in the other haploid daughter sex cell. In this case, the resultant haploid daughter cell carrying the increase in DNA would be carrying a copy of a segment of DNA it already possessed, which should not add any new functional benefit to the cell or the resultant life form if the sex cell were to unite with a second sex cell. Again, an exception would be if the shear nature of a re-alignment of nucleotide bases created by happenstance adding a fragment of genetic material to a segment of existing genetic material (as mentioned above) resulted in the creation of a unique and useable protein just by the physical coding characteristics of the new sequence of DNA and not related to some preset code or predetermined code. The thought that randomly adding nucleotides to a known quantum gene would result in a plausible and useful protein seems to take reason to the brink of logic.

There is no formal means for a 'virus' to change the genome it carries other than errors that occur to the genome when the viral genome is copied during the virus's reproduction phase. The repeated occurrence of errors would seem to logically lead to eventual failure of a working system rather than improved survivability.

There is the possibility that the human genome adds segments to viral genomes resulting in modification of viral genomes. There is also the possibility that viral genomes add segments of DNA to the human genome. If a virus were to affect the human genome of the next generation of humans, such a virus would have to influence the chromosomal material of the sex cells of the individual infected by the virus. There may be an intimate symbiotic relationship between humans and viruses that has yet to be fully understood or appreciated.

CHAPTER 27

VIRAL INFLUENCES ON DNA BY SWITCHING GENE EXPRESSION ON AND OFF

Viruses Influencing Observed Evolutionary Changes by Altering Reference Tables

Viral genomes are generally comprised of either RNA or DNA. The genome of an RNA virus, such as Hepatitis C, which bypasses the nucleus of the host cell, once separated into subunits, mimics messenger RNA and produces the proteins necessary to construct copies of the RNA virus. DNA viruses, and RNA viruses such as HIV which reverse transcribe their genome into DNA, may have a genome that either generates messenger RNAs to produce individual proteins, or functions like a reference table that is utilized to activate quantum genes that already exist in the host cell's genome. Viruses that insert their genome into the DNA may simply insert a list of instructions that at some point in the life-cycle of the cell becomes read and therefore activates a series of quantum genes that are required to produce copies of the virus.

Viruses could influence the evolution of species by inserting into the DNA of a species either new genetic material, variations to existing genetic material or much more powerfully, variations to the reference tables. Viral influence to Genome Reference Tables could affect a block of quantum genes, shutting the quantum genes off or activating a set of quantum genes.

The viral genome's influence could be either direct or indirect. A directed influence would be when the virus inserts new information such as new quantum genes into the genome or inserts genetic material that disrupts the transcription of a quantum gene. An indirect influence, which potentially produces a much greater influence of a species, is the insertion of new reference points into a genome reference table or by disrupting reference points. The most powerful affect would be if the viral genome influenced a higher order genome reference table in sex cells and activated or deactivated references to a series of quantum genes. Viral influences could be the cause of as to why the block of genes dedicated to generating a fin in a fish is deactivated and in its place a leg is permanently generated on an amphibian. The effects of viruses on animal genomes may have been responsible for the activation of genome reference tables that produced wings on birds or arms and legs on reptiles and mammals.

Genome reference tables consist of a list of addresses of the locations of quantum genes.

Dynamic Genome Reference Tables Explain Metamorphosis

Evolution has been considered a slowly progressive alteration of species morphing one form of species into another form of species. Evolution has been thought to be the result of genetic errors suffered by a species' genome that causes the morphing process, that is then subject to survival as dictated by Nature's law of 'Survival of the Fittest'. The perception of time required for a species to morph from one life form to another life form is often consider to take hundreds of thousands of years to maybe even millions of years.

The perceived concept that *'the effort and the time it takes for one species to morph into another species takes extensive time and requires a genetic error to occur'* grossly overlooks the dynamic changes that occur within species that are known to exist on the planet today.

A frog starts out its life cycle in a fertilized egg. The frog emerges from the egg as tadpole. The tadpole swims through the water propelled only by a tail. The tadpole uses internal gills to breath. Metamorphoses occurs with lungs developing, disappearance of the gills, limbs appearing including fore- and hind-limbs, the tail being absorbed and the mouth changing into a froglike mouth. The metamorphosis from tadpole to frog may take two months to two years, depending upon the species.

The frog, other amphibians and various insects such as the butterfly, exhibit dynamic alterations to their overall life form that would be considered features of evolution. To facilitate the changes in these features a series of genome reference tables are read in succession as part of the life-cycle of the frog, that first dictate the physical form of the tadpole, then as the time-line of the frog's lifecycle progresses, generate the features of the adult frog while eliminating features of the tadpole such as the tail and gills. The metamorphosis of a frog and other organisms demonstrates that genome reference tables can be very dynamic, switching the actions of quantum genes on and off, and even switching the actions of reference tables on and off during a species' own lifecycle.

CHAPTER 28

HIV: NATURE'S TEACHING TOOL

The search for a functional unique identifier related to a quantum gene is an exercise in identifying how the transcription complex actually assembles in the 5' Upstream region of a segment of transcribable nuclear DNA. The element that makes initial contact with the nuclear DNA in the 5' Upstream region most likely is interacting with the unique identifier of the quantum gene. When the portion of the nuclear DNA in the 5' Upstream region where the initial contact is made becomes a recognizable known quantity to science, the unique identifier for a specific quantum gene will become a recognized entity. The exact science of how the transcription complex assembles at a particular location along the nuclear DNA is currently on the cutting edge of medical research.

Examining the HIV genome may provide an important clue to the unique identifier of a quantum gene. The HIV virion inserts RNA into the host T-Helper cell. The HIV genome is two strands of vRNA (viral RNA) each approximately 9600 nucleotides in length. The HIV RNA genome then undergoes reverse transcription to become DNA. The resultant viral DNA is approximately the same length as the original vRNA and becomes inserted into the T-Helper cell's nuclear DNA. Later, the cell transcribes HIV's viral DNA to produce a viral RNA that resembles the original HIV RNA, except that it is 600 nucleotides shorter in length.

The HIV genome is read from the 5' region to the 3' region. The HIV DNA genome is approximately 9719 base pairs in length. There does exist variation in the HIV genome. The following therefore is intended to act as an illustration rather than to be regarded as a set standard for the design and function of the HIV genome. HIV's genome is divided into several regions including: 5' LTR (1-634), gag (790-2292), pol (2085-5096), vif (5041-5619), vpr (5559-5850), env (6225-8795), nef (8797-9417) and 3' LTR (9086-9719).

The initial portion of the HIV DNA genome is termed the Long Terminal Repeat (LTR) located at the 5' region. The LTR is comprised of the regions indentified as U3, R and U5. The LTR is comprised of the nucleotide base pairs (bp) from 1-634.

The TATA box is considered a means of signaling to the cell's transcription machinery that a segment of transcribable genetic information follows downstream from that point. At bp 427 in the 5' LTR is located the first nucleotide of a TATA box. At bp 456 starts the messenger RNA of the HIV genome. Between the TATA box and the location of the transcribable messenger RNA of the HIV genome is a space of 25 nucleotide base pairs. The nucleotides of this 25 base pair segment are 'AGCAGCTGCTTTTTGCCTGTACTGG'. This segment of 25-nucleotide base pairs may contain the 'unique identifier' of HIV to the human genome transcription machinery. See Figure 19. HIV has shown that it often utilizes mechanisms already present in the human cell, thus HIV having a unique identifier would be consistent with the identification of unique identifiers for human quantum genes.

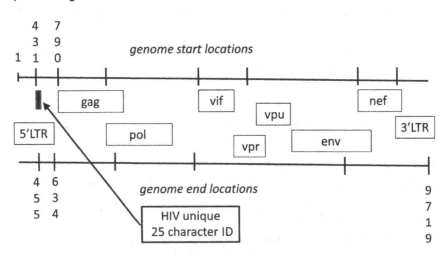

Figure 19
HIV genome with the 25-nucleotide unique identifier
demonstratable between bp 430 and 456

HIV may be mimicking a unique identifier that already exists in the human genome. When the human quantum gene is to be transcribed, the nuclear signaling protein or the control RNA that is used to identify the unique identifier is produced and seeks out the quantum gene. In some such cases, the nuclear signaling protein or control RNA locates the HIV genome and initiates the transcription process rather than locating the human quantum gene. The HIV replication process begins and takes over the normal process of the cell to produce copies of the HIV virion.

A search of the human genome of the nucleotides of HIV's 25 base pair unique identifier 'AGCAGCTGCTTTTTGCCTGTACTGG' or some unique subset, if present in the human genome, may identify the identity of a quantum gene in the human genome. If genetic information were to be found downstream from this unique identifier in the human genome, a unique human quantum gene would be identified.

The HIV genome demonstrates the presence of both 'genes' and 'quantum genes'. If a gene is considered to be a segment of DNA that once transcribed produces a ribonucleic acid, then the genome of HIV is comprised of multiple genes. Given that there is only one unique identifier associated with the HIV genome dictates that some genes are bundled together under the assignment of only one unique identifier.

Bundling more than one gene to one unique identifier demonstrates nature's effort to conserve resources. If multiple unique genes are required to perform a specific task, such as construct the proteins necessary to produce HIV virions, then only the first gene in a particular series of genes needs to be locatable. Once the unique identifier associated with the first gene is located by a transcription complex all of the genes in the series will be transcribed, producing multiple ribonucleic acids products. Such bundling of genes represents a logical approach to increase efficiency in coding genetic instructions by compacting genetic information, represents a means to reduce errors in protein construction and cell structure production, and increases the proficiency of the transcription of certain proteins required to accomplish a specific outcome.

Part 6

Origin of the Atmosphere, Water, Life

Chapter 29

THE CRUX OF THE NITROGEN CYCLE

It is well recognized that the Earth is a unique biosphere with the planet's atmosphere making it the only celestial body in the solar system capable of supporting carbon based life as we know it. However, nitrogen is also essential for life to exist. Not just human life, but all life forms. Life could not have started without an adequate supply of nitrogen to create the essential organic molecules upon which life depends. In this chapter we take a closer look at this issue as well as how the nitrogen gas came to be in the Earth's atmosphere, but not in that of the sun or the other planets, at least not to anywhere near the same level.

An Atmosphere for Life

The Earth's atmosphere is comprised of 78% nitrogen gas, 21% oxygen, and small amounts of carbon dioxide, water vapor, and argon. The Earth's atmosphere is in stark contrast with the atmospheres of the sun and all of the other planets comprising the solar system. See Table 15.

The atmosphere of the sun is comprised of 74.9% hydrogen and 23.9% helium. The planets Mercury, Jupiter, Saturn, Uranus and Neptune share similar atmospheres as the sun with hydrogen and helium being the primary components of the atmospheres of these planets.

Earth's closest neighbors Venus and Mars have atmospheres comprised of over 95% carbon dioxide and approximately 3% nitrogen. The fact that Venus, the neighboring planet closer to the sun than the Earth, and Mars, the neighboring planet farther from the sun than the Earth, have similar atmospheres with dramatically different environments prompts the question as to the mechanism of the existence of these atmospheres. It is equally curious that the sun, Mercury, Jupiter, Saturn, Uranus and Neptune have similar compositions comprising their atmospheres, while the compositions of the atmospheres of Venus, Earth and Mars pose such a stark contrast to those of the sun and the other planets.

	Hydrogen	Helium	Oxygen	Nitrogen	Carbon Dioxide	Water	Methane	Ammonia
Sun	74.9	23.9	—	—	—	—	—	—
Mercury	Primary	Primary	Primary	—	—	3.4%	—	—
Venus	—	Trace	—	3.5%	96.5%	0.002	—	—
Earth	<1	<1	21%	78%	<1	0.4%	<1	<1
Mars	—	—	Trace	3%	95.3%	0.03%	Trace	—
Jupiter	74%	23%	—	—	—	0.0004%	Trace	Trace
Saturn	96.3%	3.25%	—	—	—	Ice	<1	<1
Uranus	83%	15%	—	—	—	?	2%	Trace
Neptune	80%	19%	—	—	—	—	Trace	—
*Pluto	—	—	—	Suspected	Carbon Monoxide Identified	—	Identified	—

Table 15
Composition of the atmospheres of the sun and its planets.
*Pluto now considered a dwarf planet

It has been speculated that plant life, utilizing the process of photosynthesis, converted the carbon dioxide in Earth's early atmosphere to oxygen. Utilizing radiant energy, plants combined carbon dioxide and water to generate the sugar glucose to be used as fuel with the byproduct of oxygen also being formed.

Chlorophyll

$$6CO_2 + 6H_2O + radiant\ energy \longrightarrow 6C_6H_{18}O_6 + O_2$$

(carbon dioxide) (water)   (glucose) (oxygen)

Primordial Earth would have been much like her sister planets. The atmosphere was more than likely a combination of hydrogen, helium and volcanic gases. Volcanoes act as vents for gases trapped in the mantle and core of the planet to escape into the atmosphere. Volcanic emissions are often comprised of some measure of carbon dioxide, hydrogen sulfide, carbon monoxide, ammonia, water vapor, and methane. Earth's core was most likely very active, as it is today, and spewed large amounts of volcanic emissions into the atmosphere.

Two of the unique features of the Earth are that the vast majority of the atmosphere is comprised of nitrogen gas and 78% of the planet's surface is covered by water. The origin of the vast amount of nitrogen gas and the vast amount of water have, in the past, been a challenge to adequately explain scientifically.

A recent explanation for the presence of water on the Earth's surface has been that comets carried the water to the Earth. Overtime, the Earth was supposedly fortunate enough to be the target of enough comet and meteorite strikes to have the majority of the planet's surface covered in water. Similar accumulations of water are not seen on the other planets in the solar system though one would expect, if random circumstances were to be the sole driving force in the accumulation of water, that all of the other planets in the solar system would have suffered a similar number of meteorite and comet impacts and, therefore, would also have evidence of a similar amount of water in either a gaseous or frozen form. However, this does not seem to be the case.

Requirement for Nitrogen

Nitrogen is critical to the existence of all life on Earth. Nitrogen is a component of all amino acids, which are combined together in cells to produce proteins which are not only the building blocks of life, but carry out the cellular command and control functions as well.

There are twenty amino acids that comprise the proteins that are used in many essential functions to create and support life. Amino acids share a similar chemical composition of $NH_2CH(R)COOH$ where 'R' represents a side chain which is the variable portion of the amino acids. The simplest amino acid is glycine, where the 'R' is a hydrogen atom. The 'R' can be a variety of organic groups. In the amino acid alanine the 'R' is CH_3. Nitrogen is an essential element of all twenty amino acids. Further, nitrogen is utilized to generate the five bases that comprise nucleic acids. Nitrogen is an essential part of deoxyribonucleic acid and ribonucleic acids.

Nitrogen is essential in the construction of chlorophyll molecules. Chlorophyll is essential to the process of photosynthesis. There are four nitrogen atoms in a molecule of chlorophyll. See Figure 20. Though nitrogen is abundant in the atmosphere of today, the largest source of nitrogen, nitrogen (N_2) in a gas form, is generally unusable by plants and animals. Bacteria with nitrogenase enzymes are able to combine nitrogen gas with hydrogen to produce ammonia, which can then be further converted by bacteria to organic compounds. Some bacteria live in symbiotic relations with plants, these bacteria produce ammonia in exchange for carbohydrates.

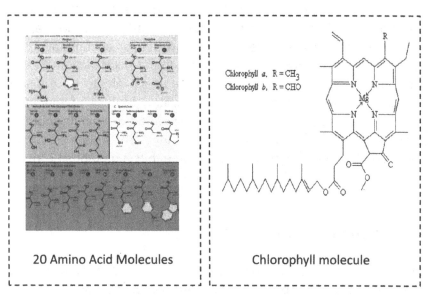

20 Amino Acid Molecules

Chlorophyll molecule

Figure 20
Amino Acids and the Chlorophyll molecule

The mechanism that created Earth's abundance of nitrogen gas present in the atmosphere remains as elusive as the origin of Earth's oceans. Yet from a molecular biology position, both the presence of water and fixable nitrogen are critically important to the existence of all forms of life.

Similar to the mechanism of photosynthesis that has converted carbon dioxide in the atmosphere into oxygen, water and nitrogen may have been purposely formed by harnessing the radiant energy of the sun. The Earth was formed approximately a billion years before it is estimated the earliest life first appeared on the planet.

The Source of Nitrogen and Water

Primordial Earth had an atmosphere dominated by the gases of hydrogen and helium similar to the sun, Mercury, Jupiter, Saturn, Uranus and Neptune. The activity of Earth's core spewed large amounts of carbon dioxide and ammonia trapped in the Earth into the atmosphere. Once enough carbon dioxide was present in the atmosphere, hydrogen and helium were pushed to the outer edges of the atmosphere. Energized by radiant energy from the sun, the lighter hydrogen and helium gases eventually separated from Earth's atmosphere and drifted into space.

Following the loss of hydrogen and helium, the abundant radiant energy emitted by the young sun created an atmospheric environment whereby carbon dioxide and ammonia could be converted to water, methane and nitrogen gas.

Extraterrestrial
Catalyst

$$3CO_2 + 8NH_3 + \text{radiant energy} \longrightarrow 6H_2O + 3CH_4 + 4N_2$$

(carbon (ammonia)   (water) (methane) (nitrogen)
dioxide)

The conditions on planet Earth were favorable for water to exist in solid, liquid and vapor forms. Water available in liquid form was critical for molecular water being made available for organic life to utilize.

The environmental conditions on Earth were favorable for nitrogen to exist in a gaseous form.

Carbon dioxide is heavier than nitrogen gas and oxygen. Therefore, carbon dioxide sinks to the level of the atmosphere closest to the surface of the planet. Thus, the highest concentration of atmospheric carbon dioxide remains available to plants to be utilized in the process of photosynthesis.

From primordial time to present day, Earth lost much of the initial hydrogen and helium gases that comprised its early atmosphere. The abundance of the carbon dioxide and ammonia emitted by primordial volcanoes was converted into water, oxygen and nitrogen gas. Oxygen in the atmosphere interacts with radiant energy at different altitudes in the atmosphere, which causes it to take on the forms of molecular oxygen, unstable ozone and molecular ozone. At the outer reaches of the atmosphere ozone absorbs radiant energy from the sun, preventing harmful levels from reaching the surface of the planet and threatening the existence of land-based life. The composition of the atmosphere transforming into 21% oxygen and 79% nitrogen made it possible for a sufficient amount of ozone to form in the atmosphere to allow animal life to leave the confines of the ocean and successfully exist on land.

The Nitrogen Cycle

The nitrogen cycle is extremely important to life on the planet. Nitrogen cycles through the atmosphere, lithosphere and hydrosphere. Ninety percent of the nitrogen gas fixed into ammonia is generated by certain bacteria utilizing nitrogenase enzymes. A small amount of nitrogen fixation occurs due to lightening strikes. Nitrogen fixing bacteria and cyanobacteria (blue-green algae) are capable of breaking the triple bonds that hold each nitrogen gas (N_2) molecule together and generate ammonia and other organic molecules. Most plants can assimilate ammonia and nitrates, but the majority of nitrogen is taken in by plants as nitrites. Plants are able to take ammonia, nitrates and nitrites and utilize the nitrogen to construct amino acids, proteins and nucleic acids. Animal obtain many nitrogen containing molecules from plants. Of the twenty amino acids humans require to generate 33,000 possible proteins needed by the body, nine are essential amino acids. An essential amino acid cannot be synthesized in the human body and, therefore, must be obtained by nutritional sources. The amino acids that are essential for humans include histidine, isoleucine, leucine, lysine, methionine, phenylalanine, threonine, tryptophan, and valine.

Denitrification refers to the reduction of nitrates back into inert nitrogen gas. Bacteria such as Clostridium and Pseudomonas in anaerobic conditions use nitrate as an electron acceptor during respiration. Bacteria participating in denitrification processes can release nitrogen gas back into the atmosphere.

Nitrogen Is Essential to Life

The harvesting of nitrogen from the environment and fixing nitrogen into organic compounds is necessary for the production of amino acids, proteins and nucleic acids. The construction of nucleic acids is critical for the generation of the genome of every species in every form of life. Without an efficient means of taking nitrogen from the environment and fixing it into organic molecules, cells could not copy their genome in the process of mitosis and divide to generate daughter cells that are exact replicas of the parent cell.

An organic means to fix nitrogen into organic molecules must have been present at the earliest appearance of life on the planet, otherwise genomes could not have been constructed, and cells could not have prospered to produce offspring.

Nitrogenase is a family of enzymes that facilitate the fixing of atmospheric nitrogen gas into organic molecules. The triple bond of gaseous nitrogen is rather stable making the nitrogen gas rather inert. Breaking the triple bond in gaseous nitrogen to produce ammonia represents a high barrier of activation without a catalyst with an E_A = 420 kj mol -1. There is no other enzyme family other than the nitrogenases, known to be utilized by organisms to harvest nitrogen from the atmosphere and fix the nitrogen into organic molecules. All nitrogen fixing organisms are prokaryotes. Organisms that synthesize nitrogenase include Cyanobacteria, Azotobacteracease, Rhizobia, and Frankia. In addition, Cyanobacteria fix carbon and account for 20-30% of the Earth's photosynthetic productivity.

153

The triple bond of nitrogen (N_2) is difficult to break. To accomplish this, the nitrogenase enzyme complex utilizes 16 ATP molecules and 8 reducing equivalents. The nitrogenase enzyme complex is comprised of two types of proteins. Nitrogenase synthetase complex is comprised of both the nitrogenase enzyme (Fe-Mo protein) as well as a nitrogenase reductase enzyme (Fe-4S protein). Without both enzymes attached to each other and functioning together the nitrogen fixing catalyst does not work.

The reductase subunit is a homodimer containing two ATP binding sites and a Fe4S4 cluster. The reductase subunit is coded by the nifH gene.

The nitrogenase subunit is a heterotetramer molecule. The nitrogenase subunit is comprised of a_2b_2 peptides. Located between the a and b domains is a FeS8 cluster. The peptides are coded in the nifD and nifK genes. The active site of the molecule contains a metallic co-factor referred to as Fe_7S_9Mo-homocitrate or simply Mo-Fe, which carries out the actual reduction of the N_2 molecule.

In the organism Azotobacter vinelandii the molecule nitrogenase molybdenum-iron protein is comprised of alpha (a) chains A and C as well as beta (b) chains B and D. The alpha chains A and C are 492 amino acids in length. The beta chains B and D are 523 amino acids in length. The nitrogenase Fe protein is homodimeric and is 289 amino acids in length. The nitrogenase molecule is sensitive to the presence of oxygen. The Fe form of the nitrogenase molecule is irreversibly damaged in the presence of oxygen, while the MoFe form of the nitrogenase molecule is insensitive to oxygen.

The nitrogenase complex converts atmospheric nitrogen to ammonia:

$$N_2 + 8\ H^+ + 8\ e^- + 16\ ATP + 16\ H_2O \longrightarrow 2\ NH_3 + H_2 + 16\ ADP + 16\ P_i$$

The two ammonia (NH_3) molecules are rapidly converted in the cell to ammonium (NH_4^+). The ammonium is directed to produce glutamate and nitrates.

There are at least fourteen genes associated with nitrogen fixation including:

(a) transcription regulators: nifA (positive) and nifL (negative),
(b) Mo-Fe cofactor synthesis: nifB,
(c) form nitrogenase component: nifD and nifK,
(d) scaffolding for Mo-Fe cofactor: nifE and nifN,
(e) forms reductase component: nifH,
(f) incorporates Mo into the Mo-Fe cofactor: nifQ,
(g) assembly of the Fe-S cluster in the reductase component: nifS and nifU,
(h) homocitrate synthase: nifV,
(i) Mo-Fe co-binding proteins: nifX and nifY.

Cyanobacteria dominate the population of the world's ocean's picophytoplankton. Two genera of unicellular cyanobacteria are Prochlorococcus and Synechococcus. The remainder of the picophytoplankton is a diverse mix of eukaryote algae. Nitrogen fixing cyanobacteria Tricodesmium are common in the oceans and thought to be responsible for half of all marine N_2 fixation.

Nitrification is the process of taking ammonia (NH_3) and oxifying it to nitrite (NO_2) and nitrate (NO_3). Nitrification is accomplished by two groups of organisms, ammonia-oxidizing bacteria (AOB) and ammonia-oxidizing archaea (AOA). AOA dominates both soil and marine environments. Ammonia monooxygenase (AMO) is the functional gene that is responsible for the oxygenation of ammonia.

The ammonia monooxygenase molecule is a cytoplasmic membrane protein. There are three subunits comprising the molecule with various metal centers. AMO is found in Nitrosomonas europaea and Paracoccus denitrificans.

The nitrogenase iron protein associated with Cyanothece, a Cyanobacteria, is 327 amino acids in length. The Cyanothece strain 51142 nitrogenase molybdenum-iron alpha chain (EC=1.18.6.1) is 480 amino acids in length, while the beta chain is 511 amino acids in length.

The nitrogenase iron protein associated with Rhizobium etli is 297 amino acids in length. The Rhizobium strain NGR234 nitrogenase molybdenum-iron alpha chain is 504 amino acids in length, while the beta chain is 513 amino acids in length.

The AMO associated with Nitrosomonas europaea is 420 amino acids in length. The nitrogenase enzymes and the AMO are molecules of significant length and complexity.

The Crux of the Nitrogen Cycle

All life requires the element nitrogen to be fixed into organic molecules such as amino acids in order to build proteins. The triple bond of atmospheric N_2 is one of the strongest bonds known to chemistry. Bacteria utilize the nitrogenase synthetase complex to break the triple bond of atmospheric N_2 and produce ammonia. Bacteria convert ammonia to more complex biosynthetic molecules.

The crux of the nitrogen cycle is the dilemma of identifying a mechanism capable of readily and efficiently fixing nitrogen into organic molecules prior to the nitrogenase protein being formed. Ammonia was present in the primordial environment due to volcanic eruptions releasing carbon dioxide and ammonia into the atmosphere, but the enzymes needed to fix nitrogen into organic molecules were not thought to exist, and have been thought to have occurred by random chance.

Further is the contradiction that to produce an enzyme may possibly occur by random chance, though remote; the process needed to generate the proper segment of DNA that produces the RNA which eventually produces the protein requires the capacity to fix nitrogen into organic molecules in order to produce the nitrogenous bases that comprise both deoxyribonucleic acid and ribonucleic acid of the genome. Without first being able to have the capacity to generate DNA and RNA, the manufacture of randomly generated enzymes could not be passed from one generation of cells to the next generation.

To expect that enzymes built themselves or that complex deoxyribonucleic acid or ribonucleic acid molecules constructed themselves is analogous to the endless argument of whether the chicken came before the egg, or the egg came before the chicken. The case of the crux of the nitrogen cycle is different, for reason dictates that it is impossible for nitrogen to be fixed into organic molecules without first the proper series of enzymes having been present to facilitate organisms to generate such organic molecules.

The Darwin theory of Evolution dominates genetic science because of a failure to appreciate and recognize the critical importance of nitrogen in molecular biology and the nitrogen cycle. If the importance of 'nitrogen' rather than 'carbon' was emphasized in the study of molecular biology, it would become obvious that evolution could not occur on the basis of random events combined with survival of the fittest. Random occurrence dramatically fails to support how complex nitrogen dependent molecules such as amino acids, proteins, deoxyribonucleic acid and ribonucleic acids could have ever been formed in the precise order that they have been formed.

Charles Darwin was a genius in his time. Darwin's theory of Evolution represented a brilliant masterpiece in the amalgamation of science and the art of scientific observation for the year 1859 when Charles Darwin published his book *On the Origin of Species*. He was undeniably courageous to stand up against the prevailing beliefs and teachings of the eighteen hundreds and assert the facts of his scientific analysis. Charles Darwin stands as a pillar of scientific ingenuity.

A century and a half later, there is available a significantly larger data base of cellular biology, genetics and biochemistry that what was available to Charles Darwin. Added to the biologic sciences, we also have the advantage of knowledge of astronomical science, computer science, electrical engineering and advances in molecular chemistry and material sciences that was not available to Charles Darwin.

One hundred and fifty three years following its debut, for a Theory of Evolution based solely on a series of random occurrences to be practical by today's scientific standards, it would have to account for the following series of critical biophysiologic events:

3.5 billion years ago with no cellular means or strategy or design present:

(1) A spherical membrane would have had to have spontaneously formed.

(2) A pool of twenty different nitrogen containing amino acid molecules would have had to randomly form inside the boundaries of the spherical cell membrane. Amino acids can be right-handed or left-handed. Biologically active amino acid molecules are all left-handed. Therefore, all twenty different amino acids would all have to have spontaneously been created as left-handed amino acids.

(3) Then amongst this pool of twenty exclusively left-handed amino acids in the case of the 327 amino acid chain necessary to generate one of the four molecules comprising the iron protein nitrogenase molecule would have had to have formed and lined up in the proper order and spontaneously attached themselves together.

(4) Given that the nitrogenase enzyme complex is a tetramer molecule this process would have had to spontaneously occurred in proper order four different times. Since there is an alpha and a beta chain, replication would have had to have occurred identically twice for the two different pairs of amino acid chains.

(5) In the same primitive cell the 'reductase enzyme' would have also had to have been spontaneously generated. Reductase is necessary for the nitrogenase enzyme to fix nitrogen. The nitrate reductase enzyme can be 741 amino acids in length, all of which would have had to have lined up in the proper order to generate the appropriate amino acid chain.

Now nitrogen can be readily fixed into organic molecules.

(6) In current day biologic cells, proteins are generated from RNA templates that originate by transcribing the DNA. The reverse process is not present in biologic cells. There is no known mechanism in a cell to take a protein and generate a gene to code for the protein.

Even if a protein spontaneously formed its gene would also have to spontaneously form without any form of assistance.

Amino acids are generally constructed in a cell by reading a code provided by linking three nucleotides together. Given now that the means to fix nitrogen gas was available to this primitive cell that lacked any sophisticated organelles by the presumed spontaneous generation of the nitrogenase enzyme and reductase enzyme, now to pass the blueprints of how to construct the nitrogenase molecule on to the next generation of daughter cells then spontaneously and independently four different nucleotides would have had to be generated then linked into the proper sequence of 981 nucleotides into a DNA molecule to create the gene for the nitrogenase enzymes.

(7) Spontaneously the machinery to transcribe the DNA, the forty proteins that comprise the transcription complex, would have had to have formed.

(8) Spontaneously the nucleic acid Uracil would have had to have spontaneously formed and be ready to be used in a sufficient amount by the transcription complex to form RNA.

(9) Spontaneously a ribosomal proteins and ribosomal RNA would have had to have spontaneously formed in order to translate the nitrogenous enzyme's RNA to produce the four protein molecules comprising the nitrogenase enzyme complex.

Now there exists in this primitive cell the chance to actively replicate the nitrogenous enzyme.

At this point there is only <u>one</u> gene.

159

This one gene is the gene to create the nitrogenase enzyme which is essential to life.

Then for genetic material to be successfully copied such that it can be passed on to daughter cells the DNA polymerase molecule consisting of 900-1000 amino acids needs to spontaneously appear. Then to generate a gene for the DNA polymerase molecule 2700 to 3000 nucleotides need to spontaneously line up properly and link themselves together so that the means to replicate the DNA polymerase molecule can be passed on to future generations of daughter cells.

It is hard to conceive that all of the above intricately complex molecules just spontaneously occurred in a single primitive cell or that even bits and pieces of the molecules spontaneously occurred in different primitive cells and somehow all by chance combined into one primitive cell.

Now the DNA for all of the proteins necessary for life must randomly-spontaneously form.

To create the human form at least 32,000 individual segments of DNA, each containing hundreds and in some cases thousands of nucleotides, had to have randomly-spontaneously formed all in their proper order of nucleotide sequencing.

The chances that such essential and intricately complex molecules spontaneously formed without some form of strategy or design is beyond human imagination and beyond the reality of statistical probability.

Oxygenic photosynthesis and nitrogen fixation are two incompatible processes, yet Cyanothece 51142, a marine species of cyanobacteria, is capable of separating and performing these two processes in the same cell. The

Cyanothece contains one large circular chromosome, four plasmids and one linear chromosome. The genome of Cyanothece is 5,460,377 bp long. Cyanothece 51142 contains the largest intact contiguous grouping of nitrogen fixing genes. The genome contains information regarding the means Cyanothece can utilize to accomplish metabolic compartmentalization and balancing incompatible processes in the same cell. Cyanothece 51142 exhibits a robust diurnal cycle with photosynthesis being conducted during the daytime and nitrogen fixation conducted at night. Thirty percent of the genes show strong cyclic expression. Cyanothece is a single cell organism that conducts incompatible biologic processes under tight control producing glycogen during photosynthesis during the day, storing the glycogen in granules, then utilizing the glycogen at night for respiration to assist nitrogenase in fixing nitrogen, the fixed nitrogen is stored in cyanophycin granules to be used during the next daytime cycle.

The mere presence of Cyanothece 51142 and the fact that over five million nucleotides had to spontaneously link together in a precise fashion to create such a complex organism, dramatically points to the fact that a new broader theory of evolution is of critical necessity.

Revisiting the composition of the atmospheres of Venus, Earth and Mars suggests a glaring pattern that indicates life may have also been attempted on Venus and Mars given the environmental factors which lead to life flourishing on the Earth. If a primordial atmosphere is comprised mostly of hydrogen and helium as suggested by the composition of the Sun, Mercury, Jupiter, Saturn, Uranus and Neptune, and this primordial atmosphere becomes converted to an atmosphere dominated by carbon dioxide and ammonia due to volcanic emissions, this intermediate carbon dioxide atmosphere eventually being converted to an atmosphere rich in nitrogen, oxygen and water vapor, Earth is obviously a testimony to the end result of this atmospheric transformation.

The atmospheres on Venus and Mars suggest two planets with atmospheres in transition between their primordial atmospheres of hydrogen and helium and Earth's atmosphere. Earth's position from the sun and the active core of the planet are the physical reasons for the atmospheric transformation to have completed its process. Venus's atmospheric transformation may have stalled due to the intense radiant energy of the sun causing surface temperatures on the planet to vaporize any water and the density of the atmosphere forcing vaporized water to the outer edges of Venus's atmosphere encouraging water vapor to escape into space. Mars's distance from the sun limits the radiant energy that reaches the planet's surface; though earlier in the history of the solar system, the sun likely burned hotter, releasing higher levels of radiation and Mars could at one time been bathed in significantly greater levels of radiant energy. Mars's greatest deterrent to atmospheric transformation being that the fires of the planet's molten core burned out; leaving Mars an inactive cold planet. The atmospheric transformation on Mars stalled due to the combination of too little radiant energy from the sun and a dead core which ceased venting carbon dioxide and ammonia gases into the Martian atmosphere. Without carbon dioxide being converted to oxygen and water, and nitrogen dominating the composition of the atmosphere, life did could not flourish due to a critical lack of the proper building blocks and a deficiency in a means to create oxidative respiration.

In Summary

Although the Earth's atmosphere may have started out the same as that of the sun and all of the other planets in the solar system, the Earth's unique position, namely its distance from the sun, allowed for its originally hostile atmosphere to be transformed into one that uniquely supports the form of life that we see today. Part of its uniqueness, its ability to support a large quantity of nitrogen, enabled our form of life to flourish. That is, the DNA provides the instruction on how to build, operate and maintain a life form. Genes contained in the DNA are used to form proteins which are the building blocks and the working elements of the cells which form the bases of the life form. Growth and maintenance of the life form depends upon the cells being able to divide. Cell division depends on nitrogen to form the DNA, RNA and amino acid strings that make up the proteins. Without the nitrogen there is no cell division. Without nitrogen, life as we know it does not exist. Nitrogen is a critical component necessary for life. The processes to integrate nitrogen into organic molecules have been essential ever since the first DNA, the first RNA, and the first protein molecules were ever produced on the Earth.

Part 7

Ecometabolous

CHAPTER 30

PRIME GENOME

The Prime DNA genome containing all of the quantum genes and reference tables necessary for all forms of organic life: more specifically The Prime Genome contains genetic design information to construct and operate all of the cell types including prokaryote, virus, and eukaryote cells; all of the cellular proteins; and the multi-cellular organic organisms comprised of eukaryote cells. See Figure 21. The Prime DNA Genome can be thought of as being arranged into branches of a tree, starting with a central trunk, with a quantum gene coding system that utilizes the base-four mathematics inherent in the DNA and branches into four major sections of information regarding instruction code and protein production. The four major branches of the Prime Genome being (1) Basic cell design and protein design, (2) Prokaryote cells, (3) Viruses and (4) Eukaryote cells.

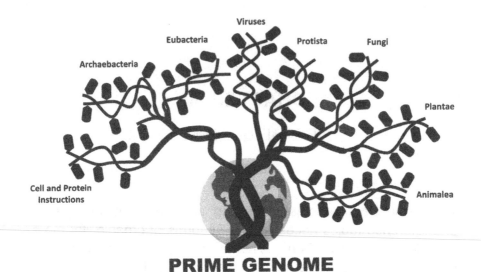

PRIME GENOME

Figure 21
Tree of the Prime DNA Genome

The Prime Genome was likely arranged in this manner, with the first major limb containing the basic information to build cells. The second major limb contains the information to generate early cell design capable of existing and flourishing in various hostile environments. Virus design exists in the third major branch of the Prime Genome. Viruses helped create changes in the genome to facilitate the orderly evolution of species and worked to control populations of unicellular organisms. The fourth major branch exists as the basic design construct of unicellular and multi-cellular eukaryote cells.

A close approximation of the original Prime Genome could potentially be reconstructed today if the DNA from all of the organic life that exists on the planet were collected together and those segments of DNA that were unique were combined and those segments that were redundant were discarded.

The Prime Genome has been the guiding genetic blueprints for the construction of all life that has existed on the planet. The Prime Genome carried the design to construct the catalyst that converted the early atmosphere from carbon dioxide and ammonia to nitrogen, water, and carbon monoxide. The Prime Genome carried the essential design for the chloroplast, utilized by plant cells to generate sugars and oxygen, and for the mitochondria utilized by prokaryote and eukaryote cells to convert sugar molecules to adenosine triphosphate molecules to drive intracellular chemical reactions.

The Prime Genome acted as a template containing all of the basic organic structural data to build cells and then to organize those cells into multi-cellular organisms. The Prime Genome was likely designed with variability as its key facilitator to achieve its primary goal of survival and secondary goal of populating the planet with a sufficient ecosystem so as to support an intelligent life form as well as to provide the genetic instruction code to generate this intelligent form of life when the environmental factors were acceptable to support such life.

Over the course of the billions of years life has existed on the planet, as the environment changed due to natural causes, the Prime Genome utilized variability as a means to structure an ecosystem that was capable of adapting to the stresses placed on the environment. Species not able to adapt to the ever changing stresses of the environment perished over time as was to be expected. Under the guidance of the Prime Genome, the environmental data was processed and species at all levels of the ecosystem evolved that were best suited for the prevailing environmental conditions. Adaptation is a dynamic process and the Prime Genome was contrived with the means to adapt the life forms it was responsible for producing to insure survival.

The Prime Genome uses various means to effect variability. HOX genes have been known to exist. HOX genes represent decision points in the genome. If a particular HOX gene is activated, genes associated with the particular HOX gene are also activated. A HOX gene may be associated with construction of options such as a fin, a wing or a leg. Activating a HOX gene to generate a fin in an animal creates the underlying bone, muscle and tendon structures necessary for the fin to appear. Activating the HOX gene responsible for a leg creates the underlying bone, muscle and tendon material required for the limb.

Quantum genes may be thought of as HOX genes. Quantum genes represent transcribable information that is associated with a unique identifier so that the transcription complexes are able to locate the genetic information. Quantum genes may be comprised of one transcribable segment or may be comprised of several transcribable segments. In the case where it is necessary that more than one RNA or more than one protein need be generated to accomplish a cellular task, it is reasonable that the transcription of certain quantum genes will result in more than one type of RNA or may generate more than one messenger RNA, each to produce a different protein.

The internal workings of genes exhibit variability. The removal of various introns or portions of introns from precursor RNAs, leaving various combinations of exons to form messenger RNA acts as a means of coding for numerous RNA options, the result of which is various options for the creation of differing proteins utilizing the same biologic coding.

CHAPTER 31

ECOMETABOLOUS VERSUS EVOLUTION

'The time has come to seek answers beyond the antiquated Theory of Evolution based on random chance mutation.'

Planet Earth has the distinct characteristics of an engine. In its raw state four billion six hundred million years ago to three and a half billion years ago, prior to the appearance of organic life, the Earth represented two very valuable resources. The first resource was an abundance of raw materials. The second resource has been the planet's potential to act as a medium for the constructive use of energy. The planet has been capable of accepting radiant energy from the sun yet far enough distant from the solar furnace as not to be overloaded by such energy. The Earth was influenced by a limited number of extra terrestrial objects including a single moon and occasional meteorite strikes. The Earth was also capable of generating its own energy in the form of heat and magnetic energy emitted by the motion of the molten core, motion related to rotation of the planet, actions of explosive chemical reactions, and movement of the atmosphere, bodies of water, and land masses.

Earth, prior to life, represented a hostile environment comprised of an igneous rock surface and volcanic ash, dotted with active volcanoes and an atmosphere being a composite of inhospitable levels of helium, hydrogen, carbon dioxide, ammonia, carbon monoxide, and sulfates. The core of the planet was a furnace of molten rock regularly expelling pressure by forcing liquid rock up through weaknesses in the crust and venting through volcanoes dotting the surface of the planet. Carbon dioxide, ammonia, hydrogen sulfates, carbon monoxide trapped in the bowels of the planet, actively bellowed out from the volcanic vents. As molten rock spewed across the surface it cooled and solidified. Deadly levels of radiant energy continuously scorched half the unprotected surface of the planet as the Earth consistently rotated on its axis while orbiting at a distance of 98 million miles from the solar furnace at the center of the solar system.

The 'definition of an engine' encompasses a device used to convert any of various forms of energy into mechanical force and motion. Certainly the Earth qualifies as an engine due to its capacity to absorb radiant energy from the sun and convert this to numerous forms of mechanical force and motion. Primordial Earth was the perfect engine from which to generate life.

Organic life has taken advantage of the rigid laws of physics and the fact that the Earth predictably acts an engine, to proactively reshape the planet in such a manner as to create an environment that eventually became capable of supporting advanced forms of life.

Possibly created before the Earth ever existed, the product of a universe that is 14 billion years old, the program necessary to create life drifted across the galaxy to this planet in the form of a Vironix particle. Harboring the seeds of life in the form of copies of a Prime Genome, the Vironix particle was carried by the solar winds created by the flux of gravity and magnetic fields that permeate through space until it was drawn to Earth by the planet's active gravitational field. Encountering the planet in its barren state, the Vironix particle introduced essential biologic programming contrived specifically to take advantage of the hostile features of the planet. The two most important goals of the Prime Genome were (i) generate forms of life that could survive given the prevailing environmental factors and (ii) survival of the genetic information at all cost. The main objective of the Prime Genome was to establish and populate the earth with layers of an ecosystem that would be sufficient to support a species that would understand the existence of this original genome and be capable of reproducing the Prime Genome. More than likely, the duty of this intelligent life form was to learn from the Prime Genome, copy the Prime Genome and perpetrate the influence of the Prime Genome further into the surrounding galaxy. These strategies have remained the most powerful driving forces of the Prime Genome.

The original elemental forms of organic life carrying the Prime Genome encountered a planet barren of water, scorched by the sun's radiant energy, and an atmosphere dominated by carbon dioxide.

Possibly spherical in shape, the original life would have settled to a low point in the terrain. Utilizing the mathematical laws of chemistry and physics, the primitive life acted as an extraterrestrial catalyst designed to utilize the sun's abundant radiant energy to convert the carbon dioxide and ammonia gases comprising the primitive atmosphere into molecules of water, nitrogen gas and methane. The accumulation of nitrogen gas and methane in the atmosphere would have served to block the intense radiation emitted by the sun allowing the planet's surface to cool, creating an environment where liquid water could pool in the low points of the surface of the planet. The passage of time being inconsequential, the primitive life would have continuously labored to surround itself in a body of water. Over time water covered 79% of the planet's surface. The atmosphere was converted from being dominated by carbon dioxide, to a mixture of nitrogen and oxygen with a scant amount of carbon dioxide and water vapor.

Once sufficiently submersed in a water environment, essential primitive life, at the direction of the Prime Genome, transformed itself into more complex forms of organic life. The Prime Genome generated the chloroplast in primitive organic life, which took advantage of the sun's radiant energy to take carbon dioxide from the atmosphere and the surrounding water to produce oxygen and glucose molecules. Glucose molecules were then used as the intracellular fuel to support complex chemical reactions. With glucose as a means of producing ATP molecules, and the Prime Genome supplying the blueprints, complex protein molecules were constructed in order to produce progressively more advanced forms of life.

The atmosphere was actively transformed by organic life from being composed of carbon dioxide and minimal nitrogen and water vapor into an atmosphere comprised of 21% oxygen, 79% nitrogen, and less than 1% carbon dioxide. The presence of a high concentration of oxygen molecules in the atmosphere provided (a) the opportunity for the development of life that could utilize oxygen in a respiratory process to breakdown glucose for fuel, which lead to the existence of a wide variety of higher order animals and (b) a natural shield to protect higher order animals from deadly levels of the sun's radiant energy.

In the stratosphere, 25 miles above the planet's surface, the subsequent naturally occurring reaction of oxygen molecules being struck by ultraviolet rays produced ozone. The accumulation of large amounts of ozone in both the stratosphere and the troposphere prevented deadly radiation of a wavelength of <290 nm from reaching the surface of the planet. The action of blanketing the globe with a protective layer of ozone eventually provided a safe environment for complex forms of life to safely leave the oceans and flourish on land.

Darwin's Theory of Evolution represents the development of life as a result of changes to DNA that were the result of a combination of chance mutation and survival of the fittest.

Though the concept of evolution has been embraced since Darwin's time there has been no cellular mechanism identified that is responsible for the generation of new genetic material . . . other than the occurrence of chance mutation or the suggestion that one bacterium ingested other bacteria. There is no organ present in the cell that has been identified as being capable of generating the DNA required to create new genes and add this newly generated DNA to an existing nuclear genome. In addition, the generation of DNA requires the sophisticated process of fixation of nitrogen into organic molecules, which is critical for a cell to be able to copy its genome and pass the genome on to daughter cells.

Mere chance mutation does occur, but such an occurrence does not adequately explain what has obviously been a progressive move of the genetic design to create an increasingly more sophisticated form of life. Specifically, 'mere chance' mutation of a species' genome does not lead to a completely new species with a larger body, improved use of the limbs, larger brain with increased intelligence. Mere chance mutation does not adequately explain the explosive diversity of life that occurred in the Cambrian period 500 million years ago. The Cambrian period generated more different types of animal life than all the rest of the history of life on Earth. Further, mere chance did not generate the numerous complex advancements present in the human body as compared to other primates including the erect stance, opposable thumb and the higher brain intellect.

The opposing theory to evolution to be considered is that an elaborate biologic program has been functioning in accordance to a distinct mission since the beginning of life on the planet. That more sophisticated forms of life have been generated according to genetic design. Advanced forms of life could not exist without first the foundation of a hospitable planet with a balanced ecosystem being established.

Preprogramming is evident all around us. Without schooling, without tools or references, birds are capable of building elaborate nests, beavers create dams, squirrels hide nuts in the ground to prepare for winter months, multi-cellular animals of most species nurture and care for their young. The capability to build a three dimensional object such as a nest is a behavior that has been referred to as 'instinct', but more accurately as a set of programming instructions that are passed down through the genetics from one generation to the next generation.

Holometabolous is a term that has been applied to the complete metamorphosis observed in some insects. Holometabola refers to a series of ten orders of insects including Coleoptera (beetles), Hymenoptera (bees, wasps, ants), Lepidoptera (moths and butterflies), Diptera (two-winged flies), and Siphonaptera (fleas), which undergo complete metamorphosis.

Ecometabolous represents the actions of the Prime DNA genome that has resulted in the complete metamorphosis of the ecosystem of the planet and the expected creation of the higher order of organic life known as homo sapiens or 'man' based on the combination of (1) a preprogrammed collection of available genetic instructions spanning all organic life and viruses that have occupied the planet since at least the inception of life on the planet and (2) selection based on survival of the fittest given the prevailing environmental factors present at the time a species has existed.

The Prime DNA Genome was arranged into four major branches emanating from a central trunk. Utilizing a quantum gene coding system that utilizes the base-four mathematics inherent in the DNA, the four major branches are arranged as (1) Basic cell design and protein design, (2) Viruses, (3) Prokaryote cells, and (4) Eukaryote cells. All life shares certain essential parts of the Prime Genome, such as biologic instructions regarding basic cell design and protein design. The Prime Genome could be reconstructed if the nonredundant portions of the genomes of all life that have lived on the Earth were combined into one genome.

Unlike the concepts underpinning the theory of evolution, survival of the fittest has not been the essential means, or the driving force, for the advancement of one sophisticated life form to another more advanced sophisticated life form. The Prime Genome has provided the preprogrammed instructions necessary to create new forms of life over the three and a half billion years based on evolving atmospheric, water and land conditions. Survival of the fittest honed the development of the new forms of life which emerged at the beaconing of the Prime Genome, eliminating the weaker physical changes and facilitating the stronger physical changes to create forms of life that have indeed possessed the best opportunity of survival given the environmental conditions concurrent at the time. The ultimate objective of ecometabolous was to create an environment that could create and sustain the human life form.

Humans, the most advanced form of life in existence on the planet, are considered the current end result of ecometabolous. Humans have occupied the planet surface for approximately 4.4 million years if the early human forms of Lucy and Ardi are included in the timeline. Human civilization has existed for approximately the 10,000 years; less than half a percent of human existence. Human existence was possible without a contrived or preplanned strategy, but human civilization is very much dependent upon an orderly existence of the history of organic life.

Without billions of years of plant life living in the seas, the toxic carbon dioxide and sulfates present in the atmosphere would not have been transformed into the oxygen and nitrogen mixture required for humans to breathe. Without the ozone layer to protect against deadly radiation from the sun, man could not have existed beyond the shelter of caves or underground dwellings. Without nitrogen fixing bacteria, including cyanobacteria, there would be no surface plants due to such plants lacking the capacity to fix sufficient amounts of nitrogen to prosper. Without millions of years of bacteria, plant and animal life cycling through life and death, the top soil of the planet would not exit, which has supported farming. Without the farmable corps and the cultivating of livestock animals, the foodstuffs needed to support a global population of human civilization would simply not exist.

Without the passage of two hundred million years of plant life slowly decaying in freshwater swamps during the Carboniferous period of Earth's history, humans would not have the coal reserves that exist. Without coal, mankind could not have heated furnaces hot enough to perform metallurgy. Successful metallurgy created the tools used to build civilization. Without coal, the steam engine would not have developed into a practical means of locomotion or the engine used in early manufacturing. Without the hundreds of millions of years of biologic activity of single celled planktonic plants starting around 540 million years ago, the oil reserves humans utilize for petroleum products would not exist. Without vast deposits of subterranean crude oil, the internal combustion gasoline engine would not have been developed; the industrial revolution would have ground to a halt and there would have been no cars, trucks, motor boats, generators, or early aircraft. In addition, without the presence of crude oil items such as lubricants, plastics and jet engine airline fuel would not have been contrived.

Human culture and technology as we know it would not have been possible if not for a well-orchestrated evolution of the many forms of organic life that have appeared, flourished and become extinct long before humans ever inhabited the planet. The mere existence of the human form, much less the advancement of humans to create and evolve the technologies of modern times is precisely dependent upon an intricately designed plan set in motion since the beginning when life first appeared on the planet.

The human genome is a sub program of the larger more complex Prime Genome. The human genome contains the essential portions of the Prime Genome necessary to generate the human life form. The human life form represents the Prime Genome's expected outcome.

The human genome is comprised of 3 billion pairs of nucleotides, which mathematically is a string of zeros, ones, twos and threes if the adenine, cytosine, guanine and thymine nucleotides are converted to numbers in a base four system. The human nomenclature of assigning names to the four differing nucleotides is arbitrary. The human genome is comprised of portions dedicated to essential protein construction, cell construction, anatomical design features of the human body and footprints of viral genomes.

Mathematical systems tend not to be arbitrary. The actual numbering system present in the genome is likely related to the size or weight of the molecule. In a system where molecular weight of the nucleotide designates the order, cytosine would represent the 'zero' since it is the lightest of the four nucleotide bases. Thymine would represent the 'one' being the second heaviest nucleotide base. Adenine would represent the 'two' being the third heaviest nucleotide base and guanine would represent the 'three' since it is the heaviest of the four nucleotide bases.

If the nomenclature of C=0, T=1, A=2, G=3 is applied to the Prime Genome, then 'C' or the number 'zero' is assigned to the first digit or primary digit of the unique identification of the initial genome that is coded for the first major branching limb, that of the building blocks of cell structure and proteins. 'T' or the number 'one' is assigned to the first digit or primary digit of the unique identification of the second major branching limb of the initial genome that is coded for the construction of prokaryote cells. 'A' or the number 'two' is assigned to the first digit or primary digit of the unique identification of the third major branching limb of the initial genome that is coded for the building blocks of viruses. 'G' or the number 'three' is assigned to the first digit or primary digit of the unique identification of the fourth major branching limb of the initial genome that is coded for the building blocks of eukaryote cells.

The limb of the eukaryote cells is further divided into four regions. 'GC' representing the base four number '30' indicates the branch for protista species. 'GT' representing the base four number '31' indicates the branch for fungi species. 'GA' representing the base four number '32' indicates the branch for plant species. 'GG' or the base four number '33' indicates the branch for animal species.

The Prime Genome was organized into four major branches. Each quantum gene in each of the four branches assigned a unique identification number comprised of 25-nucleotides. The two branches assigned to the prokaryote and eukaryote life forms shared information present in the branch dedicated to cell design and protein construction. To conserve energy and resources, as species differentiated into progressively more complex forms portions of the Primary Genome which were not necessary for current or future species were not reproduced and passed on to subsequent species.

Viruses are represented in the third branch of the Prime Genome. A virion is comprised of an outer shell, a genome and in some cases proteins that facilitate the virus's replication process. A virus often has a specific cell that it targets as its host cell for replications. Viruses have interacted with all forms of life throughout the ages. There is evidence that portions of over four hundred thousand viral genomes are present in the human genome. The interaction of viruses with plants and animals appears a likely and effective triggering mechanism to advance the intention of the Prime Genome to create more sophisticated forms of life by activating dormant genes.

Hox genes act as master control switches exerting control over a series of genes. Activating a particular Hox gene triggers a chain reaction over a specific set of genes. Hox genes direct cells to differentiate into specific cell types in order to generate the organs and limbs oriented in their proper position necessary to create a particular species. Hox genes are a subset of quantum genes.

The Prime Genome contains the design options that have been necessary to create the majority of the various species that have existed on planet Earth. Actions of the Hox genes create options in limb and organ structures for species. Introns present in genes create options in the construction of proteins. Viruses are capable of influencing the expression of genes.

Ecometabolous is defined as the directed metamorphosis of a planet per the biologic instructions of a Prime Genome to generate a balanced multi-layer ecosystem to support an intelligent higher order animal species such as the Homo sapiens.

The existence of organic life on planet Earth was distinctly planned. The Prime Genome is the mechanism that has acted to produce life, while ecometabolous represents the strategy. Together the Prime Genome and Ecometabolous are recognized as being the essential components of what is consider to be 'Nature'.

An advanced life form such as humans, are meant to achieve enough of an understanding of their existence and the ecosystem that supports them, to participate in the copying of the Prime Genome and spreading of the opportunity of life throughout the galaxy.

CHAPTER 32

ECOMETABOLOUS AND THE BRAIN

If an ancient intelligent life wrote such a sophisticated program as to have accounted for all of the species that have existed and created an environment in a stepwise pattern so as to support an increasingly sophisticated forms of life, then it is not without the possibility that this same intelligence bequeathed humans with a level of intelligence that would allow humans to develop an understanding of science and technology. Provided the correct environment, human technology has progressed significantly in the last one hundred years. Humans may possess an innate knowledge of interstellar space travel.

Computer Aided Design (CAD) software used to help designers create a wide variety of manufactured goods, facilitates the awareness that the most sophisticated manmade goods can be detailed on a computer. The design blueprints for any device can be stored in the memory of a computer hard drive or any mobile storage device equipped with adequate memory space. The mechanism used to accomplish the storage of the information is to translate the data regarding a specific subject into the binary language to facilitate storage of segments of data in a computer's memory device. Once stored in the binary computer language, data files can be transferred to other devices capable of accepting the binary data. In the blink of an eye data files can be routed per the Internet or phone line or wirelessly to a device on the opposite side of the planet. Given the proper software, blueprints for the given device can be generated and, if desired, the device can be manufactured.

We have to consider that, if an intelligent life form designed a biologic program masterful enough to have resulted in a complete metamorphosis of a dead planet into a planet capable of supporting human life, this same intelligent life form could have provided humans with the means, in the form of intelligent data files stored in their brain, to travel forth from this planet into space in an effort to insure survival of the human species. Given the environment of the earth is unpredictable and annihilation of all life could occur, it would seem logical that the intelligent life that created the primary program also provided a means for the expected outcome: the homo sapiens escaping the planet and flourish in the galaxy and possibly beyond.

Thirty years ago the SR-40 Texas Instrument calculator and other calculators like it were the rage of portable hand held technologies. At this same time a phone receiver was still tethered to the phone unit by a cord, music was played by either vinyl record or 8-track player, there were no desk top computers and flat screen imaging was science fiction. One can take the individual components of a SR-40 TI calculator and rearrange them however one wishes. If all one has are the individual components of a calculator or several identical calculators, one is not going to be able to construct the technologies of today; try as one might, one will not be able to build a portable phone, laptop computer, notebook, or simple MP-3 player. The components are not there to make more sophisticated elements; humans with their intelligence are the driving force behind the progression in technologies. This is not to ignore or downgrade the importance of the fact that the invention, manufacture and distribution of the handheld calculator was indeed a critical step in the progressive development of our current technologies. But it showcases the fact that some form of an intelligent intervention has been necessary to have generated the sophisticated human body from a planet that otherwise started out as a barren crust with volcanic rock as land masses, sterile oceans and lakes as bodies of water, and nitrogen, carbon monoxide, carbon dioxide and sulfur containing molecules as an atmosphere with the deadly radiation of the sun beating down on the already harsh foreboding environment.

Certainly what the progression of our technology has shown us is that the level of sophistication of the operating system is all important. A calculator was not programmable, so it by default had no operating system. Early desk top computers required that the operating system, generally referred to as DOS for 'disk operating system', had to be loaded by inserting a disk into the computer every time the computer was turned on in order for the electronics of the computer to function as a computer. Success or failure of the current product lines of technologies are often incredibly dependent upon how well the computer programming that acts as the primary operating system for a device interfaces with the human user. The more sophisticated the operating system which translates into the more capabilities a device has to offer to the user, often the more popular the device will be in the global marketplace.

The brain and the sophisticated nature of the DNA may have worked together in order to encourage the successful advancement of what appears to be evolution. Throughout the millions of years that life equipped with a brain has existed, the brain may have functioned not only as a means to provide the animal with a certain level of reason, instinct and subjective mobility of the organism's limbs, but the brain may have been actively sampling the environment. The rudimentary brain in every animal that has existed may have been checking its surroundings for atmospheric conditions regarding radiation and oxygen levels, as well as purity of the soil and water and the availability and integrity of the food chain. Changes to the functional aspects of the DNA may have been made by the rudimentary brain sampling the surrounding environment and making changes to future generations by altering the offspring's DNA at the level of the sex organs utilizing either nerve impulses and/or hormones.

The brains of all previous life forms may have been paving the way toward the development of the human entity. Once the prime DNA produced the human form, the human form was equipped with a brain that championed a level of intelligence to not only effectively stand upright and use the body's limbs in an effective manner, but to also reason and analyze the environment existing on the planet. What humans refer to as instinct in more primitive forms of life may simply represent innate instructions needed for an organism with a brain to survive. Humans, designed with higher brain functions, have stored memory files that can be accessed and utilized to create and develop technologies. The extent of these technology files may be vast enough to provide humans with not only locomotive transportation and air transportation, but the elements of interstellar flight. At least five times in earth's history a natural disaster has occurred to the point of reducing life down to the last ten percent of existence. Humans are the expected result of complete metamorphosis of the planet. The end game of survival of the fittest may refer to whether humanity has enough time to develop enough of an awareness of the stored library in our brains to develop technology to the point of being able to escape the confines of the planet before a natural disaster occurs that wipes clean humanity's existence from the face of the planet.

CHAPTER 33

EVIDENCE OF THE PRIME GENOME

The prevailing theory regarding the origin and progress of the development of life on the Earth has been that life is the result of an astronomical number of random events that have fortunately resulted in beneficial structural advances to create the many successful multi-layered ecosystems that inhabit the entire surface of the globe.

What is missing in this theory is that random events take an effort backward as much as they take it forward which is not seen in the development of life forms. However, a computer program designed to create life, would be capable of producing an astronomical number of alterations in a dependable and organized manner that would clearly produce the type of development life forms have under gone.

Evidence that such a program, called the Prime Genome, has existed and remains actively functioning in the form of subprograms is evident at numerous levels of the macroscopic and microscopic biologic environment that prevails across the surface of the planet.

The elements that support the presence of an organized bio computer program, the Prime Genome, include: (1) Development of a balanced ecosystem, (2) Development of Life Forms, (3) Stem cells, (4) DNA written as a base four code, (5) Existence of Hox genes, (6) Presence of programming commands, and (7) Intelligence to Carry Out Complex Functions.

Balanced ecosystem The complexity and successful existence of the global food chain demands an intricate design. Carnivorous higher order animals depend upon the existence of an adequate amount of lower order animals. Survival of lower order herbivores requires the precise orchestration of plant species and pollinating insect species. The recycling of organic material is dependent upon the actions of organisms such as insects, species of fungi and bacteria. All elements of life are necessary for higher order animals to exist. The preciseness of the ecosystem in existence on earth indicates that a script has been followed and that this is not the work of a random process.

Life Forms Life forms are often placed on charts showing the chain of life forms to which each of the life forms belong. What is interesting about this picture is that, in general, the life forms become more sophisticated the further along the chain they appear. In a truly random process this would not occur since the probability of adding capability would be the same as that of losing it—actually it would be more given the complexity of the processes carried out in a cell. However, this is not what these charts show us. They show continuous development toward higher order life forms. Further, once an action is completed it doesn't appear again. For example, fish came out of the sea 500 million years ago to become air breathing land animals. We don't still see fish coming out of the sea. That part of the development process is over. Further, if the process was random, we should see land animals going back into the sea to be fish, and we certainly have never seen that.

Stem cells The term 'stem' cell represents a cell in a multi-cellular organism that has not differentiated into a cell that has a specific duty. Research has demonstrated that a stem cell can be triggered to transform into a cell which displays features of a specific type of cell. It has been well recognized that in the bone marrow stem cells exist and are capable to differentiating into white blood cells, red blood cell and megakaryoctes, which produce platelets. The fact that with the proper chemical or hormonal trigger a cell can be transformed into a cell with a specific duty is a display that a biologic program exists in all cells in a dormant state, and in the case of the stem cell, once triggered, the biologic program transforms the potential characteristics of the stem cell into a differentiated cell with refined characteristics capable of performing a specific set of functions. This says that a cell has all of the code required to carry out any function that the body requires and that it only needs specific parts to that code, called the DNA, to be turned on or off to transform it into whatever type of cell the body is in need of.

DNA Written in Base Four Code A Transcription Complex reads the DNA and transcribes it to produce RNA. The transcription complex is comprised of approximately 40 different protein molecules and is the biologic equivalent of a desktop computer's central processing unit (CPU). The CPU in a desktop computer reads binary computer software code in the form of strings of ones and zeros. The transcription complex decodes a quaternary biologic code in the form of four elements: the nucleic acids of 'adenine', 'cytosine', 'guanine' and 'thymine'. Computers use the CPU to decode the information in the computer software. CPUs delegate mathematic calculations to logic units and graphics duties to MMX units. Once a biologic Transcription Complex transcribes a gene the resultant RNA is then modified by at least one Spliceosome. A Spliceosome is a complex comprised of a combination of small nuclear RNA molecules and protein subunits. Spliceosomes remove introns from pre-messenger RNA molecules to produce messenger RNA molecules ready for translation by ribosomes. The processing power of the Transcription Complex and the Spliceosome parallel the processing actions of binary CPUs and their ancillary units.

Cheong Xin Chan, et al[1] reports an analysis of >60,000 novel genes from mesophilic red algae. Red Algae are single cell organisms. It has been estimated that humans, a complex multi-cellular organism, possess and require 32,000 genes. The fact that a single-celled organism possesses twice the number of genes as needed to generate a human strongly suggests that the more primitive single cell organism of Red Algae possess the potential programming instructions to evolve into higher order multi-cellular organisms.

Hox Genes Hox genes are present in the genome. Hox genes control specific sets of genes and dictate the overall animal body plan. Hox genes are responsible for the development of structures such as a fin versus a wing versus an arm, or a fin versus a wing versus a leg. The presence of Hox genes in the DNA demonstrates a potential for the morphing of one species into another species. Hox genes also indicate that a design plan existed that was intended to morph aquatic life into land based species and into winged species that were capable of taking flight.

Programming Commands START, STOP, REPEAT, ADD and other commands exist in both the DNA and the RNA. That is, there are sequences of nucleotides that represent the commands of START, STOP, REPEAT, and ADD. These same types of commands are commonly used in computer programs to perform computer functions similar to those carried out by the cells.

Intelligence to Carry Out Complex Functions There are many examples of precise as opposed to randomly generated intelligence within the cells. Consider the following. Every one of the 32,000 or so proteins required by the cells of the human body is generated from its own mRNA template which in its original form had one or more Introns which had to be removed. This involves hundreds of thousands of splice sites which must be located and used with great precision less the protein be manufactured wrong and a medical problem generated, a condition which is rarely seen.

A second example is the translation of a three nucleotide code into an amino acid in a protein sequence. On one hand, this involves a polymerase II lining up correctly on the mRNA template and correctly identifying the amino acid the code calls for and then setting up a call for a tRNA carrying that amino acid. On the other hand, it also involves placing the correct complementary code on the tRNA structure and attaching the correct amino acid to it. Each of these steps must be accomplished with considerable precision less the protein be manufactured wrong and a medical problem generated, a condition which again is rarely seen.

As a third example consider the ability of cells to turn genes on and off to control both the initial development of the life form—for example how tall it is—and its maintenance. Given that the average cell has more than 10,000 command and control systems just to regulate its protein production is De facto proof that it was not developed from a random process for if it was some of these command and control systems would be malformed causing the cell to operate differently than planned.

In summary, at all levels of the macroscopic, microscopic and even submicroscopic environments, there exist the footprints of biologic programming that indicates the presence of a Prime Genome. Random mistakes in the DNA have occurred and were expected to occur. Morphing of the DNA due to copying errors during replication and damage to the genome due to radiation were also expected to occur. Survival of the fittest weeded out weaker variations that occur due to the Prime Genome versus genome copying errors versus changes due to radiation damage. An evolving genome was the critical means of surviving in an environment that has been in constant flux. The basis of the development of organic life that has filled the various levels of the multi-layered ecosystems that have existed since life began have been the result of a well organized biologic program, the Prime Genome. One of the strongest arguments for the fact that random events can guide evolution, but cannot create it, is that random events move efforts backwards to the same degree that they move them forward and we do not see things like land animals and birds returning to the sea.

1. Cheong Xin Chan, Current Biology, 27,1-6,February 22, 2011.

Part 8

Opportunities

CHAPTER 34

OPPORTUNITIES FOR MEDICAL THERAPIES

Combing the principles of the Universal Dogma of Microbiology and a cell-specific approach to delivering healthcare, such as Medical Vector Therapy, numerous new medical treatment strategies could be successfully developed.

At present, chemical drugs or protein molecules are inserted into the body through various pathways in hopes that the medication will reach its target and cause a medically beneficial effect. Medical Vector Therapy refers to the use of transport devices called vectors, which are similar in exterior construct to viruses but without their harmful capabilities, to deliver a specific payload to a specific type of cell to effect a medical therapy. Medical Vector Therapy offers a means of inserting specific chemicals, proteins and/or genetic material into specific cells types to produce medically beneficial effects in the targeted cells. Medical Vector Therapy provides a means to not only deliver a specific payload to specific cells, but offers a transport mechanism to deliver fragile molecules such as RNA molecules to cells.

The concept of the Universal Dogma of Microbiology identifies that there are numerous points in cell metabolism that could be exploited to produce medically beneficial effects. Medical Vector Therapy could be used to transport payloads such as messenger RNA, ribosomal RNAs, control RNAs, command RNAs and nuclear signaling proteins to specific cells to produce very specific effects inside target cells. See Figure 22.

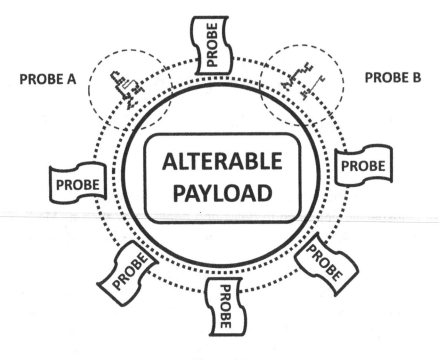

Figure 22
Medical Vector Therapy

Transporting messenger RNA molecules to specific cells provides the opportunity to generate any of the 33,000 proteins that may exist in a cell for the benefit of a specific cell type.

Transporting ribosomal RNA molecules to specific cell types provides a mechanism to up-regulate or down-regulate the production of a specific protein inside a target cell. Inserting a natural ribosomal RNA molecule into a functioning cell will interact with ribosomal proteins and enhance the translation of specific messenger RNA molecules, increasing production of the protein generated by the messenger RNA molecule. Placing in target cells, modified ribosomal RNA molecules that will combine to build a ribosome, but are dysfunctional in their capacity to translate a messenger RNA would result in a decrease in the production of a specific protein. Disease states created by an overproduction of a particular protein would be treatable by utilizing modified ribosomal RNA molecules to reduce the production of a specific protein in a target cell.

Transporting control RNA molecules or nuclear signaling proteins to specific cells offers the means to activate and deactivate the transcription of specific genes. See Figure 23. Control RNAs contain a segment that is the antithesis of a specific unique identifier associated with quantum genes present in nuclear DNA. Control RNA molecules could be used to activate the transcription of any quantum gene or DNA instruction that has a unique identifier associated with its existence. An exogenous natural control RNA molecule, once inserted into a targeted cell by a Medical Vector, would migrate to the nucleus of the cell, locate the unique identifier associated with the quantum gene the control RNA is coded for, bind with the unique identifier and initiate the construction of a transcription complex.

Modified control RNA molecules can also be utilized to block the transcription of any quantum gene or DNA instruction associated with a unique identifier. An exogenous modified control RNA molecule once inserted into a target cell by a Medical Vector, would migrate to the nucleus of the cell, locate the unique identifier associated with the quantum gene the control RNA is coded for, bind with the unique identifier and, by means of the modified construct of the RNA, block the formation of a transcription complex at that site.

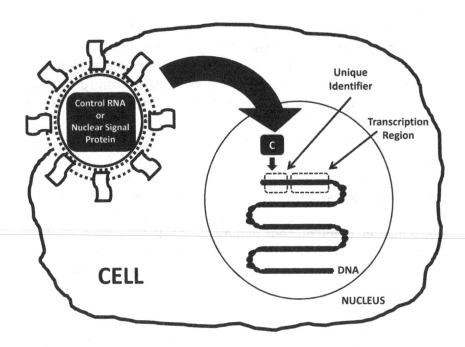

Figure 23
Using Medical Vector Therapy to Insert Control RNA
or Control Proteins into Specifically Targeted Cells

Transporting command RNA molecules to specific cells facilitates the means to generate complex molecules inside cells. See Figure 24. Medical Vector Therapy can be utilized to transport Control RNAs, Nuclear Signaling Proteins or Command RNAs into specific target cells to produce a medically beneficial result.

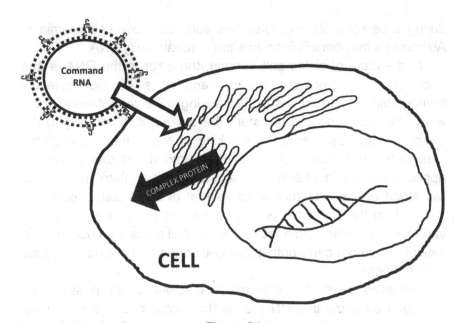

Figure 24
Using Medical Vector Therapy to Insert Command RNAs
into Specifically Targeted Cells

DNA viruses and RNA viruses that generate DNA genomes insert their DNA into a host cell's nuclear DNA utilizing the action of a protein referred to as an integrase enzyme. This process could be exploited to facilitate the insertion of medically beneficial DNA into target cells' nuclear DNA. This would give health care providers the opportunity to repair faulty DNA.

Understanding the wording and syntax of the programming language the DNA is written in facilitates knowledge of how the programming instructions present in the human genome are coded. Once the programming language comprising the DNA is understood, faults in the programming instructions in the DNA can be analyzed and determined. Faults in the human genome may be related to errors that occur due to radiation damage, errors that occur during copying of the DNA, errors introduced by malicious viruses, or errors that have occurred due to aging. Errors found in the DNA may be a fault that has occurred in the DNA that has been passed through generations as an inherited flaw in the DNA or errors present in the DNA may be acquired during a person's lifetime. Diseases such as sickle cell anemia or Alzheimer's may benefit from an effort to repair faulty DNA.

In the case of sickle cell anemia, the error in the DNA is one nucleotide that changes the characteristics of the molecule hemoglobin. The error causes the stacking of the variant hemoglobin when the red blood cell transfers the oxygen it is carrying to the peripheral tissues. Repeated stacking of the variant hemoglobin causes the red blood cell to elongate into a cell that physically appears curved in shape, like a sickle, rather than the normal red blood cell architecture which is that of a flat disc. Correcting the error in the DNA that is responsible for the production of the variant hemoglobin would prevent sickle cell crisis from occurring in individuals whom carry both sickle cell genes and are homozygous for the disease.

Diseases such as Alzheimer's disease could possibly be managed by correcting DNA faults that occur due to aging in the nucleus of neurons that comprise the brain tissues. Faulty DNA could be repaired by decoding the region of the nuclear DNA that contains the fault. Understanding the syntax of the programming language would facilitate the opportunity to insert a segment of DNA into brain cells that could act as a computer program like patch to correct errors that may have occurred in the programming instructions in the human genome present in the neurons. This approach is likened to the approach utilized by computer programmers where a small patch program is inserted into a computer to correct one or more errors found in large computer program to facilitate the computer program to run properly.

Modified viruses could be utilized to insert into target cells medically beneficial segments of DNA that would act to correct errors in the nuclear DNA or even mitochondrial DNA.

The coding principles used to generate the human body from the human genome are the same principles utilized to construct all forms of life that have existed on the planet. Lessons learned regarding identifying, activating, deactivating and repairing errors in the nuclear DNA can be extrapolated to most other forms of life that co-exist on the planet with humans. Instructions to facilitate the general construction of a cell must be universal to all life forms. Variations in cell types and how cells are physically arranged inside the parameters of a multi-celled organism are related to species specific segments of the DNA utilized by a species to create the specie's unique life form. Programming instructions vary from species to species. Data files vary from species to species.

Understanding how programming principles used to write the programming instructions to create the human body leads to the opportunity to understanding the programming language used to generate all forms of life. Understanding the programming language used by plants provides the opportunity to generate DNA code that can be inserted into plant cells to modify plants such that they will grow heartier and more proliferative crops for human consumption.

In summary, the medical treatment options discussed in the previous text include:

(1) Utilizing modified viruses to transport messenger RNA to target cells.
(2) Utilizing modified viruses to transport ribosomal RNA to target cells.
(3) Utilizing modified viruses to transport control RNA to target cells.
(4) Utilizing modified viruses to transport command RNA to target cells.
(5) Utilizing modified viruses to transport nuclear signaling proteins to target cells.
(6) Utilizing modified viruses to transport medically beneficial DNA to target cells for purposes of repairing faulty DNA. The medically beneficial exogenous DNA segment inserted in the DNA may be in the form of a segment that replaces the exact set of nucleotides that are dysfunctional in the DNA or is to be a segment of nucleotides written to produce a medically beneficial effect to replace and account for the function of the dysfunctional DNA.
(7) Lessons learned from treating human diseases can be extended to beneficially modifying plant life to grow heartier and more proliferative crops for human consumption.
(8) Lessons learned from treating human diseases can be extended to modify animals to grow heartier.

Table 16 demonstrates the options of payloads that could be transported by medical vector therapy to specific target cells and the expected outcome of having such a payload transported and inserted into target cells.

Payload Transported by Medical Vector Therapy	Expected Outcome
Messenger RNA	Generate specific protein synthesis
Ribosomal RNA	Generate specific protein synthesis
Modified Ribosomal RNA	Block specific protein synthesis
Control RNA	Activation specific gene transcription
Modified Control RNA	Block activation of specific gene transcription
Command RNA	Initiate specific complex protein production
Modified Command RNA	Block specific complex protein production
Signaling protein	Activation specific gene transcription
Modified Signaling protein	Block specific gene transcription
DNA	Correct syntax coding errors present in the genome

Table 16

Revisiting the Role of the Unique Identifier

Utilizing a unique identifier as a means of locating specific genetic material amongst the 3 billion base pairs of nucleotides comprising the human DNA supports the plausible use of gene therapy. Utilizing Medical Vector Therapy, delivering such quantum genes, which contain a unique identifier, to specific cell types provides a means of inserting specific genetic information into the cell's nuclear deoxyribonucleic acid that can be readily located by the cell's nuclear transcription complexes. These medically therapeutic quantum genes are intended to provide a wide variety of medical therapeutic options to clinicians.

The concept of the quantum gene is the key concept that opens the door to exploring the biologic software programming that comprises the DNA. Each gene acts as one or more lines of programming code containing one or more instructions or data files. Small groups of code define the series of enzymes that are necessary for biologic processes to occur. Larger groups of code define the instructions necessary to construct individual organelles inside a cell. Still larger groups of code define the construct of general and specialty cells. Much larger groups of code act as the blueprints to constructing the individual organs that comprise the body. Finally very large groups of biologic code define workings of the entity, e.g., the human body, acting to coordinate all of the biologic systems that are required to facilitate growth, development and maintenance of the body as a whole.

Identifying the existence of the quantum gene makes possible the understanding of command and control functions that occur at the cellular level. A master biologic program governs the life-cycle of a cell and the life-cycle of every multi-cellular organism. Quantum genes represent the model with which individual phenotypical instruction codes and all of the command and control instruction codes are organized with a unique identifier and the transcribable instruction linked together. Phenotypical instructions are what are identifiable as physical features of a species, while the command and control instructions are those instructions that are necessary to build the phenotypical features, arrange the phenotypical features in an organized manner to define a species, utilize the phenotypical features and maintain the phenotypical features.

Identification of unique identifiers associated with quantum genes leads to new horizons in the treatment of medical conditions. By knowing the unique identifier of a gene, small molecules can be fashioned to interface with the unique identifier of a particular gene with the intention of either activating or deactivating the particular gene. Activating a gene would be accomplished by a small molecule coded for the gene's unique identifier interfacing with the unique identifier of the gene and upon such an interaction, would stimulate the assembly of a transcription complex to transcribe the gene. Deactivating a gene would be accomplished by a small molecule interfacing with the unique identifier of a particular gene that would prevent the assembly of a transcription complex at the site of the gene, thus preventing a gene from being transcribed.

Part 9

Summary

CHAPTER 35

SUMMARY OF CONCEPTS

This text contains a significant amount of deductive reasoning. It is an attempt to take what has been a black box of genetics and cell biology and create an initial framework with which to move forward in an effort to better define the human genome and cell function. Much of the subject matter in this text has been contrived by extrapolating information from human technologies and by seeking answers to explain intricate organic life-sustaining processes that have been ongoing for hundreds of millions of years prior to man ever setting foot on the planet. Proving some of the concepts presented in this book involves parallel data analysis of the genome of numerous species, which is achievable, but beyond the scope of this text at this time. This text is meant to act as a scaffolding, from which a concrete foundation of knowledge pertaining to the biologic computer programming coded in the DNA and the biologic programming acting to control cell function can be assimilated and defined.

As discussed, the essential concepts presented in Volume 3 include:

1. A unique identification numbering system exists in the cell to direct protein manufacturing.
2. Genes are associated with a unique identification which gives rise to the term 'Quantum Gene'.
3. The unique identification associated with a gene is utilized to control transcription of the gene.
4. Messenger RNA (mRNA) molecules are associated with unique identification in the 5' region.

5. Unique identification associated with messenger RNA is used to control translation of the messenger RNA.
6. Command and Control functions are necessary features of cell growth and survival.
7. Communication occurs inside the boundaries of a cell and between cells in order to orchestrate coordinated functions necessary for growth, maintenance, survival and reproduction.
8. Ribosomal RNA (rRNA) molecules are associated with a unique identification coded to engage mRNA.
9. Control RNA (cnRNA) molecules possess a unique identification that directs the RNA to a specific gene and once contact is made the RNA's tail activates a transcription complex.
10. Nuclear Signaling Proteins, by means of their three dimensional structure which mimics the unique identification of a gene, are capable of locating a specific gene and activating a transcription complex to transcribe that gene.
11. Nuclear Signaling Proteins generate positive or negative feedback to the nucleus.
12. Command RNA molecules provide the instructions to facilitate modifications to proteins, including folding of proteins, cleaving proteins and linking of separate proteins.
13. Command RNA molecules act as instructions and interact with fixed ribosomes in smooth endoplasmic reticulum to build complex proteins.
14. The DNA is comprised of a static intelligence made up of (a) reference tables, (b) bundled instructions, (c) data files.
15. In addition to protein production, functional aspects of the DNA are contained in a programming language coded into the DNA.
16. A significant portion of the 95% of human genome considered to be redundant genetic material is comprised of the instructions needed to construct the architectural features of the cell, the organs, and the body as a whole.
17. The Universal Dogma of Microbiology states 'All protein production is a dynamic process created by a static intelligence stored in the DNA, facilitated by control RNAs

and DNA binding proteins to produce messenger RNA which are used as templates to generate proteins, the rate of production being controlled by nuclear signaling proteins and control RNAs and the construction of complex protein molecules being directed by the collaboration of static chemical processes, production rate of enzymes and command RNA molecules'.

18. The nitrogenase enzyme is essential for life since it allows certain bacteria to extract nitrogen gas from the atmosphere and combine it with hydrogen to produce ammonia, which can then be used to generate organic compounds; plants do not have this essential enzyme.

19. The nuclear DNA contains information that has acted as the means to change organic life in a manner that has been recognized as evolution.

20. Ecometabolous refers to morphing that has occurred to the ecosystem that existed on the planet with the intention that a higher order intelligent species would eventually evolve and survive.

21. The Prime DNA genome provided the basic instructions needed to generate organic life, and by manipulating the set of existing instructions created each species in a manner that best suited survival of the species given the conditions of the environment at the time and location the species existed.

22. HIV's unique identifier points research toward identifying quantum genes in the human genome.

23. When the technology described in this book is combined with that described in the first two volumes, one begins to see the vast number of diseases that could be cured and the deformities that could be corrected by bringing these technologies to bear.

24. The technologies include some simplistic approaches that could be developed and brought to bear within a few years.

POST SCRIPT ONE

Bio Programming Means to Cure
Degenerative Arthritis

The architecture of the human body is directly related to the design parameters stored in the human genome. Specific sections of the DNA are dedicated to creating the various structures that comprise the body's musculoskeletal systems. Joints are where two bones articulate. Each type of joint represents a unique design. The articular surface of each bone is comprised of a thin noncalcified surface referred to as cartilage.

Degenerative arthritis involves a reduction in the thickness of surface cartilage. The surface of the cartilage develops rough areas and pits. As degenerative arthritis advances, larger areas of the cartilage surface break down. When the cartilage surface has thinned to the point where it is no longer capable of adequately covering the articular surface of joints such as the knee, hip and shoulder, these joints may undergo replacement surgery where the bone is removed and a prosthetic device is inserted in place of the removed bone. Degenerative arthritis of the knee alone costs the United States over 180 billion dollars a year.

For bone and cartilage to have first appeared, the design of these structures must have been dictated by a set of instructions stored in the human genome. Since the human genome does not change during the lifetime of the individual the same instruction set that was originally deciphered to create the bone and cartilage remains present throughout the lifetime of an individual.

If the original section of the human genome can be reread and deciphered again, the cartilage surface comprising the surface of joints can be rebuilt.

The genes comprising the human genome are distinguished by unique identifiers.

Specific control RNA molecules can be used to trigger a transcription complex to decipher specific genes.

Since proteins can utilize their tertiary structure to also trigger a transcription complex to decipher specific genes specifically designed proteins can be developed to trigger the regeneration of specific cartilage when required.

The genes must identify the design parameters of every aspect of every bone in the body. Understanding which genes identify the various parts of the skeletal system affords the opportunity to switch such genes on by activating the genes. Cartilage was build the first time due to an active biologic process that defined where, how much and to what extent the cartilage would form on the articular surface of the bones throughout the body. Being able to define which gene represents each of the surface cartilages creates the opportunity to switch on or reactivate specific cartilage genes to generate new cartilage on bony surfaces as they are injured or as they wear with age.

HOX genes control the development of cartilage. See Figure 25. To construct the cartilage of the surface of the knee the genes utilized by the body to produce the cartilage need to be activated. Upon determining the unique identifier of the gene responsible for the cartilage layering the distal surface of the femur and the distal surface of the tibia, these genes can be preferentially activated. By activating the cartilage genes in the chondrocytes present in the distal femur and the proximal tibia bones, the cartilage can be regrown and the painful, debilitating sequelae of osteoarthritis of the knee can be averted.

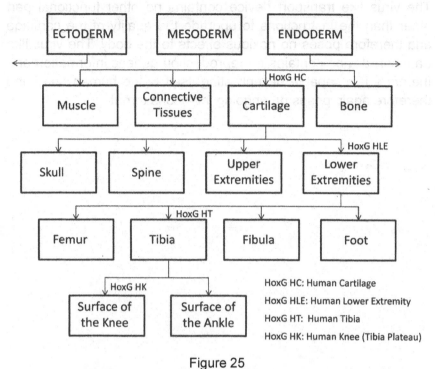

Figure 25
The sequence of HOX genes representing instructions
necessary to construct the cartilage present in the knee joint

Theoretically osteoarthritis could be cured by producing a modified virus and tasking this modified virus to transmit 'the biologic programming instructions necessary to build cartilage' to chondrocytes present in the bone at the skeletal site where the degradation of the cartilage is occurring. A virus-like transport device could be designed to be introduced into the body without stimulating the immune system, and this transport device could act like a virus and target only chondrocytes by the use of exterior probes. Once such a virus-like transport device locates a desired chondrocyte, the device inserts the biologic programming instructions to activate the chondrocyte to produce the proper array of cartilage to repair the degraded joint. The stimulant to activate the chondrocyte could be in the form of a payload that consists of either a segment of DNA, a segment of control RNA or other RNA, or a control protein.

The virus like transport device contains no other functional part other than the instructions to upgrade the quality of the cartilage and therefore poses no noxious effects to the body. The virus like transport device contains no reproduction genetic information and therefore is incapable of replicating itself in the human body and therefore again poses no ongoing infections threat.

POST SCRIPT TWO

Building Hydrocarbons To Fuel
The World's Energy Needs

The most critical problem facing the industrialized nations of the world is the shrinking natural resources of fossil fuels.

Petroleum is a hydrocarbon material formed in the sedimentary beds from animal and vegetable debris. Petroleum is present in a gaseous, liquid and semi-solid form. Crude oil refers to liquid petroleum. Gasoline, a derivative of liquid petroleum, is a fuel burned commonly in combustion engines. Gasoline is comprised of isoocatane and heptane. Isooctane is an eight carbon molecule organized as a trimethyl pentane molecule. Heptane is a seven carbon molecule. The combustion of isoocatane and heptane produces carbon dioxide, water and heat.

Known metabolic processes in biologically cells are able to take carbon and hydrogen atoms and produce a wide variety of molecules. A number of the molecules are rather complex with long chains of atoms, folds in the chains, and branching chains. Many complex molecules are comprised of two or more chains of atoms bound together.

It is known that the plants utilized the process of photosynthesis to take carbon dioxide and water to produce monosaccharides, six carbon sugars such as glucose, fructose, and galactose.

We know that Beta cells in the pancreas produce the hormone insulin and package their product in vacuoles. When triggered, the Beta cells expel their insulin, releasing the insulin from the vacuoles into the blood stream.

211

Solution to declining fossil fuel resources

Algae naturally take carbon dioxide, water and sunlight and through the process of photosynthesis generate glucose. Algae may be modified to take the intracellular glucose they produce and covert this six carbon molecule into a hydrocarbon product that can be used as a combustible fuel. Our combustible fuels are generally seven to eight carbon chains. Algae create glucose as a six carbon chain molecule by fixing carbon in series. Plants are also equipped to add glucose molecules together to generate longer chains of carbon molecules. The chemical process that would need to be engineered into the algae would be the process of removing oxygen from the carbon molecules. Glucose is represented as $C_6O_6H_{12}$. Glucose is comprised of six carbon atoms, six oxygen atoms and twelve hydrogen atoms. A hydrocarbon is comprised of only carbon and hydrogen atoms. The intriguing concept is the fact that plants such as algae are capable of fixing carbon into multi-carbon organic molecules. The factory to generate hydrocarbons is already present in nature, it only requires re-engineering to get this natural factory to produce the combustible fuel humans have become so dependent upon.

Hydrocarbons rise above a water medium and float on top of water. Algae producing hydrocarbons would release the hydrocarbons they produce. Once released, the hydrocarbon product will rise to the top of the water medium the algae are suspended in a production facility. The hydrocarbons can be skimmed from the surface of the water medium. The hydrocarbon product can be further modified into a useable combustible fuel.

Role of Command and Control

The principles of command and control reflect that plant and animal cells function due to very regulated cellular processes. Cells manufacture sugars, polysaccharides, starches, fats, proteins, amino acids, complex molecules and various chemicals. The construction of these molecules requires very deliberate and organized means to create the proper fusion of atoms, bending of molecules and branching of molecules. Biologic cells must have a means of instruction as to which molecule needs to be constructed, the amount of molecules to construct, the rate of construction of the molecules. Cells require instruction pertaining to the manner of how the structure of a sugar, protein, and chemical molecules are generated. Intracellular instructions need to address how to arrange the atoms of a molecule, where and when bending of molecules are to be made, and if branching is to occur, where and how branching is to occur in order to properly create specific isomers of molecules. Each cell must contain a specific list of instructions pertaining to the generation of each of the molecules a cell is responsible for generating in order for required molecules to be reliably created.

Command instructions are related to triggering specific events to occur in the construction of intracellular molecules. Command RNA (cmRNA) molecules, or their agents, travel from the nucleus to the smooth endoplasmic reticulum, the rough endoplasmic reticulum, the Golgi apparatus, and other structures that participate in the manufacture of sugars, proteins and chemicals.

Control instructions are related to activating genes in the DNA. Control RNA (cnRNA) molecules act as the medium that function as intranuclear instruction codes. CnRNA molecules bind to the unique identifier of quantum genes and trigger the formation of a transcription complex upstream from the RNA transcription segment of a quantum gene. CnRNA molecules cause a specific quantum gene or set of quantum genes to be transcribed.

Messenger RNA (mRNA) molecules represent one of the types of RNA molecules generated by the transcription of DNA. The mRNA molecules travel from the nucleus to the cytoplasm. In the cytoplasm, mRNA molecules bind with ribosomes. Ribosomes traverse the mRNA molecule and translate the information carried by the mRNA molecule to produce protein molecules.

The cmRNA molecules interface with the internal modifiers located inside the structure of sugar, protein and chemical manufacturing organelles. CmRNA molecules stimulate the activity of enzymes that are responsible for the construction of the structure of sugar, protein and chemical molecules. CmRNA molecules are responsible for insuring that the proper isomer of a molecule is generated.

Generation of hydrocarbons

A plant cell can be programmed to produce hydrocarbons from glucose. Photosynthesis converts carbon dioxide and water to produce glucose. The glucose product of photosynthesis can be modified intracellularly to a form of safe, but harvestable form of hydrocarbon that can be further converted extracellularly to a combustible hydrocarbon such as isoocatane.

Benefits of synthetic fossil fuel production

Utilization of a modified plant cell offer the benefit:

Generate necessary hydrocarbon fuels from the convergence of carbon dioxide, water and sunlight.

Generate relatively pure hydrocarbons; possibly of any carbon chain length that can be imagined.

Reduction in the effort required to refine the hydrocarbon product to a combustible hydrocarbon.

Production of hydrocarbon fuel encourages reduction in atmospheric carbon dioxide and an increase in oxygen content the atmosphere.

Limitations associated with synthetic fossil fuel production

Hydrocarbon producing plant cells need to have their reproduction function disabled when placed in the field so that cells do not flourish unchecked and endanger the environment.

A synthetic hydrocarbon fuel production facility would require a relatively large surface area in order to take advantage of sunlight to drive the process of photosynthesis.

POST SCRIPT THREE
Musical Key Codes

Hearing is the condition whereby a mechanoreceptor responds to the pressure, the velocity and acceleration of sound waves. The sense of hearing is limited to two types of animals including arthropods and vertebrates. Hearing is used to detect a threat, to target prey, to identify a prospective mate, to communicate in social groups and express emotions.

The significant features in complicated sounds that people perceive and differentiate correspond to the physical dimensions of frequency (the number of waves, cycles, or vibrations per second), intensity, phase, complexity of wave form, and temporal pattern. The variety of distinguishable acoustic forms is enormous.

In certain species such as bats and dolphins, sound waves are generated by the animal and used to locate objects and prey in the dark. Sound waves generated by the animal bounce off the surface of an object, are reflected back to the animal and highly refined auditory sensing structures detect the sound waves. Such sound wave detection approaches the reliability of vision in the perception of objects and spatial relations.

The outer ear consists of pinna located behind the ear opening and partially enclosing it and an auditory meatus that leads inward to the ear canal. The middle ear consists of a tympanic membrane, an ossicular chain of three elements, and two tympanic muscles. The tympanic membrane bulges inward. The elements in the ossicular chain are the malleus (hammer), incus (anvil), and stapes (stirrup). The malleus is attached to and partly embedded in the fibrous layer of the inner surface of the tympanic membrane. It connects to the incus, which connects in turn to the stapes, the footplate of which lies in the entrance to the cochlea. The inner ear is called the cochlea because in man this structure is a complex tube coiled into about 2.5 turns, thus bearing some resemblance to a snail's shell. Extending along the inside of this coiled passage is the basilar membrane, bearing on its surface the sensory structure known as the organ of Corti, which contains the hair cells.

Hearing is the process by which the ear transforms vibrations transiting through in air or water into nerve impulses. These nerve impulses are conveyed to the brain, where they are interpreted as sounds. Sounds are produced by the vibration of objects, such as the plucked string of a guitar. Vibration of an object produces pressure pulses of vibrating molecules, termed sound waves. Such sound waves can be transmitted through media such as air or water. The brain can distinguish different subjective aspects of a sound, such as its loudness and pitch by detecting and analyzing different physical characteristics of the sound waves.

Loudness is the perception of the intensity of sound. Loudness refers to the pressure exerted by sound waves on the tympanic membrane. The greater the amplitude or strength of a sound wave, the greater is the pressure or intensity, and thus the greater the loudness of the sound. The intensity of sound is measured in decibels (dB). A decibel is a unit of intensity of sound that expresses the relative magnitude of a sound on a logarithmic scale. Utilizing the decibel scale, the range of human hearing extends from 0 dB, which is inaudible, to approximately 130 dB, at which point the level of sound becomes painful.

Pitch is the perception of the frequency of sound waves. Frequency is defined as the number of wavelengths that pass a fixed point in a unit of time. Frequency is usually measured in cycles per second which is also referred to as a hertz. The human ear is most sensitive to and most easily detects frequencies of 1,000 to 4,000 hertz. Normal young ears may be capable of detecting the entire audible range of sounds which extends from about 20 to 20,000 hertz. Sound waves of still higher frequency are referred to as ultrasonic, which may be detected by other mammals.

Sound is transmitted to the central nervous system for interpretation, by the energy of the sound undergoing three transformations. First, the sound waves in the air or if submerged sound waves in water are converted to vibrations of the tympanic membrane and the three bones of the middle ear. The actions of the bones of the middle ear, vibrates the fluid inside the cochlea. Vibrations in the fluid of the cochlea travel along the basilar membrane stimulating the hair cells of the organ of Corti. These hair cells convert the sound vibrations to nerve impulses in the fibers of the cochlear nerve. The nerve impulses become transmitted to the brain stem, which from the brain stem are relayed to the primary auditory area of the cerebral cortex. Nerve impulses reaching this area of the brain are interpreted as sound.

General interpretation of sound is divided into the perception and recognition of the sound and the determination of the direction from whence the sound is coming from. It is not only important to know that a sound that signals a threat is perceived as a threat, but it is important to know from which direction such a sound might have originated. Although the two ears are not connected by mechanical means, the brain is sensitive to phase and is able to determine the phase relationship between stimuli presented to the two ears. Locating a sound source laterally in space makes use of fundamental properties of sound waves as well as the ability of the brain to identify the phase difference between signals from the two ears.

The content and existence of 'music' extends beyond traditional bounds of sound detection.

There are a number of types of music including Folk music, Marches, Ballads, Big Band, Blues, Jazz, Rock-n-Roll, Disco, Hip Pop, New Age, Rap.

Most of the time music is considered to act as (1) entertainment, (2) means to communicate a message, (3) a medium to invoke an emotional response, (4) means to cause people to act in a specific manner, such as when a march or dance is played.

Beyond the general conscious role of music includes a subconscious function to music. Music can be derived from the sounds emitted by one or more instruments, the sound emitted by the vocal cords of one or more persons or a combination of the two sources of sound.

At a subconscious level, a song that carries a musical key code is comprised of at least two elements. These two elements include the introduction and the musical key code. The introduction of a song is that part of a song that tells the brain of a listener that the sound being detected is an artificial pattern and this pattern is different than general ambient noises or general speech that may be detected by the human ear. The musical key code is that part of a song that is comprised of a unique blending of sound emitted by one or more instruments and sound emitted by one or more person's vocal cords.

The language the musical key code is in is the universal language of the brain that acts as a brain's operating system. Language is merely a form of communication used by a social network for purposes of communication between the individuals of the network. The elements of the language are assigned to acts as a meaning for symbols, objects and intentions of the language and are arbitrarily arrived at by those responsible for establishing and maintaining the language. The subconscious brain takes the elements of any language and translates them into the common base-four universal language that acts as operating system so that the element can be properly interpreted.

The operating system is comprised of an active memory to interpret language and a storage of technical files that are passed down from one generation to another.

Music that is heard by the human ear registers in the operating system first at the conscious level for enjoyment or to illicit an emotional response or a movement response, but then possibly also at the subconscious level if a musical key code is present carried by the music.

Radio and television transmission waves are generally comprised of a carrier wave, and inside the carrier wave data that the radio converts to music or speech and a television converts to visual and audio signals is carried.

The musical key code is a signal that is interpreted by the subconscious brain which acts to cause the subconscious brain to allow the conscious brain access to technical files locked in storage in the subconscious portion of the brain. The opportunity to read technical files stored in the subconscious brain spurs imagination and progress. The initial divulgence of advance technical files may present as science fiction. Those who watched the old science fiction series in the nineteen sixties never thought it possible that a communication device could actually be carried in the hand and attached to your belt when not in use; yet today a significant portion of the world's population actively uses a cell phone.

As technology advances, the construction and variation of instruments advances which leads to progression in the variety and type of music that can be created, which in turn leads to the conscious brain the opportunity to access stored technical data files in an orderly fashion, which along with problem solving, analysis, and discovery has generated a timely progress in technology over the ages.

POST SCRIPT FOUR

The Text Files Yet to be Discovered

Computer programs are written in a language that defines the syntax of the instructions and the data files. In addition to the reference tables, instructions and data files in the DNA, there may be text files. It is possible that when the DNA was created, instructions were included, in the form of text notations or files, to tell those expected to read the DNA how the developer expected the DNA to be used. If such files exist, they could provide an understanding as to the construct of the world the developer had in mind.

Computer programmers often place files inside their computer programs that are text files. Such text files are written elements that identify the intentions of the programmer to anyone deciphering the computer program.

The human genome may have text files present inside the DNA code. If humanity was the intended result of billions of years of a biologic program at work in an ever changing hostile environment, the designer of the program may have incorporated text into the blueprints of the human body. The text may identify the origin and the goal of the program.

The Earth, along with the solar system, has been estimated to have been created 4.54 billion years ago. Oldest fossil evidence suggests life started on planet earth approximately 3.43 billion years ago. Given the age of the universe is 13.75 billion years, at least part of the universe existed long before the earth was created. Intelligent life capable of traversing and exploring the universe may have existed well before the earth ever existed. Such intelligent life may have seeded new planets with a genetic program that contained the means to utilize energy to convert raw materials into life forms.

One has to consider that the human genome may represent the product of a larger, complex biologic computer program. The human genome most likely represents only a segment of the original program that was introduced to the planet. To decipher the full extent of the text present in the DNA, it may require combining the DNA of multiple species in order to gather enough text files together to assimilate an understandable amount of text.

The language the writer of the human genome would have utilized to communicate to the humans is open to speculation. It would seem that the author of the genome would have anticipated that his or her product would have developed the awareness and skill to decipher and read the text code written into the DNA. If the author wanted to communicate to humans, billions of years after the code had been written, one would have to explore how to accomplish this task.

At least three design approaches can be considered: (1) a universal nomenclature that does not change, like utilizing (i) a set of math paradigms that do not change or (ii) the periodic table of elements as the basis for the construction of a language that humans could decipher, (2) store the text in an obscure ancient language in the human brain so that when humans see the code, humans reading the DNA are capable of recognizing and understanding the text, (3) write the language in the DNA using a language stored in the human brain, a language meant to become a universal language such as English, so that those humans that decipher the text of the DNA are able to decode the meaning of the text files present in the DNA.

At first the text may be thought of as being actual written language that one reads and deciphers with their eyes. The text language written into the DNA may though be in the form of sounds such as musical notes that communicate meaning to our brains in a subconscious manner. The language of the DNA could also be representative of frequencies and quantities of light so as to produce a visual image rather than a message that is written or comprised of sound.

Still, the 3 billion pairs of nucleotides that comprise the human genome appear simply as a string of zeros, ones, twos and threes if the adenine, cytosine, guanine and thymine nucleotides are converted to numbers in a base four system. The structure of the

DNA has not changes since conception. Human nomenclature is an arbitrary assignment of names to the nucleotides. If a base-four numbering system were to be assigned to the four nucleotides, which would represent the 'zero', the 'one' the 'two', and the 'three' are unknown at this time.

Possibly the numbering system might be related to the size or weight of the molecule. In a system where weight of the nucleotide designated order, cytosine would represent the 'zero' since it is the smallest of the four nucleotide bases. Thymine would represent the 'one' being the second heaviest nucleotide base. Adenine would represent a 'two' being the third heaviest nucleotide bases, and guanine would represent a 'three' since it is the heaviest of the four nucleotide bases.

Number of bonds in the molecule is most likely not the means of designating the numbering system since adenine and guanine have the same number of bonds.

One could arbitrarily assign cytosine as 'one', thymine as 'two', adenine as 'three' and guanine as 'four', but then zero is not represented and most math systems assign an element a value of 'zero' rather than leaving zero as a null set. Since we are discussing the genome in reference to a computer program, this text will favor the mathematics approach. Therefore, for purposes of this text, cytosine is 'zero', thymine is 'one', adenine is 'two' and guanine is 'three'; in the abbreviated form C=0, T=1, A=2, G=3.

If we apply this nomenclature to the Prime Genome, then the picture presented in Figure 21 can be updated to what is presented in Figure 26. 'C' or the number 'zero' is assigned to the first digit or primary digit of the unique identification of the genome that is coded for the building blocks of cell structure. 'T' or the number 'one' is assigned to the first digit or primary digit of the unique identification of the genome that is coded for the construction of viruses. 'A' or the number 'two' is assigned to the first digit or primary digit of the unique identification of the genome that is coded for the building blocks of prokaryote cells. 'G' or the number 'three' is assigned to the first digit or primary digit of the unique identification of the genome that is coded for the building blocks of eukaryote cells. The branch of the eukaryote cells is further subdivided for illustrative purposes.

The branch of the eukaryote cells is divided into four regions. 'GC' representing the base four number '30' indicates the sub branch for protista species. 'GT' representing the base four number '31' indicates the sub branch for fungi species. 'GA' representing the base four number '32' indicates the sub branch for plant species. 'GG' or the base four number '33' indicates the sub branch for animal species.

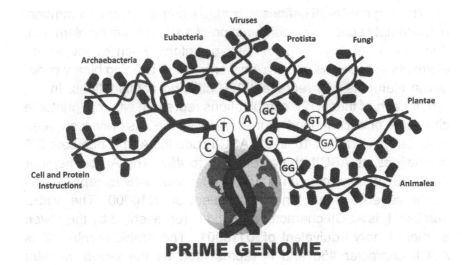

PRIME GENOME

Figure 26
The Prime Genome with branches numbered

Morse code, devised in the 1840's as means of communication utilizing the telegraph, is an entire language based off of only two differing elements. The international Morse code incorporates Roman alphabet and Arabic numbers into a standardized code of short and long dashes or 'dots' and 'dashes' that can be recognized by a trained listener or observer without special equipment.

The American Standard Code for Information Interchange (ASCII) was developed from the telegraphic code and is used for text in computers. Computers are based on transistor technology which has led to digital technology. Digital computer technology is based on machine language, which is the language of 'ones' and 'zeros' which is directly related to whether a transistor is 'on' representing a 'one' or if a transistor is 'off' representing a 'zero'. All of the most sophisticated computing power still revolves around the computer's central processing unit deciphering a strings of ones and zeros to engage in precisely accurate mind boggling mathematical computations or to generate readable text printouts or as we have come to expect, complex video images to entertain our eyes and minds.

The original ASCII defines a 'printable character' or a 'command' or the 'empty space' by a combination of a string of seven elements. This was originally used for teletypewriters. Each of the seven elements is coded as either a 'one' or a 'zero'. Utilizing binary code, seven elements can represent 128 differing combinations. In the ASCII each of these 128 combinations represent either a 'printable character' or a 'command' or the 'empty space'. As previously seen in Table 4, in Chapter 10, in the ASCII code the Arabic numbers 0-9 are defines as ASCII characters #48 to #57. The Arabic number '0' is ASCII character #48. ASCII character #48 is represented as the seven element binary equivalent of '0110000'. The Arabic number '1' is ASCII character #49 and is represented by the seven element binary equivalent of '0110001'. The Arabic number '2' is ASCII character #50 and is represented as the seven element binary equivalent of '0110011'. The progression continues for the Arabic numbers 4 to 9, which are ASCII characters #52 and #58 and represented as the binary equivalents '0110100' and '0111001'. Each of the 94 printable characters, 33 commands and the 'space' that comprise the ASCII code are defined by a unique seven digit binary equivalent. Since 1960, most pieces of electronic equipment utilize the ASCII code as the basis for communicating printable text characters.

In 1981 IBM introduced the extended ASCII code. Computers utilized a string of eight elements referred to as 'bits' to generate one 'byte'. A segment of 8 bits is considered unit of computer information. Since computers could utilize a string of eight elements this allowed for 256 differing combinations. The original ASCII code was embedded into the new extended ASCII code. The new extended ASCII code added 32 code combinations for machine and control commands, 32 combinations for numbers and various punctuation symbols, 32 combinations for upper case letters and 32 combinations for lower case letters and a few additional punctuation marks.

As represented by Morse code and ASCII, and then the extended ASCII code very sophisticated and very elaborate communication systems have been developed with a base-two binary code as the foundation of the system. The DNA utilizes a base-four system, which is capable of storing much more information while utilizing a smaller number of elements than the human base-two systems. Given biologic life is the result of this base-four system, the DNA's coding is obviously represents one of the most powerful storage and communication systems on the planet.

All languages are built on semiotics. Semiotics defines the meaning assigned to the characters utilized in the language. In the English language there are 26 letters. Each letter is assigned a place in the alphabet and a specific sound. Words are created by combining letters, then assigning one or more meanings to each word. A dictionary is a collection of words with their assigned meaning(s). Language is founded on the collection of words. Language generated by a particular group of humans is founded from an arbitrary construction of words and further an arbitrary assignment of meaning to the words used in the language. The meaning of language is also dependent upon the rules or syntax of how verbs, nouns, and adverbs are used in collections referred to as sentences. Language is an arbitrary process and there are an estimated 3000-6000 differing languages in use by humans today.

Given humans have so many variations in language, it is a monumental task to take the 3 billion base pair of nucleotides build on a base-four language, which humans are not generally efficient at working in, and make sense of a language written at least 3.5 billion years ago, if not longer.

It must be assumed that the author of the language in the DNA meant for humans to decipher the meaning of the DNA. Understanding the rules or syntax of any language is paramount to understanding a language. Where would the syntax be stored, such that it could be found?

The rules of the language stored in the DNA could be arranged in one segment of the DNA or distributed in differing locations throughout the DNA. Since the rules of the language are necessary for those that might read the language to understand what the material written in the language contained, it would be imperative for a potential reader of the language to locate the rules without much trouble and to clearly understand the rules. Not being able to find the rules would lead to the meaning of the text in the DNA remaining undecipherable. Locating only a portion of the rules would lead to either not being able to decipher the text or lead to misinterpretation of the text.

If the rules were present in one location in the DNA, the site of the location would need to stand out. There are 3 billion base pairs. One might think the rules would be listed at the beginning of the DNA. Given there are 46 chromosomes, it would be anyone's guess as to which one of the chromosomes is considered the first chromosome. Possible the smallest chromosome is the first. Possible one of the sex chromosomes is the first. The 'y' chromosome is possible the most unique chromosome since it only appears in men, where all of the other chromosomes including the 'x' sex chromosome appear in both sexes. Possibly the 'y' chromosome is the site of the collection of text rules since it is the most unique chromosome and the original writer of the text might have guessed humans would have recognized the uniqueness and started looking at such a site first.

If the collection of language rules is located on one chromosome, the question is where might such documentation of language syntax be located on the chromosome? It might be most obvious to start the rules on one of the two ends of the chromosome, but then which end is chosen? One might consider the centromere, the center of each chromosome, to be the site where the rules of the language have been located.

Rather than placing the rules in one location, there is the possibility that the rules of the language were spread out over the 46 chromosomes that comprise the human genome. Possibly located at the beginning and end of each of the chromosomes there are sections of DNA that acts as keys to deciphering the syntax of the DNA's language. If the beginning and end of each chromosome did possess a segment that acted as a keycode, there would be at least 92 elements in the keycode. American Morse code had 37 defined meaningful elements in its keycode. By comparison, the original ASCII code defined 128 characters. The original ASCII code was based on the fact that the value of 2 to the power of seven equaled 128. Of the 128 combinations available in the original ASCII code 94 were printable characters. Given that if the two ends of a chromosome were used to store the characters and syntax of the language and therefore there are 92 possible sites, this is remarkably close to the 94 printable characters humans which have defined in the English version of the ASCII code.

Utilizing the binary language, again it takes eight elements, each element being able to represent a 'one' or a 'zero, to provide the 256 different combinations that comprise the extended ASCII code. In a base-four system it would take only four elements, each element being able to represent a 'zero' or a 'one' or a 'two' or a 'three' to be able to provide a total of 256 different combinations. A segment of four nucleotides could easily encompass 92 different combinations, with 164 options remaining available to be utilized to communicate additional information.

The objective for deciphering the text files would be to read the intentions and comments made by the designer(s) of the design code responsible for all of life that has inhabited the planet. Knowing what the writer(s) of the biologic code, whom created the ecosystem that has populated the planet, intended the product of their creation to be aware of regarding the origin of life, would be priceless to all of humanity. Recognizing that one author or a single group of authors wrote the Prime Genome genetic code, which is responsible for Human existence, would unify the diverse populations residing across the globe and help to culminate world peace.

POST SCRIPT FIVE

The Fabric of Space:
Sub^2 Atomic Particle Physics Theory

A visitor stands feet planted at the edge of a vast canyon. The visitor peers over the great distance to the opposing side. The gap between the majestic canyon walls is at least half mile across. Mimicking an artist's canvass, beautiful hues of red, gold, tan and brown are seemingly whimsically painted across the tall rocky walls of the canyon. Over the right shoulder and left shoulder the visitor spies that the canyon extends many miles into the distance and eventually disappears into the horizon.

A quarter mile below the cliff where the visitor's feet reside an unbridled river winds through the basin of the canyon. As it has for millions of years, the river snakes its way across the sparse terrain ever so slowly, meticulously cutting its way deeper into the bedrock of the canyon.

It is a clear day. The noon sun warms the visitor's cheeks. The heavens overhead are a vivid tropical blue color. The sky is amazingly crystal clear.

Being a practical person the visitor realizes the canyon cannot be crossed without considerable effort requiring scaling down the canyon wall, hiking across the canyon bedrock and then climbing the rugged stone wall on the opposing side. The distance separating the edge where the visitor's tennis shoes stand and the opposite side of the canyon is too great to leap. If the visitor knows nothing of science, it would appear the gap between the two opposing steep canyon walls is empty, void of any matter.

The clue that there is matter which fills the void is that a crisp warm wind blows across the visitor's face. As the visitor inhales and exhales each breath creates a force that can felt on the raised palm.

Swatting at a fly that is in a mood to bite, an artificial breeze brushes the cheeks alerting the senses that there is mass comprising what appears to be nothingness.

Before the visitor's eyes, across the distance, a red tailed hawk gracefully takes flight from a tree located on the canyon floor and effortlessly rides a warm updraft of the invisible wind gusting up from the canyon floor and rising into the sky above.

Prior to Einstein's time the scientific community thought the universe was comprised of an ether. Such an 'ether' was considered to be a substance that connected all things from one end of the cosmos to the other end. At one time it was thought to reach the distant edge of the ether was to reach the limits of the universe.

Einstein dismissed the idea that an 'ether' existed. Since Einstein has been revered as the father of the atomic age and understood the atom, space and time better than anyone of his day, it has been acceptable to ignore that there may be such a fabric of space.

We stand at night and peer up at the heavens in the sky above. We see the light of stars from our own galaxy. Some of the light emitted has traveled 90 million light years distance, from the opposite side of the disc shaped, spiral Milky Way to our planet. Some of the light we see originated in distant galaxies, which are billions of light years away. To our perception such light energy crosses the great distances through an empty medium, void of any form of matter. One ponders the question as to how does light that originated from a galaxy billions of light years away, make it across an empty void to Earth? What actually is 'light' that it can accomplish the task of traversing billions of light years of distance passing through 'no conductive medium'? Or is there in fact a conductive medium?

Like a person standing on the edge of a canyon wall knowing that one cannot leap across the vast expanse of the canyon because there is no medium to support the human body, how can light travel such great distances between galaxies if there was no medium to conduct the travel of light? Yet, this same visitor to the canyon appreciates that a heavier than air object such as a bird is able to seemingly effortlessly fly across a expanse of the canyon with wings adapted to taking advantage of the invisible medium of air that fills a person's lungs and fills the gap between the canyon walls. Such an experience begs the question: Mustn't there also be an 'ether', a 'fabric of sorts', that acts as a medium to effortlessly conduct light energy over great distances? If energy is conserved, it may truly travel long distances without dissipating, if there was a medium to conduct its travel.

We peer at the planets in the solar system endlessly marching in orbit around the sun. We accept that centrifugal force is exerted on the planets, yet our perception is that there is no physical connection between the planets and the sun. So how does this centrifugal force exist? For all practical purposes some medium must exist through which the invisible force that connects the planets is able to exhibit such power.

An electron circles the nucleus of an atom. What is the means that causes the electron to orbit the center of the atom? An electron jumps from a closer orbit to a more distant orbit about the nucleus dependent upon how much energy is absorbed by the electron or atom. Why doesn't the electron just escape the atom? Upon release of a quantum of energy, which is represented as radiant energy, the electron falls from the distant orbit to a tighter orbit around the nucleus of the atom. There is no perceived mechanical connection between the electron and the protons and neutrons comprising the nucleus of the atom. But logic suggests a connection does exist. Like the invisible force that affects the planets orbiting the Sun, some medium must be present that allows a force to be exerted between the electrons in orbit about the proton center of an atom.

The known quantities of gravity and magnetism are physical forces that are present to the most casual observer, yet the essence of these forces remains a scientific mystery teasing our intuition, yet defying our intellect. As one stands at the canyon's edge the body does not drift up and out into space because the invisible elusive force of gravity gives weight to the body and holds one's feet firmly on the ground. If one lifts their foot and peers at the tread on the bottom of their shoe, there is no physical attachment, no tether line connecting one to the earth, yet due to an unexplained gravitational force, one's body is connected to the earth.

Holding a single bar magnet in one's hand, one cannot detect the magnetic force surrounding the piece of metal. Placing the bar magnet on top of a desk and sprinkling the area surrounding the magnet with metal shavings reveals the presence of bands of invisible energy that surround the magnet. These bands of energy connect the positive and negative ends of the magnet. The bands of energy are powerful enough that by turning the magnet in proximity of coiled wire, an electrical current can be created in the wire.

The experience of scuba diving introduces one to the concept that with the aid of buoyancy, gravity can be defied. Maneuvering through a three dimensional water medium introduces one to an enhanced perception of density as water becomes a defined means to exploit in order to successfully traverse from one location to another. The concept of an 'ether' becomes distinctly visible when one is submerged in a body of crystal clear water sixty feet below the surface.

Underwater, if an explosion were to occur in the direction one was looking, as a diver one would see the flash of light with the eyes. Following the flash, one would hear the sound of the explosion in the ears as the sound wave passed through the water. The diver would also feel the wave created by the explosion strike the human body and pass around and through the human body.

Returning to the edge of vast canyon, hovering over the distance horizon is a magnificent thundercloud. The cumulonimbus cloud rises 20,000 feet up into the velvet blue sky. Dark plumes of dense water vapor hover at the clouds base stretching several miles across. The unbridled energy swirling about the heart of the monstrous storm cloud creates flashes of lightning. Thirty-thousand amp electrostatic discharges of pure energy periodically escape from the base of the great rainmaker, appearing to mercilessly strike a wicked blow to the canyon floor.

Standing at the brink of the canyon with a thundercloud hovering in the distance, and witnessing a flash of lightning, depending upon the distance, there would be a delay in perceiving the sound of thunder created by the lightning strike. But eventually, a rumble of thunder would be detected by the ears. If the storm cloud were at a great distance, as an observer one would not expect to feel the air stir due to simply the lightning strike alone. The stirring of the air would be related to turbulence in the atmosphere caused by the approach of the storm, if the thundercloud were to overrun the position where the observer stood.

On this day, the great storm cloud lazily drifts southward, away from the observer. The air remains calm. The temperature warm and arid. The sky clears.

As the sun sets in over the western horizon and darkness ensues, the blue canopy above fades to black. As the night deepens and the sparkle of a myriad of stars poke through the onyx black shell above, the sense of great distance magnifies. One never senses a pushing force from space; nor does one ever hear sound traversing through space such as when great spiral galaxies collide. Yet, the light originating from trillions of celestial bodies, some located billions of light years distant from Earth, can be detected by the human eye on a clear night.

Summing up the observations, the obvious conclusion is that there exists some form of fabric that comprises the blackness of space. Smaller than an electron, proton or neutron, there exists a sub-sub atomic particle, from which, all other atomic particles are constructed.

Physics has been coaxed into dividing the universe into 'positive' and 'negative' charges. It has been assumed that the universe is dependent upon the absolute of equilibrium between the positive constituents of the universe and the negative constituents of the universe. But instead of seeing the universe as two absolutes, the concept of the matter of the universe could be broadened into the concepts of positive and negative simply being 'states' of energy and matter. When the perception of positive and negative is shifted to consider them as states, a third state, that of 'neutral' can be added without too much reservation. The construction of an atom hints at the presence of three states of matter/energy given the components of an atom can be consist of a proton, an electron and a neutron. Three states of matter/energy facilitate the physical phenomena we see with matter and energy.

The essential sub^2 atomic particle is constructed similar to three egg-like shapes fused together, existing in a tripolar structure such that one projection or pole is a positive side, one projection or pole is a negative side and one projection or pole is a neutral side. See Figure 27. Thus, the essence of sub-sub atomic particle physics can account for all three states of electrical charge including positive, negative and neutral. This, the most fundamental of all particles, comprising the 'ether' of space, is the 'tritron'.

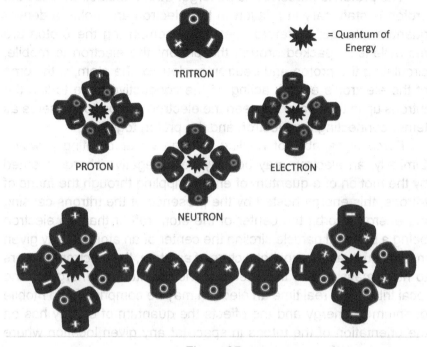

Figure 27
Tritrons are a sub-sub atomic tripolar particle that are combined to create the electron, proton and neutron

A proton, therefore, is a sub atomic particle comprised of sub² atomic tripolar particles known as tritrons. These tritrons arranged in a shell-like shape with the positive state pointed outward and the negative and neutral states pointed inward, the center of the collection of tritrons harboring at least one quantum of energy. A neutron, is a sub atomic particle comprised of sub² atomic tripolar tritrons, these tritrons arranged in a shell-like shape with the neutral state pointed outward and the positive and negative states pointed inward, the center of the collection of tritrons harboring at least one quantum of energy. An electron, is a sub atomic particle comprised of sub² atomic tripolar tritrons, these tritrons arranged in a shell-like shape with the negative state pointed outward and the positive and neutral states pointed inward, the center of the collection of tritrons harboring at least one quantum of energy.

The proton is perceived to be larger than the electron since the proton is stationary in relation to the electron and holds a denser quantum charge, therefore, the tritrons comprising the proton are more densely packed around the proton; the electron is mobile, circulating the proton and neutron nucleus of the atom, with some of the electron's energy acting as the conductive force to line the tritrons up in the space between the electron and proton to serve as tether connecting the electron and the proton together.

Force is capable of rippling through water creating a wave. Similarly, an electron may actually be a negative charge created by the motion of a quantum of energy rippling through the fabric of tritrons, this energy hosted by the presence of the tritrons causing the energy to orbit the center of the atom rather than an electron being a physical particle circling the center of an atom. At any given instant, such as a snapshot picture of an atom, the electron appears to have mass due to the effects of the quantum of energy on the local tritrons. In real time an electron may be comprised of a mobile quantum of energy and the effects the quantum of energy has on the orientation of the tritrons in space at any given location where the quantum of energy exists.

Having the capacity to collect together into a spherical shape and hold quantums of energy, tritrons can form to make a proton, an electron and a neutron. When not collected together and holding a charge, tritrons are ubiquitous in the universe. In effect the universe is a vast ocean of sub^2 atomic tritrons. Energy uses tritrons to act as its invisible medium for transfer. When not collected together as a sphere-like structure to store energy, the tritrons fill the ether of space and act as a potential gate or pathway to conduct energy from one location in space to another location in space.

Thus, the universe consists of a vast space filled with a nearly equal volume of ether. There exists a void, but interspaced in this void exists a sea of tritrons, these tritrons being the simplest of particles, exhibiting the properties of three different states of charge. Therefore, all matter is comprised of these essential sub^2 atomic particles, the tritron particles. Tritron particles form to make electrons, protons, neutrons and other sub atomic particles. The electrons, protons and neutrons combine to produce atoms. The number of electrons and protons comprising an atom define the element the atom represents. The number of neutrons helps define the behavior of the atom. Individual atoms combine to produce materials. The properties of a material are dependent upon the composite of the number of types of atoms comprising the material. At the sub-sub atomic level, both energy and tritrons are conserved, neither being consumed nor produced. The actions of energy and the organization of tritrons are responsible for all of physical phenomenon we are able to see and appreciate at the macroscopic level.

Similar to water and air mediums, density of the tritrons varies in the universe. The closer to a source of gravity, the denser, more compact the particles become. Air and water represent molecular or atomic mediums, tritrons represent a sub-sub atomic medium. Light behaves different than sound energy. Light energy uses tritrons as its conductive medium. Light travels at a constant speed due to being conducted at the sub-sub atomic level, therefore, density of matter is inconsequential to light energy since light energy travels through a medium that is smaller than an atom and permeates the components of an atom. Light energy may become absorbed by sub atomic particles in packet units of quanta, in some cases the pathway of light energy can be redirected, but where free tritons exist, light can travel unimpeded across great distances since energy is a constant neither being created, nor destroyed; only in motion or locked in storage in atoms.

Tritons acting as the medium by which light travels across the universe also explains some of the peculiar properties of light. Some experiments suggest light behaves as a wave, while other experiments suggest light acts as a particle. The concept of a substance acting both as a particle and a wave is generally incompatible with our current understanding of atomic physics and material science. But if a sub-sub atomic tripolar particle acts as the medium for light to be conducted from one location to another, then similar to the properties of water which can act as a wave or a column, the behavior of light acting in some situations as a particle and in some situations as a wave can easily be explained. Light is packed into discrete quanta of energy. A single quanta of energy passing in one direction would contain properties of a particle.

Numerous quanta of energy being released simultaneously from a single origin directed in different directions would behave similar to a wave.

A sun represents a great central density of free tritrons, emitting light energy outward along the spherical dimensions of the density of tritrons surrounding the sun. A black hole represents the opposite physical phenomenon. It has been thought that light is unable to escape a black hole due to the light energy not being able to travel fast enough to escape the gravitational force the black hole.

The theory that light is unable to escape the gravitational pull of a black hole contradicts a fundamental belief of light, that light travels at a constant speed. If a black hole is able to trap light, then clearly gravity can affect the speed of travel of light, which would lead to the conclusion that varying the gravitational field strength would vary the speed of light. Since the fundamental physical mechanism explaining the presence of the force of gravity remains unknown, and therefore if it is unknown, science is unable to accurately explain how this would affect the flight path of light, which the fundamental principles explaining the existence of light remain equally unknown beyond the vague explanation that light represents quanta of energy.

Further, Einstein provided the world the equation $E = MC^2$, and based the equation on light exhibiting a constant speed. Somewhat paradoxically, Einstein won the Noble prize by identifying that light passing near the vicinity of a Sun would have its flight path deviated toward the Sun due to the gravitational pull of the Sun. Again, Einstein appears to contradict himself. If light passes through space at a constant speed, and gravity is able to exert a force on light which causes light to change direction, then the speed of light is potentially no longer a constant. The fact that it was demonstrated during a solar eclipse, that the path of light from a distant source did indeed bend toward the Sun as it passed by the vicinity of the Sun, helped to usher in the age of quantum mechanics. Quantum mechanics being the scientific study of the behavior of light and matter on the atomic and subatomic scale.

An alternative manner by which to explain the effects of a black hole on light and the effects of a star's gravity on light, without the above-mentioned contradiction, is by analyzing the properties of the sub-sub atomic tritron. Light is unable to escape a black hole due to the intense gravitation field drawing a majority of the tritrons in the region of the black hole into the center of the black hole and therefore the density of tritrons drops to the point that there is an insufficient amount of tritrons available to conduct light energy, therefore, 'light' cannot use tritrons as a conduction medium to escape the black hole. Light energy is thus trapped in the center of the black hole because the conductive medium used by light is clustered at the center of the black hole. The fabric of space resumes at the edges of the influence of the gravitational field of the black hole, which is the distance from the center of the black hole where tritrons are no longer being actively sucked into the center of the black hole by gravity.

Einstein was awarded the Noble prize for predicting that the path of light could not only be impeded, but bent by the gravitational forces of a star. The efforts by scientists examining the a solar eclipse in an attempt to prove or disprove Einstein's theory, demonstrated that the path of light from distant stars was indeed altered as the light from these distance sources deviated from their original path taking a path closer to our Sun as the light passed near the perimeter of the Sun, briefly distorting the visible position of the distant light source to the observer on Earth. Light energy is conserved. Light follows the path of greater density of tritrons rather than a path of less dense tritrons. Since a sun represents a density of free tritrons compared to open space, visible light traveling from one location to another would curve toward a star rather than pass through a less dense section of tritrons in open space.

What would be the end of the universe if there were no ether? One reaches the end of a pool when one reaches the edge of the water. Outer space is reached when the limits of the atmosphere are breached. The edge of the ether is the final boundary of the universe.

Like the invisible breeze that brushes your face as you stand at the edge of canyon to let you know air exists, the tug of the invisible hands of gravity that hold your feet firmly to the ground lets you know that an ether that represents the fabric of the universe must truly exist.

POST SCRIPT SIX

The Enigma of the Magnet Solved

The existence of the magnet and magnetic energy has defied human understanding for all time, until now. A magnet is a material object that produces a magnetic field. Materials that can be magnetized are called ferromagnetic materials and include iron, nickel, cobalt, alloys of rare earth metals and lodestone.

Examining a bar shaped magnet one recognizes a positive pole on one end of the bar and a negative pole on the opposite end. Sometimes the opposite ends of a magnet are referred to as the north end and south end. The poles are a property of the material comprising the bar magnet, such that if the bar magnet is separated into two pieces, each resultant piece becomes its own bar magnet with a positive and negative pole.

If one takes a clear plastic cylinder, places a smaller clear plastic cylinder in the center of the first cylinder and seals one end, then into the space between the two clear plastic cylinders adds metal shavings, then finally the opposite end of the two cylinders is sealed such that the metal shavings are trapped in the space between the two clear plastic cylinders, this provides an experimental tool to observe the behavior of a magnetic field. Through the smaller clear plastic cylinder a bar magnet is introduced. The metal shavings line up along what appears to be bands of energy traversing from the positive pole of the magnet to the negative pole of the magnet.

Without the aid of the metal shavings to illustrate the bands of energy traversing from the positive end of the bar magnet to the negative end of the bar magnet, the bands of energy are invisible and appear to have no physical substance.

If one takes two equal sized bar magnets and places the positive pole of one magnet in proximity to the negative pole of the other magnet an attraction of the two poles is detected. If one takes the positive pole of one bar magnet and attempts to position the positive pole of the second bar magnet together a repulsive force is detected. If the two bar magnets are strong, the force of attraction and the force of repulsion can be substantial. Ferromagnetic materials generally respond to the presence of a magnetic field in a manner that is observable; all other substances also respond to the presence of a magnetic field but to some lesser degree. Despite the strength a magnet might have, to the human senses a magnetic field is invisible, tasteless and generally has no density or substance.

The presence of a magnetic field may be explained similar to the existence of light energy. Like light energy, a magnetic field exists and functions at the sub atomic level. A magnetic field is capable of generating a powerful force because it is being created by the actions of sub-sub atomic tripolar particles referred to as tritrons. Tritons exist as the medium that is smaller than an electron, proton or neutron. Tritrons occupy the space between protons and electrons in an atom and between atoms in a material. A magnetic field, in of itself, does not register to human senses because it exists at a level that is smaller than the molecular or atomic level.

It is believed energy is neither created, nor destroyed. Tritrons: tripolar particles carrying a positive, negative and neutral charge, which act as the building blocks for electrons, protons, neutrons and other sub atomic particles are neither created, nor destroyed. See Figure 27. Tritrons act as the transfer medium for energy.

The various arrangements of tritrons and the trapping of quanta of energy produces the sub atomic particles of the proton, electron, and neutron. Combining protons, electrons, and neutrons produces atoms. The hydrogen atom is comprised of one electron orbiting a proton. See Figure 28. A quanta of energy becomes trapped in atomic structure. Depending upon the arrangements of protons, neutrons, and electrons present in atoms different elements are generated. Each element exhibits a unique physical behavior and electrical properties based on number of protons and neutrons present in the core, and the compatibility of the electrons orbiting the core. The construction of an atom dictates whether the element will behave more as a negatively charged atom, a positively charged atom or a neutrally charged atom.

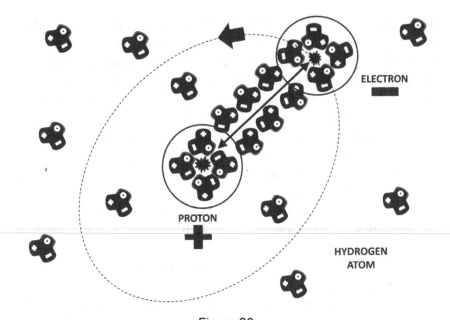

Figure 28
The hydrogen atom is comprised of one electron
orbiting one proton

Given that energy is conserved throughout the universe, some atomic structures are able to trap energy. Energy can be trapped at the sub atomic level inside a shell of tritrons, or energy can be trapped between the actions of protons and electrons, or energy can be trapped in a material that allows the energy to circulate the material.

At the macroscopic level energy is conserved. Energy is known to be stored and released. A clear example of stored energy is typified by an explosive device. An explosive device is harmless until the energy stored in the material is activated. Once an explosive device is detonated, the once harmless material one moment may create a deadly percussive force with a release of light, heat and sound following detonation. Generally, at the macroscopic level, energy seeks a path of least resistance and greatest stability; whenever possible water flows from a higher altitude to the lowest altitude possible in a gravitational field. We also generally appreciate that for energy to produce work, work must be involved in the transfer of energy from one macro medium to another. Millions of years of work by trees created the fossil fuels, which were the result of transferring the Sun's radiant energy into combustible oils, natural gas and the gasoline that powers our combustion engines.

A magnet seemingly defies our general perception and knowledge of what energy is and how energy behaves; yet a magnet also portrays one of our fundamental scientific beliefs: that *energy is neither created nor destroyed*. A bar magnet will exhibit the same magnetic field twenty-four hours a day indefinitely without apparently any stimulus or input of energy. The invisible force emitted by a magnet is capable of performing work by interacting with other objects that can be attracted or repulsed by the magnetic field. Yet, there is seemingly no defined cause for this capacity of the magnetic field to engage in work.

The atomic properties of the material comprising a bar magnet create the opportunity for a positive and negative pole to be present inside the same material. Energy is trapped in the magnet, but because of the two poles being present, energy also has the opportunity to flow in a circular manner about the exterior of the magnet. The circular flow of energy generates one or more bands of energy that can be demonstrated to surround the bar magnet.

The circular flow of energy creating a magnetic field is facilitate by the alignment of tritons surrounding the bar magnet. See Figure 29. Energy flows from one pole of the magnet to the other pole within the atoms of the bar magnet. This energy then flows out of the magnet from one end and circles back to the opposite end facilitated by tritons creating a pathway for the energy to return to the opposite pole of the bar magnet.

241

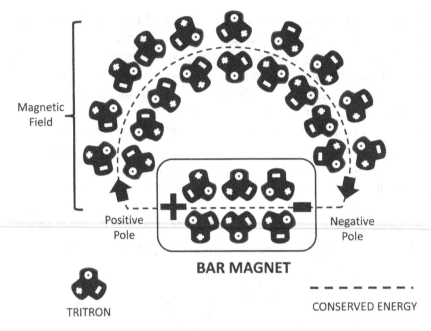

Magnetic Field

Positive Pole

Negative Pole

BAR MAGNET

TRITRON

CONSERVED ENERGY

Figure 29
Tritrons create the pathways for energy to continuously circulate
around the two poles of the magnet

If two bar magnets are placed in proximity to each other, if the poles are opposite poles then the energy circulated both between the two opposing poles of the two bar magnets and between the two poles of each bar magnet creating an attraction. When the like poles of two bar magnets are placed in proximately to each other the outgoing flow of energy from the bar magnets is suppressed and repulsion occurs. Similarly, if the open end of two water hoses were pointed at each other and water flowed outward from each hose, a repulsive force would be generated if the rate of flow of the water was substantial enough.

To facilitate the flow of energy in the magnetic field, the tritrons line up in a specific manner with regards to their tripolar polarity with the negative pole of the tritron pointed outward on the negative end of the bar magnet, a transition phase to neutral where the neutral pole of the tritron is pointed outward in the center of the band of the magnetic field and the positive pole of the tritron is pointed outward in the proximity of the positive end of the bar magnet. The like ends of two bar magnets oppose each other because the tritrons facilitating the magnetic field surrounding the ends are of similar polarity and resist each other's presence. Similarly, there is little resistance when the centers of two bar magnets are placed in close proximity because the neutral state exists, but does not attract or resist. The presence and function of tritrons makes it physically possible for a magnet to exist.

POST SCRIPT SEVEN

Principles of Gravity:
From the Atom to the Black Hole

Formal Definition

Gravity: a fundamental physical force that is responsible for interactions which occur because of mass between particles, such a photons, aggregations of matter, such as planets and starts, and between particles and aggregations of matter. The definition lacks substance since it actually does not identify what the physical force is that creates the physical phenomenon referred to as 'gravity'. The challenge is that no definition has be put forth to explain the presence of the phenomenon of gravity.

The Mystery of Gravity

The lessons learned when one first encounters the unforgiving and relentless force of gravity can lead to life-long emotional and/or physical scars. The first time the novice climbs onboard a bicycle, pedals the wheels, rattles the handlebars and frantically shifts their weight in a attempt to defy gravity, the result can be just a tragic as it can be exhilarating. There is no feeling quite like conquering gravity by successfully riding a bike for the first time; as well as there is no feeling comparable to skidding a knee or an elbow across the asphalt when the bike crashes to the ground, the rider a victim of gravity. When one falls from grace by losing their balance off a bike, off a fence, or falls from any height, and crashes to the ground, the thud the body makes as the muscle and bone structures strike the ground activates sensors that send a panicky alert to the brain, informing the conscious mind that the invisible bonds which tie the human body to the surface of the planet, indeed exist and are relentless.

Gravity presents a particularly challenging puzzle to the analytical prowess of the human brain. Gravity clearly exists. The invisible force of gravity paradoxically is a dominant force in the universe. The escape velocity for a rocket to leave the confines of the Earth is approximately 11 km a second. The greater the volume and mass of a celestial object the greater the force of gravity it exerts on objects in the universe. Yet, despite many millennia of mathematical calculations regarding this physical phenomena, human science is no closer to understanding the etiology of the force that shapes the universe than when Sir Isaac Newton witnessed an apple falling from a tree, which sparked him to surmise his Law of Gravity.

Sir Isaac Newton's Law of Universal Gravitation:

Every object in the universe attracts every other object with a force directed along the line of centers for the two objects that is proportional to the product of their masses and inversely proportional to the square of their distance:

$$Fg = G \frac{M1 \; M2}{R^2}$$

Fg is gravitational force
G is the universal gravitational constant
M1 is mass of the first object
M2 is mass of the second object
R is distance

Newton describes the gravitational phenomenon by a mathematical formula, but he does not derive a cause for the phenomena.

245

To begin to unravel the perplexing mystery that shrouds the most basic of forces known to man it is important to examine how the universe is constructed. Similar to the Russian Matryoshka Nesting Dolls, the universe is built on five differing states of matter, each state built from the constituents of the state preceding it. See Table 17. The initial sub^2 atomic state comprised of tritrons is used to construct the sub atomic state of protons, electrons and neutrons. The sub atomic state is used to build the atomic state which is comprised of 118 differing elements as listed in the periodic table. The elements are combined to create molecules. Molecules combine to produce materials.

State	Constituents	Energy
I Sub^2 atomic particles	Tritrons	Electromagnetic energy including Light energy Magnetic Field energy Gravity
II Sub atomic particles	Proton, Electron, Neutron	Electromagnetic energy
III Atoms	118 Elements	Electromagnetic energy including Light energy Heat energy Sound energy Percussive Force energy
IV Molecules	Proteins, carbohydrates, fats, various chemicals, etc.	Electromagnetic energy including Light energy Sound energy Percussive Force energy Heat energy
V Materials	Wood, plant and animal tissues, alloy metals, etc.	Electromagnetic energy including Light energy Sound energy Percussive Force Energy Heat energy

Table 17
States of Matter

There are five levels of matter in the universe. The smallest level is the sub-sub atomic level comprised of tritrons. See Figure 30. The next level is the sub atomic level comprised of the constituents of an atom. The third level is the atomic level comprised of the elements of the Periodic Table. The fourth level is the molecular level. The fifth level is the level of material which is comprised of various combinations of molecules.

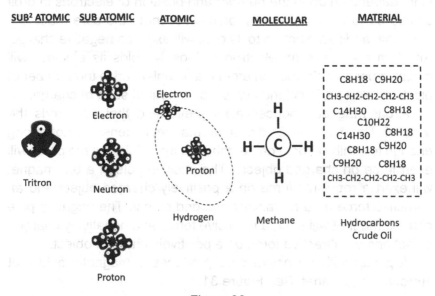

SUB² ATOMIC   SUB ATOMIC   ATOMIC   MOLECULAR   MATERIAL

C8H18   C9H20
CH3-CH2-CH2-CH2-CH3
C14H30   C8H18
C10H22
C14H30   C8H18
C8H18   C9H20
C9H20   C8H18
CH3-CH2-CH2-CH2-CH3

Tritron

Electron
Neutron
Proton

Electron
Proton
Hydrogen

Methane

Hydrocarbons
Crude Oil

Figure 30
The five levels of matter

Gravity is generally considered an invisible force of attraction that causes objects to have weight and causes objects to fall toward the center of the earth. Gravity is also thought to be responsible for the attraction existing between heavenly bodies such as the Sun and the planets comprising the solar system. Further gravity is thought to be present at the center of the galaxy in the form of a black hole, which is of sufficient magnitude to prevent light escaping the boundaries of the black hole.

There exist at least five models common to most observers that appear to exert similar behaviors. The atom, a bar magnet, the Earth, the Sun and planets comprising the solar system, and Milky Way galaxy behave similarly.

The atom is comprised of at least one electron orbiting at least one proton, such as in the hydrogen atom. As the atomic number of an atom increases from two (helium) to 118 (ununoctium), each atomic number adds one electron to the electron cloud orbiting the central mass and adds one proton and one neutron to the central mass of the atom. The atom exhibits a positive, negative and neutral state depending upon the number and position of electrons in orbit compared to the number of protons present in the core mass. An atom that adds an electron to its orbit will exhibit a negative charge. An atom that loses an electron or loosely holds its electron will exhibit a positive charge. An atom that is balanced in the number of electrons and protons tends to exhibit a neutral state of charge.

A bar magnet produces a magnetic field that surrounds the magnet. The magnetic field of a bar magnet is generally not strong enough to exhibit a force on neighboring materials, but the poles will exert force on charged objects. The positive pole of a bar magnet will exert a repulsive force on a positively charged object and an attractive force on a negatively charged object. The negative pole of a bar magnet will exert a repulsive force on a negatively charged object and an attractive force on a positively charged object.

A planet with an active core produces a magnetic field that surrounds the planet. See Figure 31.

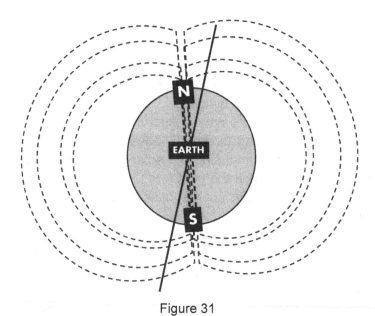

Figure 31
The magnetic field that surrounds a planet with an active core

The symbol for the tritron can be abbreviated by the illustration present in Figure 32.

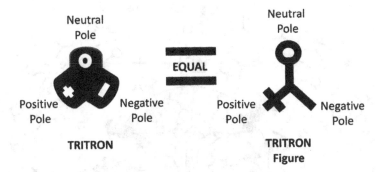

Figure 32
Symbol illustrating a tripolar tritron and a short-hand symbol for the tritron

Energy passes through the core of the Earth from the magnetic South Pole to the magnetic north pole. The energy that has passed through the core of the planet then exits through the North Pole wraps around the planet and enters back into the planet through the south pole of the planet. The energy that surrounds planet Earth is recognized as the magnetic field that protects the Earth. See Figure 33.

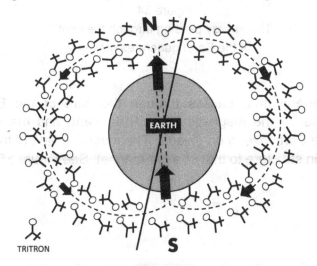

Figure 33
Illustration of the magnetic field that surrounds the Earth

As the energy passes through the center of the Earth it creates the phenomenon of gravity. See Figure 34.

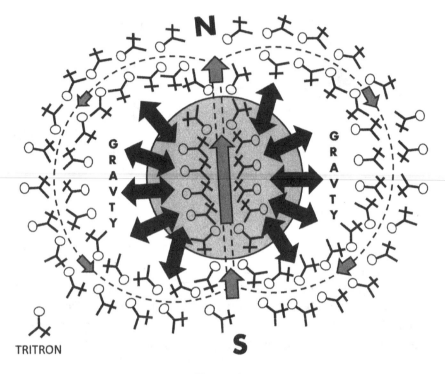

Figure 34
The energy passing through the core
of the Earth generates gravity

The energy that passes through the core of the Earth is responsible for the magnetic field of the Earth and the force of gravity the Earth exerts on objects. The magnetic field of the Earth is similar in structure to that of a bar magnet. See Figure 35.

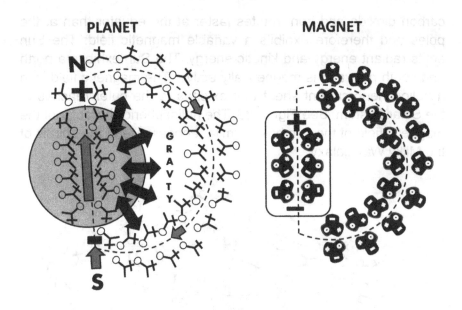

Figure 35
The magnetic field exhibited
by the Earth is similar to a bar magnet

In the center of a solid planet such as the Earth, the tritrons line up between the positive and negative pole of the planet. The tritrons act as a conduit for the passage of energy from the positive and negative pole of the planet. The tritrons course between the positive and negative poles of the planet with the positive end of the tripolar particle pointed toward the positive pole of the planet and the negative end of the tripolar particle pointed toward the pole of the planet. The neutral portion of the tripolar particle is pointed outward. As energy passes through the corridor of tritrons lined up between the positive and negative poles of the planet, the neutral portions of the tritrons attract the positive and negative charges indiscriminately toward the center of the planet, resulting in an attractive force for all charged atoms and molecules, which is recognized as gravity.

In our solar system, a single star, the Sun, resides at the center. The Sun represents more than 99% of the mass of the entire Solar System. The sun, being a gaseous body comprised of 73% hydrogen, 25% helium and 1.69% other gases including oxygen, carbon dioxide and iron, rotates faster at the equator than at the poles and therefore exhibits a variable magnetic field. The Sun emits radiant energy and kinetic energy. The Sun exhibits a north and south pole and is magnetically active. The magnetic field is in a heliospheric current sheet that extends to the outer reaches of the Solar System. See Figure 36. The heliospheric character of the magnetic field of the sun has a similar appearance to the spirals of the Milky Way galaxy.

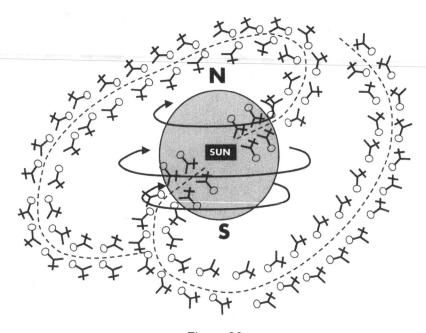

Figure 36
Heliospheric magnetic field generated by the poles and equator
of the Sun rotating at differing speeds

The existence of tritrons explains two of the odd behaviors of light. The first behavior of light that tritrons explains is the phenomenon that Albert Einstein predicted. Dr. Einstein stated that light would be attracted to a star if light passed in the vicinity of a star. Photos taken as a solar eclipse took place demonstrated in fact that light from a distant star indeed did bend toward the Sun as it passed in close proximity to the Sun. The second behavior that tritrons explain is the existence of black holes.

Dr. Einstein was awarded the Nobel Prize for surmising that the gravity of a star would cause light to change course as it traversed through space. Stars act as a powerful source of gravity. This attractive force exhibited by a star results in a concentration of tritrons in the vicinity of a star. See Figure 37.

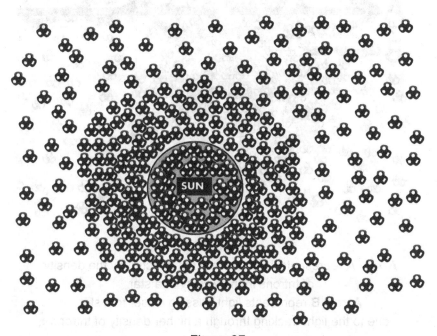

Figure 37
The density of tritrons is greater in the vicinity of a star
than in open space

Since light uses tritrons as the medium by which it traverses any distance, light follows pathways of higher densities of tritrons as opposed to pathways comprised of lesser concentrations of tritrons. The more dense the field of tritrons the easier it is for a quanta of light to travel from one location to another location. Since light favors the density of tritrons, and the space surrounding a star will exert a gradient of increasing concentration of tritrons as you get closer to the star, light will flow closer to a star as it passes by a star. See Figure 38.

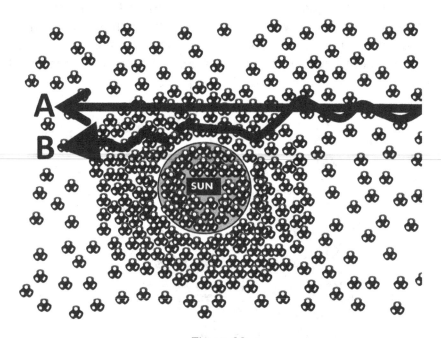

Figure 38
Arrow A represents light if it were not affected by the density
of tritrons in the vicinity of a star.
Arrow B represents light passing closer to a star
due to the light tracking through a higher density of tritrons

The Sun and the accompanying solar system are but one small component of a large mass of stars known as the Milky Way galaxy. See Figure 39. The name is derived from the appearance of a milky density that courses across the night sky that is created by the galactic plane of the disc like galaxy of stars that surrounds the Earth. The Earth is located in the galactic plane approximately 27,000 light years from the center of the galaxy.

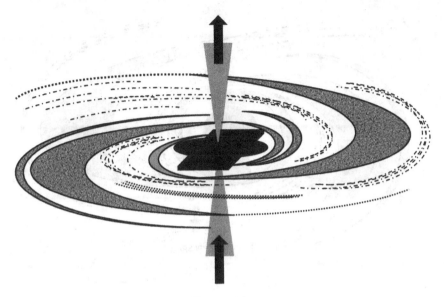

Figure 39
Illustration of the Milky Way galaxy

The Milky Way galaxy is a spiral galaxy estimated to be approximately 120 million light years in diameter. Our galaxy contains an estimated 200-400 billion stars. The center of the galaxy is located in the direction of the constellation Sagittarius. At the center of the Milky Way is a bar shaped core. See Figure 40. The disc shaped spiral galaxy is comprised of several prominent arms and several minor arms. The Scutum-Centaurus Arm and the Perseus Arm originate from opposite ends of the bar shaped center of the galaxy. Smaller arms include the Sagittarius Arm, Norma Arm and the Outer Arm. The Sun is located in the Orion spur in the Sagittarius Arm, a relatively small cluster of stars. The Milky Way is rotating and has a velocity of approximately 600 km a second and takes 15 to 50 million years to complete a rotation.

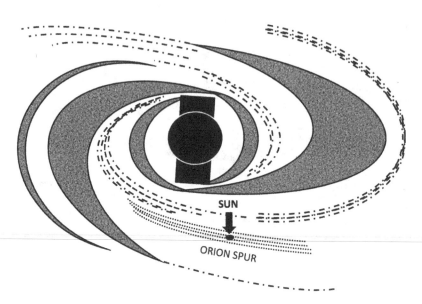

Figure 40
The Milky Way is a bar shaped spiral galaxy

The center of the Milky Way is considered to be a super massive black hole. Observations suggest most galaxies have a black hole located at their center. The Milky Way's black hole is equivalent to 4.1 million solar masses. A solar mass is equal to the mass of our Sun, which is 1.988 x 10^{30} kg.

The term black hole has been the identifier of the phenomenon that exists at the center of some galaxies, including the Milky Way galaxy. Black hole has been a term synonymous with light not being able to escape the region of space where the black hole resides. The theory of the existence of a black hold is thought to be the result of the implosion of a star. As a star collapses it is though the matter of the star condenses into an extremely dense core that exhibits a very strong gravitational field. The core or center of a black hole has been termed a gravitational singularity. It is theorized that a singularity has a volume of zero but infinite density. It is the powerfully attractive nature of the gravitational field of the black hole that is thought to project enough of an attractive force to the surrounding space to prevent the escape of light itself.

The above mentioned description of a black hole is contradicted by the description of some galaxies with black holes have been observed to have light and matter spewing out of one end of the black hole. Either a black hole exerts a spherical shaped force of gravity such as a star or it doesn't. The understanding of the mechanics of a black hole is limited due to the lack the capacity to directly observe a black hole on one side and then directly observe the same black hole on the opposite side. If a black hole were spinning, our level of technology would not be able to detect if a black hole was rotating or not, since theoretically it would be void of a light signature.

Black Hole: a term of description

The term 'black hole' may simply be a term of 'description' to explain the observation that light is void in the region of space that a black hole encompasses, rather than its traditional role as the 'explanation' of the phenomena.

A black hole refers to a region of space that nothing can escape including light. See Figure 41. A gravity field where light could not escape is not a new idea, being first speculated by John Mitchell and Pierre-Simon Laplace in the 18th century. The simplest black holes have mass, but no electric charge, no angular momentum.

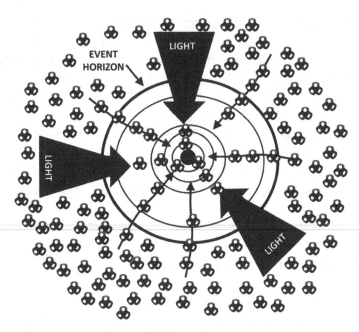

Figure 41
Black hole created by a vortex

The edge of the black hole is termed an event horizon. The event horizon refers to the perimeter around the center of a black hole were light becomes attracted to the center of the back hole and is not able to escape the black hole. Since light is not able to escape the black hole, light is void inside the defined boundaries of the event horizon. See Figure 42.

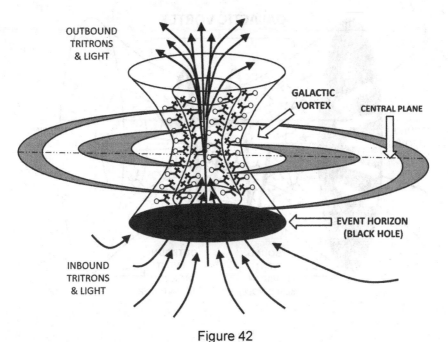

Figure 42
Light and matter that cross the event horizon of a black hole
are drawn into the black hole

The black hole of some galaxies have been observed to attract light and matter from one side into the center of the black hole and spew light and matter out the opposite end of the black hole. See Figure 43.

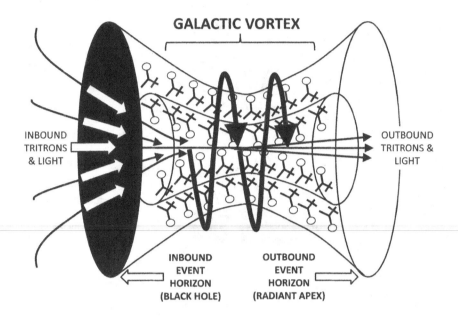

Figure 43
A galaxy's black hole may draw light and matter in one end
and spew light and matter out the opposite end

The concept of a 'gravitational singularity' is predicated on the concept that a black hole has been generated by the collapse and implosion of a star. Zero volume, infinite density and nearly infinite magnitude of gravitational attraction all seem to describe a black hole when the point of observation is looking at the circular view of the black hole. This same array of descriptive terms is 'incompatible' with the observed behavior of a black hole when the point of view is from the side of a black hole located at the center of a disc shaped spiral galaxy.

A more coherent description of the phenomena of a black hole is to state that the observed black hole with its event horizon, represents one end of a funnel or tube shaped vortex. Light and matter become sucked into the inbound end of the vortex called a black hole due to the extreme forces of gravity located at the center of the galactic vortex. Unlike the concept of a gravitational singularity, which is described as having no measurable volume, a galactic vortex has a defined length and the inner diameter of the passage through the vortex may nearly be infinitely small, such as one tritron wide or a few tritrons in width, but there is a width. Leading into the center of the galactic vortex, the vortex takes on the shape of a cone with the smallest point of the cone leading to the center of the vortex. This is the intake funnel. The opening of the intake funnel is considered the event horizon of the black hole. Almost as a mirror image, on the opposite side leading away from the center of the vortex is also a cone, similar in size and shape to the cone that acts as the intake funnel. This connecting and opposing cone leading away from the center of the vortex is the outbound funnel. The outbound funnel leads to an outbound event horizon.

Gravity rotates unevenly inside the center of the galactic vortex similar to the Sun's gravitational field rotating in an uneven pattern. The uneven rotation of gravity in the center of the galactic vortex sets up a twisting pattern that acts like an atmospheric tornado, but the galactic vortex contains enough attractive force such that it is capable of sucking light and matter from the boundaries of the event horizon of the black hole and propel this light and matter through the center of the galactic vortex and to the opposite side of the central plane of the galaxy. Light and matter which traverses the vortex is ejected out the opposing end of the galactic vortex.

Light and matter exiting a galactic vortex exhibit opposite behavior than that of the black hole. The light exiting the outbound horizon of a galactic vortex causes the outbound horizon to be brilliantly radiant. The galactic vortex as seen from the side of the outbound horizon is termed a radiant apex to describe the radiant brilliance of the light escaping the galactic vortex. Therefore, the term 'black hole' refers to the region of space comprising the inbound event horizon of a galactic vortex and the 'radiant apex' describes the region of space comprising the outbound event horizon of a galactic vortex.

Tritrons explain the behavior of the galaxy

A galaxy's vortex generates a strong enough gravitational field that it is capable of displacing tritrons by sucking tritrons into the vortex on one end and spewing tritrons out the opposite end. Since light uses tritrons as the medium by which is traverses any distance, light follows the flow of tritrons. The side of the vortex where tritrons are sucked into a galactic vortex is void of light since light follows the tritrons into the vortex. See Figure 44.

Tritons are the medium that quanta of light use to traverse the universe. Though tritrons act as the primary fabric of the three dimensional universe, the density of these tripolar objects varies throughout space. The attractive force of gravity will cause changes in the density of tritrons dependent upon the magnitude of the gravitational field. In the vicinity of a source of gravity, such as a star, the density of tritrons increases. The difference between a star and a black hole is the gravitational power of the black hole is much greater than a star. A star attracts a greater concentration of tritrons to its local vicinity than the surrounding region of space. A black hole attracts tritrons, but due to the greater magnitude of gravity, the black hole attracts both tritrons and electromagnetic energy such as light due to the physical displacement of tritrons in space.

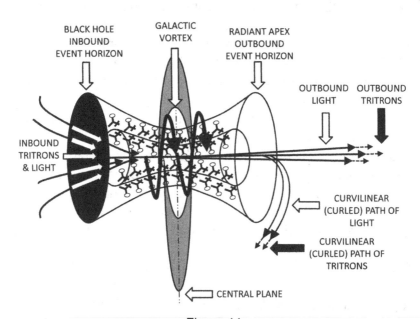

Figure 44
Light follows the flow of tritrons into a galactic vortex,
which creates the black hole phenomena

The opposite end of a vortex is very bright since tritrons are spewing out of the vortex and light is following the flow of tritrons and therefore escaping the vortex. Our capacity to view very distant galaxies may be related to our capacity to view the light escaping the bright side of a vortex. This bright side of a galactic vortex is termed a radiant apex.

The flow of tritrons out of the radiant apex of a galactic vortex may provide the propulsive means for a galaxy with an active vortex. Galaxies with an active vortex will therefore move from one part of the universe to another part of the universe by their own power, making a galactic vortex the largest engine in the universe. If this is the case, the Big Bang theory may be in question. The universe may not be in perpetual cyclic expansion and contraction as theorized by the Big Bang theory, but instead the galaxies may simply be in perpetual motion due to the propulsion provided by each galaxy's vortex. In addition, the actual size and age of the universe may need to be recalculated if the Big Bang theory is determined not to be as correct as previously surmised.

Newton's Laws of Motion

Sir Isaac Newton's laws of Motion are as follows:

1. Every object persists in its state of rest or uniform motion in a straight line unless it is compelled to change the state by forces impressed on it.
2. Force is equal to the change in momentum (mV) per change in time. For a constant mass, force equals mass times acceleration.
3. For every action, there is an equal and opposite re-action.

Newton's First Law of Motion, also referred to as the Law of Inertia, needs further discussion when applied to sub-sub atomic physics. Tritrons are the primary or essential component of matter. Tritrons fill the three dimensional volume of space and extend out to the very boundaries of the universe. A void exists between tritrons. At the sub-sub atomic level there exists the tritron tripolar particles, void or emptiness, and the quanta of energy that utilizes free tritrons as a conductive and organized tritrons as a storage medium.

The density of tritrons varies across the universe. Tritrons are denser near a source of gravity. The density of tritrons in the proximity of a gravitational field is proportional to the magnitude of the gravitational force exerted by the field. Gravity is variable and in special instances such as black holes, when the magnitude of the gravitational force is high enough, gravity is capable of causing tritrons to move from one point in space to another point in space. Motion of tritrons and the density of tritrons can affect the apparent motion of electromagnetic energy, such as visible light.

A Newtonian fluid is a fluid whose shear stress is linearly proportional to the velocity gradient in the direction perpendicular to the plane of shear. Water is considered a Newtonian fluid because it continues to display properties of a fluid no matter how much it is stirred or mixed.

There is a difference between the Laws of Motion in a body of fluid such as a pool of water and the space that exists between planets and stars. In a body of fluid such as water, atomic and molecular objects displace water. If a diver under water moves his hand in a direction away from his body, he will displace a volume of water due to the hand being more solid than the water. The displaced water moves in the direction the hand moved. The diver might expect to see a reaction in the water around him such as displacement of an object such as seaweed if the seaweed were in the path of the displaced water. In space, if an astronaut moved his hand in a direction away from his body, the astronaut would not expect to witness any reaction by the void of space that surrounds the astronaut. Given the two scenarios, it is easy to conceptualize that in space, Newton's first law of motion is correct. Most logical people would expect that in space if an object is set in motion, this object will continue to move in the direction of its motion unless acted upon by another force.

At the sub-sub atomic level of the tritron particle, the size of a tritron is trivial in comparison to the volume of even the simplest atom. There exists a vast volume between the nucleus of an atom and the orbital path of the atom's most distant electron in comparison to the size of the tritrons that occupy the same volume. Free tritrons occupy the volume of every atom and the space surrounding the atoms, and between the atoms comprising the atomic matter of the universe.

So much like a screen door closing and the surrounding air does not become appreciably displaced by the movement of the door, material objects do not displace the volume of tritrons filling space. Free tritrons move through objects and objects move through space occupied by free tritrons. The only place in the universe where this in not true is in a galactic vortex. The density of tritrons is of such a magnitude, energy is separated from tritrons. In the heart of a galactic vortex all materials are broken down into the basic elements of pure tritrons and quanta of energy. This product of energy and free tritrons is projected out of the radiant apex of a galactic vortex.

Proof Tritrons Exist

To prove that tritrons indeed exist, an approach similar to Albert Einstein's strategy to discern that gravity affected the flight path of visible light could be embarked upon. The existence of tritrons could be extrapolated from observing the heavens. Sometimes solutions to micro problems can be seen being played out on a galactic scale for all to witness.

Once set in motion, quanta of light travel in one discrete direction. Dr. Einstein predicted, which was proven, that the path of light can be altered or bent by the forces of gravity. Traditionally, it has been thought that light could even be stopped by gravity, since light is thought not to be able to escape the clutches of the extreme magnitude of gravitational force exhibited by a black hole.

The path of light in free space is not expected to curl. Artificially, with aide of a fiber optic fibre, the pathway of light can be curved. Traveling in free space, light should follow a straight path unless acted upon by gravity.

Tritrons will spew out of a galactic vortex like water jutting forth from the mouth of a fountain. The trajectory of some tritrons being ejected from a galactic vortex will arch or even 'curl'. The trajectory of tritrons following a curled path is related to tritrons ejecting from the center of the galactic vortex encountering other tritrons in space. In free space, tritrons generally do not appreciably interfere with each other. The concentration of tritrons existing outside the outbound event horizon of the galactic vortex is unusually dense with tritrons given that tritrons are constantly being displaced and ejected by the galactic vortex. The tritrons exiting the outbound event horizon collide with the volume of tritrons that already exist in space. Some of the tritrons exiting from the galactic vortex will stream forward and continue on a path that is perpendicular to the central plane of the galaxy in which the galactic vortex exists. Some of the tritrons exiting the galactic vortex will have their path blunted. The tritrons exiting the galactic vortex that have their path blunted on a curvilinear course, the arch depends upon the density of tritrons encountered by the tritrons exiting the galactic vortex. The greater the density of free tritrons outside the galactic vortex that the ejected tritrons encounter, the more arched the trajectory of the ejected tritrons. The trajectory of ejected tritrons can be arched to the point the ejected tritrons exhibit a curled flight path.

If no tritrons were to exist, light exiting a galactic vortex should exhibit only a linear trajectory away from the center of the galactic vortex until such light encounters a significant gravitational source some distance from the galactic vortex.

If tritrons exist, light exiting the galactic vortex will follow the paths the tritrons take exiting the galactic vortex. Some of the tritrons being ejected out the outbound event horizon will follow a perpendicular trajectory, while some of the tritrons will follow an oblique trajectory. If tritrons exist, then a portion of the light exiting the galactic vortex will demonstrate a linear trajectory perpendicular to the central plane of the galaxy, while other tritrons will exit on an oblique trajectory. If tritrons exist, light will follow the path of tritrons that demonstrate a curvilinear trajectory exiting the galactic vortex. In circumstances where the density of tritrons outside the outbound horizon is particularly high, tritrons will demonstrate an arched and even a curled trajectory. See Figure 44. Light may exhibit a gentle curvilinear trajectory when acted upon by a gravitational force, but typically light in free space will not demonstrate a curled trajectory. Light demonstrated to exit a galactic vortex on an arched or curled trajectory is significant circumstantial evidence that tritrons indeed exist.

In Summary

There are four different forms of attractive expressed in the universe. The first form of attractive force (referred to as magnetism) is exhibited by a magnet. The second form of attractive force (referred to as gravity) is exhibited by a planet. The third form of attractive force (referred to as gravity) is exhibited by a star. The fourth form of attractive force (termed gravity) is a black hole. The four different forms of attractive force are dependent upon the intensity of quanta of energy passing through the vortex at the core of the phenomenon.

In the vortex of a magnet the neutral side of the tritrons point outward. The vortex of a magnet is the center point of the magnet on the line between the positive and negative poles of the magnet. Energy passes from the negative pole of the magnet through the vortex in the magnet to the positive pole, then out the positive pole. The energy leaving the positive pole of the magnet will follow a pathway created by the alignment of tritrons back to the negative pole to complete a circuit since energy is conserved. This mechanism, which is based on the conservation of energy, creates the magnetic force exhibited by a magnet. The amount of energy passing through the vortex of the magnet is generally not enough to have a visible effect on neighboring objects. The positive and negative poles of the magnet are able to attract and repel materials depending upon the magnitude of the material's negativity or positivity. The weak gravitational force of a magnet is termed magnetic force or magnetic attraction.

In the vortex of a planet the neutral side of the tritrons point outward. The vortex of a planet is the center point of the planet on the line between the positive and negative poles of the planet. The positive and negative poles of the planet may be referred to as the north and south pole respectfully, such as respect to the Earth. Energy passes from the negative pole of the planet through the vortex in the center of the planet to the positive pole, then out the positive pole. The energy leaving the positive pole of the planet will follow a pathway created by the alignment of the tritrons back to the negative pole of the planet. This mechanism, which based on the conservation of energy, creates the magnetic field that surrounds the planet. The planet is a solid mass and rotates as one body. The magnetic field remains constant due to the planet acting as one relatively uniform mass. Due to the extent of the energy passing through the vortex of a planet with an active core the neutral ends of the tritrons are able to indiscriminately attract both positive and negatively charged particles, atoms and molecules drawing these toward the center of the planet; this attraction is recognized as gravity.

In the vortex of a star the neutral side of the tritrons point outward. The vortex of a star is the center point of the star on the line between the positive and negative poles of the star. The positive and negative poles of a star may be referred to as the north and south pole respectfully, such as respect to the Sun. Energy passes from the negative pole of the star through the vortex in the center of the star to the positive pole, then out the positive pole. The energy leaving the positive pole of the star follows a pathway created by the alignment of tritrons back to the negative pole of the sun. As with the Sun, the poles of a star rotate at different speeds than does the equator of the star. The differing rotational speeds of the Sun produce a magnetic field that is heliospheric in nature. The variation of the magnetic field created a solar system where the planets orbit in a common plane rather than the planets orbiting in a spherical fashion around the Sun.

Within the galactic vortex at the center of the galaxy the neutral side of the tritrons is pointed outward. The vortex of a galaxy is the center point of the galaxy on the line between the positive and negative poles of the galaxy. The positive and negative poles of the galaxy may be referred to as the north and south pole respectfully, or may be referred to as the radiant apex and the black hole respectfully. The center of the galaxy has a mass that has been approximated to be 4 million times that of the sun. Energy passes from the negative pole of the galaxy (the black hole), through the vortex in the center at the central plane to the positive pole, then out the positive pole (the radiant apex). See Figure 44. Energy leaves the positive pole spewing out into space like a fountain, but then follows a pathway created by the alignment of tritrons back to the negative pole of the galaxy to complete the circuit; similar to that of a magnet, a planet such as the Earth and a star, such as the Sun. See Figure 45. Due to the corkscrew rotation of the galactic vortex, the magnetic field produced by the galactic vortex is heliospheric in nature and rotational. The attractive force, referred to as gravity, of the galactic vortex is of such a magnitude that tritrons are physically displaced. Tritrons are drawn into the galactic vortex on the side of the black hole, the tritrons pass through the center of the galactic vortex in a corkscrew like manner, to be ejected out the opposite end of the galactic vortex through the radiant apex. Light and other frequencies of electromagnetic energy follow the flow of tritrons into the black hole, follow the flow of tritrons through the vortex, then follow the flow of tritrons out of the radiant apex.

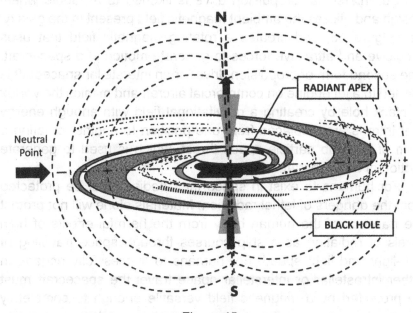

Figure 45
A magnetic field is generated by the galactic vortex
surrounds the entire galaxy

There are many bands to the magnetic field produced by the galactic vortex. Similar to a bar magnet, the magnetic field is neutral at the center plane of the galaxy.

The central plane of a spiral galaxy with an active galactic vortex, such as the Milky Way, represents the linear plane where the gravity exerted by the galactic vortex is the greatest magnitude. The central plane is also the point where the magnetic field reaches a neutral point between the positive (or north) pole of the galaxy and the negative (or south) pole of the galaxy.

Navigating the Galaxy

Given the construction of the galaxy, two forms of spacecraft propulsion drives present themselves for consideration. The first form of interstellar propulsion drive is likened to a paddle wheel design and utilizes the ambient magnetic field present in the galaxy, see Figure 45, and creates a rotating magnetic field that uses repulsive and attractive forces to generate motion of a spacecraft. The second form of propulsion drive for an interstellar spacecraft is likened to a jet engine on commercial aircraft and mimics the vortex of black hole by creating a gravitational field with enough energy that tritrons are displaced from one position to another creating a form of sub-sub particle space thrust, which is used to generate motion of a spacecraft.

For humans to exist in space their bodies must be protected from the dangers of lethal radiation. Materials alone will not protect the frailness of the human body from the harmful effects of high levels of radiation as a ship courses through space traveling at sub-light and light speed. For humans to successfully engage in either intrastellar or interstellar space travel the spacecraft must be protected by a magnetic field versatile enough to completely surround the spacecraft and strong enough to repel any dangerous levels of radiation that might course through space. See Figure 46. Without a magnetic shield to protect human occupants the fragile cells of the human body would be irrevocably damaged and humans would not successfully survive a flight through space and would die of radiation sickness.

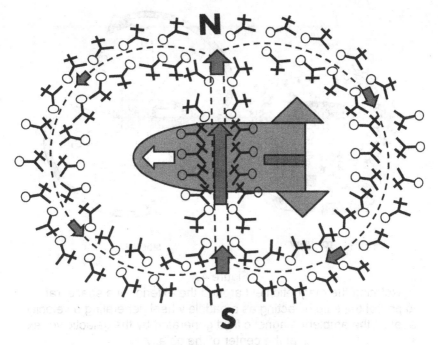

Figure 46

Artificial magnetic field to surround spacecraft
to protect human occupants

If a space ship needs to be designed with a magnetic bubble surrounding the craft to protect the human occupants, then the next logical action is to incorporate the protective force of the magnetic field as a means of propulsion for the space ship. Similar to the paddle wheel of a steam boat, the magnetic field of the magnetic bubble surrounding the ship could be rotated around the exterior of the ship. See Figure 47. The rotation of the magnetic field would interact with the ambient magnetic field generated by the galactic vortex at the center of the galaxy and create motion for the spacecraft. Similar to a boat equipped with a paddle wheel, rotation of the magnetic field around the spacecraft could move the ship forward or backward through space.

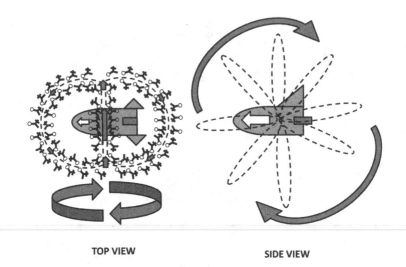

TOP VIEW   SIDE VIEW

Figure 47
Rotating the magnetic field around the exterior of a spacecraft
to propel the ship by acting as a paddle wheel generating a velocity
against the ambient magnetic field generated by the galactic vortex
at the center of the galaxy

Generating a magnetic field with the vortex present in the central portion of the spacecraft would also generate an artificial gravitation field that would anchor the human occupants to the ship and provide a comfortable work and living environment, while maintaining the health and strength of the human occupants.

Mimicking the design of a galactic vortex, a jet engine like propulsion drive could be devised. Instead of igniting combustible gases through a jet engine to turn turbine blades to generate thrust, such as the case of jet engine equipped aircraft, an engine could be devised that incorporates a heliospheric shaped gravitational field of enough magnitude to displace tritrons. The displacement of tritrons from one position through the vortex of the engine to another position would create a sub-sub particle space thrust, which would be used to generate motion for spacecraft. Since the motion of tritrons is at the sub-sub space level the movement of such particles would not be damaging to humans. The speed of the space craft could theoretically reach light speed depending upon the magnitude of the gravitational field that is generated by the spacecraft.

POST SCRIPT EIGHT
The Great Albatross of Physics: 'LIGHT'

The very existence of light has been befuddling to science since the dawn of time. Paradoxically, light behaves in some ways as a particle and in some ways as a wave. To science, it has been challenging to think of quanta of light energy behaving in two vastly different physical manners.

Yet, we believe and understand that water can behave in a number of ways. If a pebble is dropped into a pool of perfectly still water, once the pebble strikes the surface of water a circular wave radiates outward from the point of impact where the pebble made initial contact with the body of water. If the pool of water is cooled to the point where the water freezes and the same pebble is dropped onto the same location, the pebble may not even break the surface of the frozen body of water. If water freezes as it falls through the atmosphere and becomes snow, and this snow is collected into a ball, water behaves not as a wave, but as a particle when thrown as a snowball through the air.

The Great Albatross for Physics is the existence of LIGHT. The equation $E=MC^2$ represents that 'E' is Energy which is equal to 'M' the Mass of an object multiplied by 'C' the value of the speed of light which is again multiplied by 'C' the value of the speed of light. The equation $E=MC^2$ is dependent upon light traveling at a constant speed of 186,000 miles a second. Albert Einstein's theory of special relativity as of 1905 states that the speed of light in a vacuum is always measured the same 299,792.458 km/s or 186,000 m/s. Einstein stated, "*The velocity c of light in a vacuum is the same for all inertial frames of reference in all directions and depend neither on the velocity of the source nor the velocity of the observer*".

273

Later, to explain the existence of a black hole, the 'constant' speed of light needed to be modified, which Albert Einstein himself wrote that 'special relativity holds only so long as we are able to disregard the influence of gravitational fields'. In 1915, Albert Einstein developed his theory of General Relativity, in which the velocity of light varied by the presence and intensity of a gravitational field. In the presence of gravity, the speed of light becomes relative.

The reason LIGHT is the great Albatross of Physics is that light surrounds us, and in essence is essential for life, however, the existence of light has yet to be adequately explained. Light has no apparent density, yet light is reflected. If one stands at the edge of a pond and throws a flat stone sideways, such that the flight path of the stone is intended to have the flat edge of the stone strike the surface of the water, with appropriate thrust, the stone will skip off the surface of the water. To the casual observer, the stone has density and the water has density and therefore when the stone makes contact with the surface of the water on a tangential flight path, if there is sufficient speed and the angle to the water's surface is sufficiently obtuse, instead of penetrating the water, the stone will be reflected off the surface of the water.

An object that possesses density that strikes another object with sufficient density generates a variance in the path of the first object. Billiard balls on a pool table, the ricochet of a bullet off a steel door, a tennis ball traveling from an outstretched racket, to a brick wall and back at the tennis player are all examples of masses with density striking an object with a density and the object that is traveling exhibits an alteration in its trajectory.

A slightly different, less clear example is standing at the edge of a canyon and shouting out a 'name' in the direction of the canyon wall on the opposing side of the gully. If the air is still enough, the person who did the shouting can hear the spoken 'name' echoing off the distant canyon wall. The echo represents the sound wave initiated by the person's vocal cords traveling through the air molecules striking the canyon wall and being reflected back to the speaker through the air. To the casual observer, the voice is a force produced by the muscles of the speaker's neck, which stimulates a wave of resonance in the air molecules filling the atmosphere, which provides an explanation as to why the echo occurs. In a vacuum, the same vocal cords would produce no sound.

If not exposed to a substantial gravitational force, light is theorized to travel at a constant speed. Light is considered to have an 'optical density' which is related to the absorbance that occurs when light passes through a material. As mentioned above, light sometimes displays the quality of behaving like a particle, suggesting light itself has mass. 'Light' though generally is not considered to have mass. If one stands in the brilliant luminescence of a high-powered floodlight and one might become temporarily blinded by the intensity of the light, but one would not expect to feel any form of pressure on the skin due to the luminance of the light source no matter how intense the light is shining, beyond heat possibly generated by the light source.

The Albatross created by the existence LIGHT is the paradox of how does an energy phenomena such as light, which has no substantial mass, become reflected off objects? We see color because white light supposedly strikes an object and the surface of the object reflects back to our eyes the visible light component that makes up the color we see and appreciate. At first the question seems intuitive. We have all been led to believe that light behaves like sound. If one stands at the edge of a canyon and projects their voice toward an opposing canyon wall, one will hear the sound of their voice echoing off the canyon wall if the ambient noise that surrounds us is low enough and the air is still. But light energy is not sound energy. Light energy behaves different than sound energy. Light travels vast distances through the vacuum of space; sound travels only through a medium where sound energy can sufficiently vibrate molecules comprising the medium to propagate the sound energy through the medium.

Light is theorized to be comprised of discrete packets of energy referred to as quanta. Atoms are comprised of one or more electrons orbiting a nucleus comprised of one or more protons and some quantity of neutrons depending upon the type of atom. In relation to the size of the proton(s), neutron(s) and electron(s) that comprise an atom, the space existing between the electron(s) and the nucleus of the atom is theorized to be quite considerable. Likened to our solar system, the sum of the volume all of the planets combined is miniscule when compared to the three dimensional volume of space that comprises the solar system. All materials are comprised of atoms. Therefore, analyzed at the atomic level, if a quanta of light energy, which has no substantial mass, encounters an atom in a material, what is 'it' that light is reflect off of in an atom in order to produce reflected visible light?

The electromagnetic spectrum represents the range of frequencies of electromagnetic energy. The electromagnetic spectrum is comprised of low frequency long wave length electromagnetic energy such as radio waves to high frequency short wave length electromagnetic energy such as gamma rays. Light is the visible portion of the electromagnetic spectrum.

Visible light refers to the phenomenon that the human eye can detect electromagnetic energy in the wavelength range of 380 nm to 760 nm. The color blue has an approximate wavelength of 400 nm, green 500 nm, yellow 600 nm and red 700 nm.

In addition to visible light, other forms of electromagnetic energy include radio waves, microwave radiation, infrared energy, ultraviolet energy, x-ray radiation and gamma rays. The human eye is equipped with a lens in the front of the eyeball for focus and a retina in the back of the eyeball for detection of the light energy. The retina is equipped with a specialized set of cells to convert light energy into chemical energy and by use of the optic nerve, send nerve signals to the back of the brain and produce images in the occipital lobes of the cerebellum. 'Language' provides an individual with an arbitrary convention of names for the various colors the occipital lobes are able to detect given the input signals collected by the eyes.

So white light, which is comprised of the entire spectrum of frequencies of visible light, is emitted by the Sun along with various other forms of electromagnetic energy. White light travels the 93 million miles through space to the Earth. This white light traverses the atmosphere during daytime hours, strikes the objects on the surface of the earth where objects are not shaded from the radiant energy of the sun. The human eye detects visible light that traverses from an object in the presence of a light source to the human eye.

In a windowless room void of any amount of visible light, the human eye is unable to detect the image of any object that might be in the room. In a room lit with a light, if the intensity of the light reached the point the sensors in the retina of the eye were overloaded, such as if a flash bomb were to be set off, filling the room with intense white light, the human eye would become blind to the image of any object present in the room. Therefore, the conditions of no light and an excessive amount of light both lead to an inability to visually detect objects. To properly view an object the object must be illuminated by the presence of electromagnetic energy within the visible light spectrum at an adequate but reasonable intensity for the human eye to detect the image of an object that is gazed upon.

Again, though light may behave as if it were comprised of matter, generally light is not considered to have a detectable density. An object traveling at the speed of light is theorized to have no measurable mass. So if light has no detectable mass, how does shining white light at an object able to produce the effect where visible light of a particular color is transmitted from the surface of the object back in the direction of the eyes of a human observer? How does a quanta of energy with essentially no density ricochet off an atom containing miniscule subatomic particles with such precise regularity such that there is never a flaw in the color of an object, unless the composition of the material or the light source is altered?

We all believe that light is reflected off of objects. Part of the reason for the propagation of this belief is due to the common imagery of white light passing through a prism and the path of the visible light being altered or bent as it passes through differing materials. A prism can be used to refract light, changing the direction of the light by changing the speed of the light. But if a white light is shined on an object, and this object appears scarlet red to the human eye, has the red component of white light really been reflected off the object and transmitted back to the human eye, or is there actually another phenomenon which is occurring?

If one observer holds a white light source and shines white light at an object and the object appears red in color to the observer, interestingly to other observers who may be in the vicinity, the object will also appear red in color. The phenomenon of where all observers see the same color, even if the object is irregular in shape is generally explained away as due to scatter of the white light energy which originated from the white light source.

An alternative explanation for a white light source to produce the existence of individual colors that the human eye is able to detect is that light is not physically reflected off an object, but that when white light strikes an object and is absorbed by the atomic structures comprising the surface of the object, depending upon the composition of the atoms of the material, the material is able to absorb a portion of the white light, but becomes overloaded with the frequency of visible light that is the 'visible color' of the object. Therefore, when white light strikes the visible surface of an object, the atoms comprising the surface of the material emit energy at the frequency where the material's surface atoms are overloaded and the atoms emit radiant energy related to the properties of the material; the original white light energy is in fact not reflected back to the observer. The light being reflected back is the result of energy being emitted that represents the overload threshold of the atoms comprising the material.

Tritrons are tripolar sub-sub atomic particles that act as the most fundamental building blocks of the universe. Light travels from a light source to the object conducted by tritrons. Light emitted from objects to give the appearance of color is conducted by tritrons from the object to the human eye.

An example of the concept that atomic constituents of materials emit radiant light energy is seen with combustible objects. A piece of fire wood may appear as some shade of brown when not in a state of combustion. Once a piece of dry firewood is set ablaze, this otherwise dull object may produce and become a brilliant source of the full spectrum of white light. The fact that fire light exists has been explained by the chemical forces comprised in the combustion process. Still the fact remains, that an otherwise dark, quiescent object can become a source of light points directly at the fact that the atoms comprising a combustible material contain a measurable amount of inherent energy that can be emitted and detected by the electromagnetic sensors in the human eye. The signals acquired by the light sensors present in the retina are then constructed into images in the occipital lobe of the brain and analyzed for meaning and movement.

Any object, exposed to radiant energy, in the presence of free floating tritrons will undergo four levels of energy: Light, Heat, Deformation, Explosion (release of light and percussive force which affects both molecules and atoms). See Table 18.

Response of Material	State of a Material	Action when exposed to radiant energy
Origin of Light	Atomic level	Matter emits light energy at the wavelength where the combination of atoms is overloaded by the radiant energy striking the surface of the matter
Light	Sub^2 Atomic Level	Tritrons act as the medium for the transference of light and other electromagnetic energies
Heat	Molecular level	Vibration of the molecules comprising the matter
Deformation	Molecular level	Separation of molecular bonds
Explosion	Atomic level	Separation of inter atomic bonds

Table 18

Light of a particular color is the result of matter emitting light energy at the wavelength where the combination of atoms is overloaded by the radiant energy striking the surface of the matter. Heat is the result of vibration of molecules present in a material. Deformation occurs when molecular bonds are disrupted. Explosive energy occurs when inter atomic bonds are disrupted and atomic bond energy is released in sufficient magnitude.

POST SCRIPT NINE

Polymyalgia Rheumatica Explained

Polymyalgia rheumatica (PMR) is a mysterious illness that appears in a small subset of people over 60 years of age. There has been no known etiology formally identified as the cause for this affliction. Most often patients present to a physician complaining of muscle stiffness involving the shoulders, the neck muscles and the thigh muscles. People diagnosed with PMR will report difficulty lifting their arms to comb their hair, difficulty with movement of the neck and a progressively difficulty rising up out of a chair. Often this medical condition is accompanied by lack of appetite, weight loss, mild fever, and fatigue. Infrequently there may be a low red blood cell count or even a low platelet count. The most reliable serum study is the sed rate, which is regarded as being a serum marker of inflammation. A normal sed rate can be as high as thirty and as low as zero. When a patient is suffering from a serious bout of PMR, the sed rate is often above sixty. There is no other radiologic study or blood study that assists the doctor in making the diagnosis as to whether PMR is present or not. Specifically the muscle tests, the CPK and the aldolase are indeed normal in this disorder which presents as muscle stiffness. Even a biopsy of the muscles is generally found to be normal in patients suffering from PMR.

The cause of PMR, which can evolve into a very debilitating condition, remains unknown. Once the diagnosis is made, the treatment for PMR is generally oral corticosteroids. Corticosteroids or glucocorticoids (sugar-steroid) are a form of steroid that reduce inflammation in the body and are often used as a medical therapy to treat adverse inflammatory conditions. The intravenous form of glucocorticoid is hydrocortisone. Common oral forms of glucocorticoids include prednisone and methylprednisolone.

Providing a patient with PMR prednisone at a dose of 15 to 30 mg a day routinely will result in near complete resolution of the PMR symptoms within 5-10 days.

In the normal healthy adult, there are present two adrenal glands. The adrenal glands appear as slivers of tissue, positioned superior to the kidneys, one present on each side. The blood supply of the adrenal gland is married into the blood supply of the perspective kidney that the adrenal gland sits above. Since the blood supply of the adrenal gland and the kidney are joined, it is difficult to isolate and assess the output of the adrenal gland. It is approximated that the sum of the output of the two adrenal glands is equivalent to an oral dose of 7.5 mg of prednisone a day. The production of the glucocorticoids by the adrenal glands is rather minute at any given time and spread over a twenty-four hour cycle. Quantifying of the amount of glucocorticoids produced by the adrenal glands is challenging given the small amount that is in the blood stream at any given time.

If the adrenal glands make an excessive amount of glucocorticoids, such as in the case of a tumor present in one of the adrenal glands, this condition is referred to as Cushing's disease. Cushinoid patients often develop weight gain as they preferentially swell the face, trunk and abdomen. Glucocorticoids are considered a master hormone, which is necessary for life. When both adrenal glands shut down and fail to make any glucocorticoids, the body goes into crisis, which left uncorrected can lead to death. Adrenal failure is referred to as Addison's disease.

The behavior of the adrenal glands is poorly understood. The glucocorticoid output is difficult to measure. The absolutes of too much production of glucocorticoids or the lack of production of glucocorticoids can be determined, but how close a patient is making the equivalent of 7.5 mg of prednisone a day is difficult to measure and is a test that is not available to the clinician in general medical practice.

Most patients with PMR respond very quickly and successfully to the initial burst of prednisone. There are a number of conditions that mimic the symptoms of PMR, including some cancers, and therefore not all patients respond to treatment. Following the resolution of the patient's symptoms, when the dose of prednisone is slowly tapered, if the diagnosis is correct, the majority of patients usual continue to report they feel well.

Once the daily dose of prednisone is decreased below 5 mg a day, some of the patients report a recurrence of their symptoms. Clinical experience suggests that approximately 30-40% of the patients are able to successfully taper off the glucocorticoid supplement if the tapering is performed slow enough, such as in the order of deceasing the daily dose by 1 mg a month. Approximately 60% of the patients are not able to completely wean off the daily corticosteroid treatment. Some of the patients will identify that a chronic dose of 5 mg of prednisone a day is necessary for them to feel well. Other patients with PMR will identify that they require a daily dose of either 4 mg or 3 mg of prednisone a day in order to feel normal. Infrequent cases require 10 mg or 2 mg of prednisone on a daily basis in order for the treatment to be successful.

PMR remains an enigma of medicine. The etiology of the symptoms of PMR remains one of medicine's mysteries. Yet, if the treatment of this condition is almost exclusively the use of prednisone, then it could be extrapolated that the body lacks an adequate amount of glucocorticoid production. If the adrenal glands produce the equivalent of 7.5 mg of prednisone a day, half of this amount would be 3.75 mg a day. The amount of absorption of any oral form of medication varies from person to person. When a patient swallows a given dose of prednisone, they do not absorb all of the dose, a portion of the dose passes unused through the gastrointestinal tract. Therefore it makes sense than that if one of the two adrenal gland fails in a patient, the patient may require supplement of what the adrenal gland would normally produce in order to feel healthy since corticosteroids function as a master hormone and is necessary to the proper function of the human body. Further, it makes sense that a dosing range of 5 mg a day to 3 mg a day exists and is representative of successful treatment in patients since there is no control over the absorption of oral prednisone.

Medical conditions that cannot be precisely measured often remain mysteries. In the case of partial failure of the adrenal glands due to interruption of the blood supply to one or both of the adrenals or a disease state infiltrating the adrenal tissues or failure of adrenal cells due to factors related to aging, the clinician is blind to this phenomenon due to an inability to properly measure the glucocorticoid output of the two adrenal glands. Deductive reasoning suggests that the condition of PMR is a problem directly related to dysfunction of one or both adrenal glands.

Permanent loss of glucocorticoid production by one of the adrenal glands necessitates a chronic supplement of low dose oral corticosteroids. Brief loss of partial glucocorticoid production by the adrenal glands necessitates supplementing the patient with symptoms consistent with PMR during the time segment the adrenal gland(s) is recovering. Denying a patient with PMR their corticosteroid treatment may place the patient in a state of grave ill health.

As with any treatment, the use of chronic corticosteroids can lead to unwanted side effects. Consulting and being monitored by a trained healthcare professional before and during chronic corticosteroid treatment is advisable. Unwanted side effects may still occur despite close observation by a healthcare professional; in some cases adverse outcomes are unavoidable, but ideally can be minimized.

POST SCRIPT TEN

A Systems Engineer's Approach to a Cure for HIV

The Human Immunodeficiency Virus's (HIV) genome is read from the 5' region to the 3' region. The HIV DNA genome is approximately 9719 base pairs in length; like most genomes variation exists with HIV's genome. The following is an example since variation in Nature does exist. HIV's genome is divided into several regions including: 5' LTR (1-634), gag (790-2292), pol (2085-5096), vif (5041-5619), vpr (5559-5850), env (6225-8795), nef (8797-9417) and 3' LTR (9086-9719).

The initial portion of the HIV DNA genome is termed the Long Terminal Repeat (LTR) located at the 5' region. The LTR is comprised of the regions indentified as U3, R and U5. The LTR is comprised of the nucleotide base pairs (bp) from 1-634.

The TATA box is considered a means of signaling to the cell's transcription machinery that a segment of transcribable genetic information follows downstream from that point. At bp 427 in the LTR is located the first nucleotide of a TATA box. At bp 456 starts the messenger RNA of the HIV genome. Between the TATA box and the location of the transcribable messenger RNA of the HIV genome is a space of 25 nucleotide base pairs. The nucleotides of this 25 base pair segment are 'AGCAGCTGCTTTTTGCCTGTACTGG'. **See Figure 19 in Chapter 28.** Differing strains of HIV may have this 25-nucleotide segment in differing locations in the viral genome.

This segment of 25-nucleotide base pairs has been compared to the human genome. No such 25-character segments have been found to exist the human genome.

At first glance this may appear to be a setback. If the 25 base pair segment are 'AGCAGCTGCTTTTTGCCTGTACTGG' truly represents a unique identifier then one might expect that HIV uses this identifier because the identifier mimics a naturally occurring identifier already present in the human genome. That when the life-cycle of the cell naturally activates the human gene using this 25 character identifier, the HIV genome is also simultaneously activated. This sharing of a human gene's unique identifier would explain the dormant state the HIV genome appears to experience prior to the HIV genome becoming active and taking control of cellular functions.

On the other hand, the observation that the segment 'AGCAGCTGCTTTTTGCCTGTACTGG' does not appear in the human genome suggests that this segment is indeed unique to HIV. Meaning that this segment, which appears at the beginning of the transcribable portion of the HIV genome, is a vulnerability of the HIV genome. Treatment strategies can be directed at this segment and not affect the human genome because there appears no 25 character segment in the human genome identical to this segment. See Figure 48.

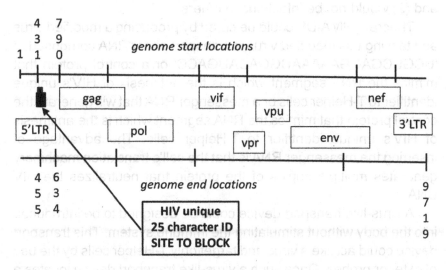

FIGURE 48

Inserting a RNA or a nuclear signaling protein that would attach to the unique identifier in the HIV genome to prevent the HIV genome from being transcribed

Treatment strategies include either an RNA or a nuclear signaling protein that would permanently attach to this unique segment of HIV, following exposure to HIV, either while the segment was present in the cytoplasm or after the segment has been spliced into the human DNA in a T-Helper cell. The RNA segment 'UCGUCGACGAAAAACGGACAUGACC' would represent the antithesis of the DNA segment 'AGCAGCTGCTTTTTGCCTGTACTGG'. An RNA composed of 'UCGUCGACGAAAAACGGACAUGACC' or a control protein that mimics the RNA segment which is the antithesis of HIV's unique identifier would attach to the DNA along the HIV DNA genome and block the ability for the HIV genome to be transcribed. If the HIV genome cannot be transcribed the threat of HIV to the infected T-Helper cell has in effect been neutralized. Not being capable of being transcribed, the HIV genome is then unable to take control of the T-Helper cell and redirect the T-Helper cell's internal mechanisms to produce copies of the HIV virion. Such a patient would (1) not succumb to the deleterious effects of the presence of the HIV virion and (2) would not be infectious to others.

Theoretically AIDS could be cured by producing a modified virus and tasking this modified virus to transport either RNA composed of 'UCGUCGACGAAAAACGGACAUGACC' or a control protein that mimics the RNA segment which is the antithesis of HIV's unique identifier to T-Helper cells or a messenger RNA that will generate the control protein that mimics the RNA segment which is the antithesis of HIV's unique identifier to T-Helper cells. The advantage of inserting the messenger RNA is that the cell's translation machinery generates multiple copies of the protein that neutralizes the HIV DNA.

A virus-like transport device could be designed to be introduced into the body without stimulating the immune system. This transport device could act like a virus and target only T-Helper cells by the use of exterior probes. Once such a virus-like transport device locates a desired T-Helper cell, the device inserts the either RNA composed of 'UCGUCGACGAAAAACGGACAUGACC' or a nuclear signaling control protein that mimics the RNA segment which is the antithesis of HIV's unique identifier into T-Helper cells. An alternative to inserting an RNA or nuclear signaling protein would be to insert a messenger RNA coded to generate the nuclear signaling control protein. Conceivably, a segment of DNA that would produce an mRNA that could be transcribed to produce the nuclear signaling control protein could be inserted into T-Helper cells that would continuously produce the nuclear signaling protein that would block the functionality of the HIV genome if present in the T-Helper cell.

The virus-like transport device contains no other functional part other than the means to block transcription of the HIV genome and therefore poses no noxious effects to the body. The virus-like transport device contains no reproduction genetic information and is incapable of replicating itself in the human body and therefore again poses no ongoing infections threat. This approach could be very effective in eliminating the noxious effects of HIV DNA in some patients infected with the AIDS virus.

Given there is variability in the HIV genome amongst differing strains of HIV, a fully effective strategy would need to take in account the presence of the 25-nucleotide strand and location of the strand in the various genomes infecting the population. In circumstances where the 25-nucleotide strand is not present, or it is present but the location is such that blocking its functionality would not deter the transcribability of the HIV genome, possibly another 25-nucleotide strand could be utilized in such strains of HIV. To effectively cure HIV, more than one segment of the HIV genome may need to be targeted by an RNA or nuclear signaling protein designed to physically adhere to the HIV DNA genome to prevent the genome from being transcribed, thus neutralizing the action and therefore the threat of HIV.

POST SCRIPT ELEVEN

Mars Proof-of-Origin Project

Hypothesis: The Milky Way galaxy is estimated to be 13.2 billion years old. Primordial Earth offered the ideal environment comprised of an abundance of raw materials and a fiery natural engine on which to cultivate life. Between 4.6 billion years ago and 3.5 billion years ago the seeds of life, referred to as Vironix particles, migrated through the solar system carried along by the solar winds. The Vironix particles were impervious to the low levels of radiation present in deep space. The seeds present in the Vironix particles were designed to travel extreme distances and remain in hibernation indefinitely, until the proper conditions were encountered in our galaxy, sufficient for the genetic programming contained in the seeds to flourish properly and produce life.

Analysis of the atmosphere of the planets in our solar system suggests the atmospheric characteristics of Venus, Earth and Mars were artificially altered. Ammonia (NH_3) is a naturally occurring component of an atmosphere often seen in volcanic emissions. The presence of nitrogen gas (N_2) in an atmosphere of a planet is a component of an atmosphere that is artificially placed in the atmosphere by the presence of an extraterrestrial catalyst. Where the conditions on Venus were too hostile, on Earth life flourished, the environmental conditions present on Mars may be preserving evidence of the earliest proof of origin of life in the form of seeds that contain the Prime Genome.

Objective: To prove that life on Earth was due to the work of an extraterrestrial genome, that has acted as a catalyst and that evidence of this can be found as specimens of the Prime Genome still present in the atmosphere or soil samples on Mars.

Project: Mars Lander spacecraft to conduct experiments on the surface of Mars to demonstrate the presence of the Prime Genome on Mars.

Description: On Earth, the Prime Genome can only be estimated. Reconstruction of the Prime Genome by combining the genomes of all of the life currently on the planet lacks segments lost due to extinction of previous forms of life. The genomes present on the Earth represent fragments of the original Prime Genome.

Examination of the contents of the atmosphere of the Sun and the planets comprising the solar system suggest five stages of development of the atmospheric conditions. See Table 19. The most primitive atmosphere (Stage 1) is comprised predominantly of hydrogen and helium gases such as seen in the atmosphere of the Sun, Mercury, Jupiter, Saturn, Uranus and Neptune. A slightly more advance atmosphere is comprised of carbon dioxide and ammonia gas (Stage 2). The next phase of atmospheric development (Stage 3), capable of supporting primitive life, is comprised of carbon dioxide, nitrogen gas and water vapor. Water vapor is converted to liquid water due to cooling of the temperatures on the surface of the planet caused in part by the alterations to the composition of gases in the atmosphere partially protecting the surface from the radiant energy of the sun. Venus and Mars contain predominantly carbon dioxide and a small amount of nitrogen gas. The fourth stage is comprised of predominantly nitrogen, oxygen, water vapor and a progressively dwindling amount of carbon dioxide. Carbon dioxide is actively being consumed by a large variety of ocean dwelling life. The final phase (Stage 5) atmosphere, capable of supporting animal life, is comprised predominantly nitrogen, a significant amount of oxygen, water vapor, ozone present in the upper layers and <1% carbon dioxide. On Earth the atmosphere is comprised of 79% nitrogen and 21% oxygen.

If a Prime Genome of extraterrestrial origin labored to create environmental conditions sufficient to support organic life, then the analysis of the atmosphere surrounding Venus and Mars suggests two planets that progress from the most primitive form of atmosphere, but stalled at the second phase of atmosphere. The atmosphere of both Venus and Mars transformed from hydrogen and helium, to the second stage atmosphere of carbon dioxide and nitrogen, but failed to advance to the mixture of nitrogen and oxygen which could support oxidative respiration, necessary for life as we know it.

Venus and Mars appear to be locked in Stage Three of the planetary atmospheric transformation process. Earth advanced to Stage Five of the transformation process.

Venus failed to advance to a life supporting atmosphere most likely due to an excessive amount radiation from the Sun scorching the surface of Venus due to the second planet's close proximity to the Sun.

Mars failed to advance to a life supporting atmosphere most likely due to an insufficient amount radiant energy from the sun due to the fourth planet's distance from the sun. Mars also failed to advance to a life-supporting planet due to the planet's molten core becoming inactive, which terminated the release of volcanic gases and volcanic energy into the atmosphere. Given that Mars is a cooler neighbor due to the greater distance from the sun and there is a lack of volcanic activity, Mars may be harboring traces of primordial life-generating seeds caught in a state of perpetual suspended animation.

Stage	Phase	Dominant Atmospheric Gases	Description
1	Primordial Phase 1	Helium and Hydrogen	Primordial Earth
2	Primordial Phase 2	Carbon dioxide and ammonia	Volcanic eruptions emit carbon dioxide and ammonia gas into atmosphere, hydrogen and helium pushed to outer atmosphere and drift into space
3	N_2 Photosynthesis	Carbon dioxide, Nitrogen, water	Extra terrestrial catalyst introduced, converts CO_2 and NH_3 to N_2 and H_2O
4	O_2 Photosynthesis	Nitrogen, oxygen, water, carbon dioxide	Photosynthesis converts carbon dioxide and water to oxygen and glucose. Mass transformation of the primary genome occurs in the oceans. Primary genome causes a wide variety of life to begin to appear. Survival depends upon best species design to adapt to prevailing conditions.

5	Ozone Synthesis	Nitrogen, oxygen, ozone, water, carbon dioxide	Ozone naturally occurs creating the final phase. Due to protection afforded by ozone, life is capable of existing on land. Primary Genome continues to generate mass replication of the life. Survival depends upon best species design to adapt to prevailing conditions.

Table 19

The Five Stages of Atmospheric conditions.

If such primordial seeds do exist on Mars, the existence of such seeds may not be in a form that is generally expected given the state of transition the planet's atmosphere is in at this time. Such primordial seeds, if they exist, would potentially behave in a manner that may not generally be expected for one seeking direct evidence of organic life. Primordial seeds containing the Prime Genome may be primarily engaged in converting carbon dioxide gas and ammonia gas into nitrogen gas, oxygen and water rather than engaged in replication. Unlike organic life present on the Earth, which in the case of a chlorophyll-containing plant would utilize carbon dioxide to produce oxygen and glucose, or an animal that would utilized oxygen and glucose in aerobic respiration, the biologic programming in primordial seeds would recognize that the conditions of Mars's atmosphere could not support glucose as a medium of energy transfer and could not support nitrogen fixation to support organic life as we know it to exist on Earth.

In the mid seventies NASA sent the Viking lander to Mars. NASA's Viking lander analyzed material from the Martian surface. Life detecting experiments indicated the presence of oxidized organic material near the surface, though this oxidation was thought to be the result of a chemical reaction caused by naturally occurring hydrogen peroxide present on Mars. The NASA Phoenix lander touched down on Mars's north pole on May 25, 2008. The Phoenix lander sent back information for five months. The unit went silent presumably due to ice buildup on the solar arrays which irreversibly damaged the solar arrays. Without the solar arrays functioning, the Phoenix lander lost its capacity to generate electricity, which led to the space probe going dark. The Phoenix lander did verify

291

that there does exist water in the form of ice in the Martian surface soil. Phoenix also recorded snow falling on Mars. Evidence for the existence of life or the potential to produce organic life has yet to be discovered on Mars.

The Experiment:

To engage in an experiment to investigate for evidence of the presence of seeds that contain the Prime Genome, a landing craft would be sent to Mars. See Figure 49. Such an intra-planetary landing craft would act as a platform for a number of experiments. The tests are listed in Table 20.

Test	Conditions: Heat cycling between 80-110 degrees F. Radiant energy cycling to mimic night/day cycles.	Expected Results if Primordial Seeds containing Prime Genome exist on Mars in the atmosphere or in the soil.
1	Carbon dioxide gas + Nitrogen gas	Increase in nitrogen gas content. Formation of oxygen gas. Formation of water.
2	80% Carbon dioxide gas + 20% Ammonia gas	Increase in percentage of nitrogen gas content. Formation of oxygen gas. Formation of water.
3	79% Nitrogen gas + 21% Oxygen gas	Evidence of the formation of cell structures. Formation of carbon dioxide.
4	Carbon dioxide gas + Nitrogen gas + Water	Increase in percentage of nitrogen gas content. Formation of oxygen gas.
5	80% Carbon dioxide gas + 20% Ammonia gas + Water	Increase in nitrogen gas content. Formation of oxygen gas.
6	79% Nitrogen gas + 21% Oxygen gas + Water	Formation of carbon dioxide. Evidence of the formation of cell structures.
7	Carbon dioxide gas + Nitrogen gas + Water and glucose	Increase in percentage of nitrogen gas content. Consumption of glucose.
8	80% Carbon dioxide gas + 20% Ammonia gas + Water and glucose	Increase in nitrogen gas content. Consumption of glucose.
9	79% Nitrogen gas+ 21% Oxygen gas + Water and glucose	Formation of carbon dioxide. Consumption of glucose. Evidence of the formation of cell structures.

Table 20
Types of testing and expected outcomes to measure.

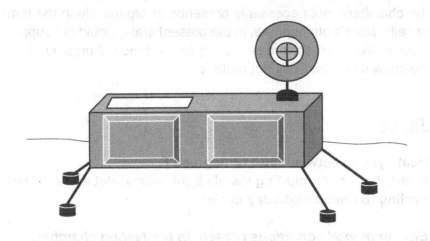

Figure 49
Mars Lander to seek out Prime Genome

The primordial seeds may be submicroscopic, having dimensions of between a bacteria and a virus. Most Earth viruses range in 5 to 300 nanometers (10^{-9} m). Eukaryote cells are typically 10 times larger than prokaryote cells. Prokaryotes average 1-10 micrometers (10^{-6} m), while eukaryotes 10-100 micrometers. The diameter of a DNA alpha helix is 2 nm. The average cell in the human body is 50 micrometers or 0.05 mm. The unaided human eye can see up to 0.1 mm long. The light microscope is limited by the wavelength of visible light which is about 500 nm. Electron microscopes are used to investigate objects less than 500 nm in size. Since the primordial seeds of life may be between 5 to 500 nm in diameter, simple light microscopy may not detect their presence. The primordial seeds of life may be present in either the atmosphere of Mars or in the soil of Mars.

All tests would be conducted in separate testing chambers inside the Mars landing craft that are sealed once air samples and soil samples are retrieved from the planet's surface. A sample of the Martian soil would be present in each testing chamber and exposed directly to atmospheric conditions inside the testing chamber.

Testing would be seeking evidence of changes in the conditions of the chambers, not necessarily presence of organic life in the form of cells. Mars's atmosphere, in the present state, would not support organic life and therefore searching for evidence of organic life as we know it is most likely not realistic.

Test 1

Heat cycling between 80-110 degrees F.
Radiant energy including visible light, ultraviolet and infrared, cycling to mimic night/day cycles.

Environmental conditions present in the testing chamber:
Carbon dioxide gas + Nitrogen gas

Description: A sample of the atmosphere present on the surface of Mars would be introduced into the test chamber. A sample of Mars's soil would be placed in a well in the testing chamber. The chamber would be incubated.
Expected results to be monitored for include:

  (1) Increase in nitrogen gas content.
  (2) Formation of oxygen gas.
  (3) Formation of water.

Test 2

Heat cycling between 80-110 degrees F.
Radiant energy including visible light, ultraviolet and infrared, cycling to mimic night/day cycles.

Variable environmental conditions present in the testing chamber:
80% Carbon dioxide gas + 20% Ammonia gas

Description: A sample of the atmosphere present on the surface of Mars would be introduced into the test chamber. A small portion of ammonia gas would be added to the Martian atmosphere. A sample of Mars's soil would be placed in a well in the testing chamber. The chamber would be incubated.

Expected results to be monitored for include:

(1) Increase in percentage of nitrogen gas content.
(2) Formation of oxygen gas.
(3) Formation of water.

Test 3

Heat cycling between 80-110 degrees F.
Radiant energy including visible light, ultraviolet and infrared, cycling to mimic night/day cycles.

Environmental conditions present in the testing chamber:

79% Nitrogen gas + 21% Oxygen gas

Description: A sample of the atmosphere present on the surface of Mars would be sucked into the test chamber. The Martian atmosphere would be mixed with a gaseous mixture of 79% nitrogen and 21% oxygen. The carbon dioxide would be removed from the gas mixture. A sample of Mars's soil would be placed in a well in the testing chamber. The chamber would be incubated.

Expected results to be monitored for include:

(1) Evidence of the formation of cell structures.
(2) Formation of carbon dioxide.

Test 4

Heat cycling between 80-110 degrees F.

Radiant energy including visible light, ultraviolet and infrared, cycling to mimic night/day cycles.

Environmental conditions present in the testing chamber:
Carbon dioxide gas + Nitrogen gas + Water

Description: A sample of the atmosphere present on the surface of Mars would be introduced into the test chamber. A sample of Mars's soil would be placed in a holding chamber inside the testing chamber. Liquid water would be introduced into the holding chamber together with the Martial soil. The chamber would be incubated.

The expected results to be monitored for include:

(1) Increase in percentage of nitrogen gas content.
(2) Formation of oxygen gas.

Test 5

Heat cycling between 80-110 degrees F.
Radiant energy including visible light, ultraviolet and infrared, cycling to mimic night/day cycles.

Environmental conditions present in the testing chamber:

80% Carbon dioxide gas + 20% Ammonia gas + Water

Description: A sample of the atmosphere present on the surface of Mars would be sucked into the test chamber. A small portion of ammonia gas would be added to the Martian atmosphere. A sample of Mars's soil would be placed in a holding chamber inside the testing chamber. Liquid water would be introduced into the holding chamber together with the Martial soil. The chamber would be incubated.

Expected results to be monitored for include:

(1) Increase in nitrogen gas content.
(2) Formation of oxygen gas.

Test 6

Heat cycling between 80-110 degrees F.
Radiant energy including visible light, ultraviolet and infrared, cycling to mimic night/day cycles.

Variable environmental conditions present in the testing chamber:
79% Nitrogen gas + 21% Oxygen gas + Water

Description: A sample of the atmosphere present on the surface of Mars would be introduced into the test chamber. The Martian atmosphere would be mixed with a gaseous mixture of 79% nitrogen and 21% oxygen. The carbon dioxide would be removed from the gas mixture. A sample of Mars's soil would be placed in a holding chamber inside the testing chamber. Liquid water would be introduced into the holding chamber together with the Martial soil. The chamber would be incubated.

The expected results to be monitored for include:

(1) Formation of carbon dioxide.
(2) Evidence of the formation of cell structures.

Test 7

Heat cycling between 80-110 degrees F.
Radiant energy including visible light, ultraviolet and infrared, cycling to mimic night/day cycles.

Environmental conditions present in the testing chamber:

Carbon dioxide gas + Nitrogen gas + Water and glucose

Description: A sample of the atmosphere present on the surface of Mars would be introduced into the test chamber. A sample of Mars's soil would be placed in a holding chamber inside the testing chamber. Liquid water mixed with glucose would be introduced into the holding chamber together with the Martial soil. The chamber would be incubated.

Expected results to be monitored for include:

  (1) Increase in percentage of nitrogen gas content.
  (2) Consumption of glucose.

Test 8

Heat cycling between 80-110 degrees F.
Radiant energy including visible light, ultraviolet and infrared, cycling to mimic night/day cycles.

Environmental conditions present in the testing chamber:
80% Carbon dioxide gas + 20% Ammonia gas + Water and glucose

Description: A sample of the atmosphere present on the surface of Mars would be introduced into the test chamber. A small portion of ammonia gas would be added to the Martian atmosphere. A sample of Mars's soil would be placed in a holding chamber inside the testing chamber. Liquid water mixed with glucose would be introduced into the holding chamber together with the Martial soil. The chamber would be incubated.

Expected results to be monitored for include:

  (1) Increase in nitrogen gas content.
  (2) Consumption of glucose.

Test 9

Heat cycling between 80-110 degrees F.
Radiant energy including visible light, ultraviolet and infrared, cycling to mimic night/day cycles.

Environmental conditions present in the testing chamber:
79% Nitrogen gas+ 21% Oxygen gas + Water and glucose

Description: A sample of the atmosphere present on the surface of Mars would be introduced into the test chamber. The Martian atmosphere would be mixed with a gaseous mixture of 79% nitrogen and 21% oxygen. The carbon dioxide would be removed from the gas mixture. A sample of Mars's soil would be placed in a holding chamber inside the testing chamber. Liquid water would be introduced into the holding chamber together with the Martial soil. The chamber would be incubated.

Expected results to be monitored for include:

(1) Formation of carbon dioxide.
(2) Consumption of glucose.
(3) Evidence of the formation of cell structures.

Time to Achievement of Expected Results:

The conversion of Earth's atmosphere spanned at least from 4.6 billion years ago to 3.5 billion years ago when life first appeared. Once life first appeared the first animals did not appear until 600 million years ago, suggesting Earth's atmosphere could not support oxidative respiration prior to 600 million years ago. Oxidative respiration in animal cells facilitates the efficient conversion of glucose to ATP, with ATP molecules utilized to energize many cellular chemical reactions. To support oxidative respiration in animals, the atmospheric levels of carbon dioxide would have had to been dramatically reduced from levels of the primordial atmosphere, and the levels of oxygen would have had to have dramatically increased.

299

Analyzing the information suggests it took four billion years for the Earth's atmosphere to be converted to a form that could support organic life that utilizes oxidative respiration to obtain energy. Therefore, the expected results of the above-mentioned experiment may take a while to become measurably apparent.

Expected Outcome for Proof of Origin

If any of the above-mentioned outcomes are observed, the presence of an extraterrestrial catalyst is proven. See Table 21. The extraterrestrial catalyst would be the Prime Genome in the form of seeds, otherwise referred to as Vironix particles.

Test	Variable Test Conditions	Interpretation of results
1	Sample Mars atmosphere: 96% Mars's carbon dioxide gas + 3% Mars's Nitrogen gas	If the Prime Genome is present in the atmosphere or soil and is set between the N_2 photosynthesis mode and the O_2 photosynthesis mode, there should be observed an increase in nitrogen gas content and formation of water or formation of oxygen and possibly the formation of early cell structures.
2	80% Mars's Carbon dioxide gas + 20% Ammonia gas	If the Prime Genome is present in the atmosphere or soil and is set in the N_2 photosynthesis mode there should be observed an increase in nitrogen gas content and formation of water.
3	79% Nitrogen gas + 21% Oxygen gas + trace Mars's carbon dioxide gas	If the Prime Genome is present in the atmosphere or soil and is set in the O_2 photosynthesis mode, there may be evidence of the formation of cell structures; though without the presence of water this is less likely.
4	Sample Mars atmosphere: 96% Mars's carbon dioxide gas + 3% Mars's Nitrogen gas + water (H_2O)	If the Prime Genome is present in the atmosphere or soil and is set between the N_2 photosynthesis mode and the O_2 photosynthesis mode, there should be observed an increase in nitrogen gas content and formation of water or formation of oxygen and possibly the formation of early cell structures.
5	80% Mars's Carbon dioxide gas + 20% Ammonia gas + water (H_2O)	If the Prime Genome is present in the atmosphere or soil and is set in the N_2 photosynthesis mode there should be observed an increase in nitrogen gas content and formation of water.

6	79% Nitrogen gas + 21% Oxygen gas + trace Mars's carbon dioxide gas + water (H_2O)	If the Prime Genome is present in the atmosphere or soil and is set in the O_2 photosynthesis mode, there may be evidence of the formation of cell structures. If the Prime Genome is present in the atmosphere or soil and is set in the O_2 photosynthesis mode, there may be evidence of the formation of cell structures.
7	Sample Mars atmosphere: 96% Mars's carbon dioxide gas + 3% Mars's Nitrogen gas + water (H_2O) and glucose	If the Prime Genome is present in the atmosphere or soil and is set between the N_2 photosynthesis mode and the O_2 photosynthesis mode, there should be observed an increase in nitrogen gas content and formation of water or formation of oxygen and possibly the formation of early cell structures. Consumption of glucose.
8	80% Mars's Carbon dioxide gas + add 20% Ammonia gas + water (H_2O) and glucose	If the Prime Genome is present in the atmosphere or soil and is set in the N_2 photosynthesis mode there should be observed an increase in nitrogen gas content and formation of water. Consumption of glucose.
9	79% Nitrogen gas+ 21% Oxygen gas + trace Mars's carbon dioxide gas + water (H_2O) and glucose	If the Prime Genome is present in the atmosphere or soil and is set in the O_2 photosynthesis mode, there may be evidence of the formation of cell structures. If the Prime Genome is present in the atmosphere or soil and is set in the O_2 photosynthesis mode, there may be evidence of the formation of cell structures. Consumption of glucose.

Table 21

Expected Results from the Mars Experiments.

If an extraterrestrial catalyst is determined to be present on Mars, then additional studies including collection of soil and air samples for the purpose of electron microscopic studies would be in order. Understanding how the Prime Genome was structured would lead to evidence of origin of life as well as be a monumental achievement in understanding how life flourished on Earth. The medical opportunities afforded by understanding such genetic information would be astronomical.

Mapping Out Origin of Life

The solar system the Earth resides in located in the Milky Way Galaxy. The Milky Way is considered to be a disk-shaped spiral galaxy with a bar-shaped center measuring approximately 120 light-years in diameter. The Milky Way is thought to be comprised of two major spiral arms, the Peseus arm and the Scutum-Centarous arm. There are a number of smaller spiral arms. Earth's solar system is located in a smaller adjunct arm known as the Orion-Cygnus arm, located between the two major arms. The location of our solar system is approximately 28,000 light years from the center of the Milky Way and 25,000 light years from the outer rim of the galaxy. The Milky Way is thought to contain between 200 to 400 billion stars. The estimated age of the Milky Way is 13.2 billion years. It is estimated that it takes 250 million years for Earth's solar system to make one complete orbit around the center of the Milky Way.

Considering that a significant amount of nitrogen gas (N_2) is generated in the atmosphere of a planet as the result of the presence of an extraterrestrial catalyst, then nitrogen gas becomes the perfect biomarker with which to explore the universe from our fixed perspective on the Earth. Planets with atmospheres containing nitrogen gas are planets that have been influenced by the Prime Genome. As technology becomes further refined, astronomers will be able to detect the possible presence of life on distance planets by identifying the presence and the percentage of nitrogen gas in the atmosphere of planets. By doing such an analysis, the path the Primary Genome has taken through the Milky Way galaxy can be plotted. See Figure 50. The percentage of nitrogen gas present in the atmosphere of planets in neighboring solar systems will indicate what state of influence of the Prime Genome on planets in neighboring solar systems.

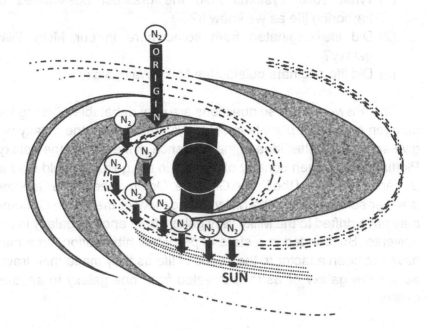

Figure 50
Plotting the Origin of Prime Genome

The composition of atmosphere of planets (1) Primordial State 1: helium/hydrogen, (2) Primordial State 2: Carbon dioxide and ammonia, (2) Prime Genome State 1: Carbon dioxide, Nitrogen, water vapor, (4) Prime Genome State 2: Nitrogen, Oxygen, water vapor, <1% carbon dioxide, and (5) Prime Genome State 3: Nitrogen, Oxygen, Ozone, water vapor, <1% carbon dioxide. Plotting out the pattern of atmospheric conditions of planets across the galaxy may point toward the origin of the Prime Genome in the galaxy, with planets that contain Prime Genome State 3 consisting of Nitrogen, Oxygen, Ozone, water vapor, <1% carbon dioxide being planets that have the highest likelihood of sustaining life.

Plotting the nitrogen content of the atmospheres of planets around our galaxy will lead to answering the timeless questions of:

(1) What solar systems hold the greatest possibilities of harboring life as we know it?

(2) Did life originated from somewhere in our Milky Way galaxy?

(3) Did life originate outside the Milky Way galaxy?

The answers to these questions are very debatable. Plotting the nitrogen content of planets in solar systems around the galaxy will give science a better idea of the presence of life across the galaxy. Plotting the nitrogen content of planets in the galaxy should lead to evidence of origin of the Prime Genome. Origin of the Prime Genome is either somewhere in the Milky Way galaxy or the Prime Genome may have drifted to the Milky Way galaxy from another galaxy in the universe. Suspended in a state of perpetual hibernation, time may have not been a factor to the seeds of life as they made their travel across the galaxy or as they traveled from one galaxy to another galaxy.

Conclusion

We witness the work of seeds throughout the environment. A sperm cell unites with an egg cell and from the union a zygote appears, and from this single fertilized egg cell the entire human body is constructed. The helicopter appearing Dandelion seed takes flight and drifts off in the wind migrating aimlessly in search of fertile ground in which to lay roots and, if the conditions are just right, produce a copy of the parent plant that originally produced the seed. Plants of all sorts fill the air with seeds in hopes that like the Dandelion, they too will produce offspring that will continue the circle of life. The giant Redwood coniferous evergreen timber tree, that can reach 300 feet in height, starts as a single seed. Many aquatic and amphibians species produce thousands to millions of fertilized eggs in hopes that a few will survive the hostile conditions of the planet, mature and live long enough to repeat the life-cycle. The concept that our galaxy was seeded with the opportunity to generate life is not beyond the imagination if we study what nature is trying to teach us.

Charles Darwin's theory of evolution was brilliant at the time it was contrived, and Darwin was epic in his effort to stand by his theory against the prevailing teachings of his time. The importance of the nitrogen cycle on the existence of life is undeniable. Like a caterpillar undergoing metamorphosis and transforming into a butterfly, the time has come to incorporate new data and transcend our current perspective of evolution, that is Darwin's Theory of Evolution, to a new updated perspective the Prime Genome Theory of Evolution and Ecometabolous.

Prior to stepping foot onto a distant planet or retrieving any substance from one of our neighboring planets it becomes imperative that we fully understand the programming principles of the human genome, viruses and bacteria. Though the Prime Genome may have facilitated the emergence of the human form on Earth, this same program may have facilitated the existence of viruses, bacteriophages and bacteria on other planets that could pose a deadly threat to humans. An alien pathogen may possess the means of circumventing our natural immune defense mechanisms, creating a plague of biblical proportions. Before we send humans to other planets we need to insure that we can protect our genome and that we understand how to sufficiently defend ourselves from pathogens that could be laying in wait in the extraterrestrial soil of some distant planet.

Final Collective Thought:

The entire universe can be summarized into the Universal Primary Equation:

Universe[1] = Energy (conserved) + Tritrons (conserved) + Space to be occupied

GLOSSARY & ABBREVIATIONS

Black Hole: Term of description that identifies the side of a galactic vortex that acts as the inbound event horizon where electromagnetic energy such as light and tritrons are drawn into a galactic vortex.

Carbohydrate: The general name for simple sugars as well as complex sugar molecules.

C³i: Command, Control, Communications, and Intelligence

Command RNA (cmRNA): A RNA molecule that provided command instructions to the endoplasmic reticulum or the Golgi apparatus to facilitate how a protein is to be constructed.

Control RNA (cnRNA): A small RNA molecule that acts as the antithesis of a unique identifier such that when a gene is transcribed, a cnRNA is generated that points to a sequential gene to be transcribed by the cnRNA physically migrating to the site of the unique identifier and attaching to a unique identifier of a gene, thus activating the construction of a transcription complex at the site of attachment and thus causing the gene to be transcribed.

Crux of the Nitrogen Cycle: It is virtually impossible to readily fix life-promoting quantities of nitrogen into nitrogen containing organic molecules without the presence of an extraterrestrial catalyst.

DNA: Deoxyribonucleic acid

Ecometabolous: The intention and action of the Prime DNA Genome which has resulted in the complete metamorphosis of the ecosystem of the planet with the expected outcome being the creation of the higher order of organic life known as homo sapiens or 'man' facilitated by the combination of (1) a preprogrammed collection of available genetic instructions spanning all organic life and viruses that have occupied the planet since the inception of life on the planet and (2) a selection of successful genomes based on survival of the fittest given the prevailing environmental factors present at the time.

Electron: A sub atomic particle comprised of sub-sub atomic tripolar particles known as tritrons, these tritrons arranged in a shell-like shape with the negative state pointed outward and the positive and neutral states pointed inward, with the center of the collection of tritrons harboring a quantum of energy.

Extraterrestrial Catalyst: A sub program in the Prime Genome that promoted the alteration of the atmosphere by means of N_2 Photosynthesis transferring the dominant carbon dioxide and ammonia atmosphere to an atmosphere comprised of nitrogen gas, methane and water; further, the genetic instructions contained in the Prime Genome provided the templates for the construction of enzymes and other molecules to fix nitrogen into nitrogen containing organic molecules.

Exon: A segment of the transcribable portion of a gene that, following RNA splicing, becomes a segment of the messenger RNA.

Galactic Vortex: A galactic engine represented by a region of infinitely high density located at the center of a galaxy where the magnitude of gravity is sufficient to attract (1) tritron particles and (2) electromagnetic energy, including light, such that tritrons and light are displaced from one location to be drawn into the galactic vortex through the event horizon known as a black hole, passed through a spiraling funnel located in the central plane of the galaxy to a location on the opposing side of the central plane to be ejected out of the galactic vortex through the radiant apex.

Gene: Unit of inheritance that contains transcribable genetic information that will produce messenger RNA that can be translated to produce a protein.

Genetic Reference Table (GRT): A segment of genetic material present in nuclear DNA associated with a unique identifier that is comprised of a series of transcribable sequences that when such sequences are transcribed result in one or more control RNA molecules.

Gravity: The attractive force between planets, stars, and galactic vortexes and charged atomic objects, generated by passage of energy through a core in the center of a planet, a star or a galactic vortex created by the alignment of tritrons such that the neutral end of the tritrons attracts positive and negatively charged objects.

HIV's Unique Identifier: 25 character bp string: 'AGCAGCTGCTTTTTGCCTGTACTGG' located in HIV's genome from 431 bp to 455 bp.

Holometabolous: Complete metamorphosis. This is a term that has been applied to the complete metamorphosis observed in some insects. Holometabola refers to a series of ten orders of insects including Coleoptera (beetles), Hymenoptera (bees, wasps, ants), Lepidoptera (moths and butterflies), Diptera (two-winged flies), and Siphonaptera (fleas), which undergo complete metamorphosis.

Hox gene: Genes that act as master control switches exerting control over a series of genes to direct cells to differentiate into specific cell types in order to generate the organs and limbs oriented in their proper position necessary to create a particular species.

Intron: A segment of the transcribable portion of a gene that, following RNA splicing, is removed before the exons contained in the gene are spliced together to form the resultant messenger RNA.

Ligand: A ligand is a molecule that acts to convey a signal by binding to one or more other molecules to form a molecular complex. The presence of a ligand causes the resultant molecular complex to perform an intended function; the absence of the ligand prevents the molecular complex from performing the intended function.

Magnetic Field: An energy field capable of work created by energy passing between the positive pole and negative pole of a magnet facilitated by the alignment of tritrons inside and outside the boundaries of the magnet through which conserved energy continuously flows, this conserved energy flowing in a circular manner out of the positive pole of the magnet around the perimeter of the magnet and back into the magnet through the negative pole of the magnet to flow back to the positive pole in a perpetual cycle.

Medical Vector Therapy: The use of transport devices such as modified viruses to deliver a specific payload to a specific target cell to effect a medical therapy.

Neutron: A sub atomic particle comprised of sub-sub atomic tripolar particles known as tritrons, these tritrons arranged in a shell-like shape with the neutral state pointed outward and the positive and negative states pointed inward, with the center of the collection of tritrons harboring a quantum of energy.

N_2 Photosynthesis: Catalyst driven conversion of carbon dioxide (CO_2) gas and ammonia (NH_3) gas to nitrogen (N_2) gas, methane (CH_4) and water (H_2O).

N_2 Photosynthesis equation:

$$3CO_2 + 8NH_3 + \text{radiant energy} \xrightarrow{\substack{\text{Extraterrestrial} \\ \text{Catalyst}}} 6H_2O + 3CH_4 + 4N_2$$

(carbon dioxide)   (ammonia)   (water)   (methane) (nitrogen)

Nucleotide bps: Nucleotide base pairs.

Prime DNA Genome or Prime Genome: Collection of all the genomes that have existed on the planet containing all of the quantum genes and reference tables necessary for all forms of organic life; more specifically contains genetic design information to construct the cell, all of the cellular proteins, viruses, prokaryote cells, eukaryote cells and the multi-cellular organic organisms comprised of eukaryote cells.

Proton: A sub atomic particle comprised of sub-sub atomic tripolar particles known as tritrons, these tritrons arranged in a shell-like shape with the positive state pointed outward and the negative and neutral states pointed inward, with the center of the collection of tritrons harboring a quantum of energy.

Quantum Gene: Genetic material associated with a unique identifier.

Radiant Apex: Term of description that identifies the side of a galactic vortex that acts as the outbound event horizon where electromagnetic energy such as light and tritrons are ejected out of a galactic vortex.

RNA: Ribonucleic acid

TBP: TATA box Binding Protein

Tritron: The fundamental tripolar sub-sub (or sub^2) atomic particle shaped as a combination of three conjoined elliptical spheres, with one elliptical sphere exhibiting a positive state, one pole exhibiting a negative state, the third exhibiting a neutral state, this sub^2 particle comprising the ether of space from which all sub atomic particles are constructed.

Unique Identifier: A sequence of nucleotides used as an identification code for quantum genes, messenger RNAs, ribosomal RNAs and transport RNAs; in the case of the quantum gene the unique identifier may be comprised of a series of 25 nucleotides.

Universal Dogma of Molecular Biology: 'All protein production is a dynamic process created by a static intelligence stored in the DNA, facilitated by control RNAs and DNA binding proteins to produce

311

messenger RNA which are used as templates to generate proteins, the rate of production being controlled by nuclear signaling proteins and control RNAs and the construction of complex protein molecules being directed by the collaboration of static chemical processes, production rate of enzymes and command RNA molecules'.

Universal Genetic Reference Table: The genetic reference table in the Prime Genome

Universal Primary Equation: The entire universe can be summarized into the Universal Primary Equation.
Universe[1] = Energy (conserved) + Tritrons (conserved) + Space to be occupied

Vironix Particle or Pod: Contained the original seeds of life, each seed carrying a Prime DNA Genome.

PATENT APPLICATIONS BOOK III

1. QUANTUM UNIT OF INHERITANCE VECTOR THERAPY

2. QUANTUM UNIT OF INHERITANCE VECTOR THERAPY METHOD

3. CONFIGURABLE MICROSCOPIC MEDICAL PAYLOAD DELIVERY DEVICE TO DELIVER **NUCLEAR SIGNALING PROTEINS** TO SPECIFIC CELLS TO MANAGE DIABETES MELLITUS AND GENETIC DEFICIENCY DISORDERS

4. CONFIGURABLE MICROSCOPIC MEDICAL PAYLOAD DELIVERY DEVICE TO DELIVER **CONTROL RNAs** TO SPECIFIC CELLS TO MANAGE DIABETES MELLITUS AND GENETIC DEFICIENCY DISORDERS

5. CONFIGURABLE MICROSCOPIC MEDICAL PAYLOAD DELIVERY DEVICE TO DELIVER **COMMAND RNAs** TO SPECIFIC CELLS TO MANAGE DIABETES MELLITUS AND GENETIC DEFICIENCY DISORDERS

PATENT APPLICATION
SPECIFICATION NUMBER 1

TITLE OF THE INVENTION:

QUANTUM UNIT OF INHERITANCE VECTOR THERAPY

BACKGROUND OF THE INVENTION

1. Field of the Invention

This invention relates to any medical device intended to correct a protein deficiency or genetic deficiency in the body by utilizing a configurable microscopic medical payload delivery device to insert one or more quantum genes into one or more specific type of cells in the body to improve cell function.

1. Description of Background Art

[0001] The central dogma of microbiology dictates that in the nucleus of a cell, genes are transcribed to produce messenger ribonucleic acid molecules (mRNAs), these mRNAs migrate to the cytoplasm where they are translated to produce proteins. One of the great unknowns that has challenged the study of microbiology is the subject of understanding of how the genes, comprising the genome of a species, are organized such that the nuclear transcription machinery can efficiently locate specific transcribable genetic information and instructions that the cell requires to maintain itself, grow and conduct cell replication. Decoding the means as to how the genetic information contained in the nuclear deoxyribonucleic acid (DNA) of a cell is organized, helps to further the efforts to produce an effective gene therapy treatment strategy. Understanding the basis of genetic instruction code information stored in a cell's DNA and utilizing such knowledge of labeling and cataloging of genetic information, makes inserting biologic instruction into the DNA of cells a practical and effective means of treating a wide scope of medical conditions.

[0002] The human genome is comprised of deoxyribonucleic acid (DNA) separated into 46 chromosomes. The chromosomes are further subdivided into genes. Genes represent units of transcribable DNA. Transcription of the DNA refers to generating one or more of a variety of RNA molecules. Regarding the human genome, currently it is estimated that 5% of the total nuclear DNA is thought to represent genes and 95% is thought to represent redundant non-gene genetic material. The DNA genome in a cell is therefore comprised of transcribable genetic information and nontranscribable genetic information. Transcribable genetic information represent the segments of DNA that when transcribed by transcription machinery yield RNA molecules, usually in a precursor form that require modification before the RNA molecules are capable of being translated. The nontranscribable genetic information represent segments that act as either points of attachment for the transcription machinery or act as commands to direct the transcription machinery or act as spacers between transcribable segments of genetic information or have no known function at this time. A segment of nontranslatable DNA that is coded as a STOP command, under the proper circumstances, will cause the transcription machinery to cease transcribing the DNA at that point. A segment of DNA coded to signal a REPEAT command, will cause the transcription machinery to repeat its transcription of a segment of genetic information. The term 'genetic information' refers to a sequence of nucleotides that comprise transcribable portions of DNA and nontranscribable portions of DNA. In the DNA, four different nucleotides comprise the nucleotide sequences. The four different nucleotides that comprise the DNA include adenine, cytosine, guanine, and thymine.

[0003] Computer programs, commonly utilized in desk top computers, laptop computers, mainframe computers are comprised of a series of software instructions and data. In order for a computer program to run its digital programming in an orderly fashion, each software instruction and each element of data is assigned or associated with a unique identifier such that the software instructions can be carried out in an orderly fashion and each element of data can be efficiently located when there is a need to process the data elements. Similarly, each unit of genetic information, often referred to as a gene, comprising the nuclear DNA of a species genome, must have a unique identifier assigned to it such that the genetic information can be readily located by the transcription machinery and utilized when needed by a cell.

[0004] When a gene is to be transcribed, approximately forty proteins assemble together into what is referred to as a transcription complex, which acts as the transcription machinery. The transcription complex forms along a segment of DNA, upstream from the start of the transcribable genetic information. The transcription complex transcribes the genetic information to produce RNA. It is vital to the cell that the transcription complex is able to locate a specific gene amongst the 3 billion base pairs comprising the human genome in an orderly and efficient fashion to enable it to perform functions the cell requires to operate, survive, grow and replicate.

[0005] For purposes of this text there are several general definitions. A 'ribose' is a five carbon or pentose sugar ($C_5H_{10}O_5$) present in the structural components of ribonucleic acid, riboflavin, and other nucleotides and nucleosides. A 'deoxyribose' is a deoxypentose ($C_5H_{10}O_4$) found in deoxyribonucleic acid. A 'nucleoside' is a compound of a sugar usually ribose or deoxyribose with a nitrogenous base by way of an N-glycosyl link. A 'nucleotide' is a single unit of a nucleic acid, composed of a five carbon sugar (either a ribose or a deoxyribose), a nitrogenous base and a phosphate group. There are two families of 'nitrogenous bases', which include: pyrimidine and purine. A 'pyrimidine' is a six member ring made up of carbon and nitrogen atoms; the members of the pyrimidine family include: cytosine (C), thymine (T) and uracil (U). A 'purine' is a five-member ring fused to a pyrimidine type ring; the members of the purine family include: adenine (A) and guanine (G). A 'nucleic acid' is a polynucleotide which is a biologic molecule such as ribonucleic acid or deoxyribonucleic acid that allow organisms to reproduce. A 'ribonucleic acid' (RNA) is a linear polymer of nucleotides formed by repeated riboses linked by phosphodiester bonds between the 3-hydroxyl group of one and the 5-hydroxyl group of the next; RNAs are a single strand macromolecule comprised of a sequence of nucleotides, these nucleotides are generally referred to by their nitrogenous bases, which include: adenine, cytosine, guanine or uracil. The term macromolecule refers to any very large molecule. RNAs are subset into different types which include messenger RNA (mRNA), transport RNA (tRNA), ribosomal RNA (rRNA) and a variety of small RNAs. Messenger RNAs act as templates to produce proteins. A ribosome is a complex comprised of rRNAs and proteins and is responsible for the correct positioning of mRNA and charged tRNA to facilitate the proper alignment and bonding of amino acids into a strand to produce a protein. A 'charged' tRNA is a tRNA that is carrying an amino acid. Ribosomal RNA (rRNA) represents a subset of RNAs that form part of the physical structure of a ribosome. Small RNAs include snoRNA, U snRNA, and miRNA. The snoRNAs modify precursor rRNA molecules. U snRNAs modify precursor mRNA molecules. The miRNA molecules modify the function of mRNA molecules.

[0006] A 'deoxyribose' is a deoxypentose ($C_5H_{10}O_4$) sugar. Deoxyribonucleic acid (DNA) is comprised of three basic elements: a deoxyribose sugar, a phosphate group and nitrogen containing bases. DNA is a macromolecule made up of two chains of repeating deoxyribose sugars linked by phosphodiester bonds between the 3-hydroxyl group of one and the 5-hydroxyl group of the next; the two chains are held antiparallel to each other by weak hydrogen bonds. DNA strands contain a sequence of nucleotides, which include: adenine, cytosine, guanine and thymine. Adenine is always paired with thymine of the opposite strand, and guanine is always paired with cytosine of the opposite strand; one side or strand of a DNA macromolecule is the mirror image of the opposite strand. Nuclear DNA is regarded as the medium for storing the master plan of hereditary information.

[0007] Genes are considered segments of the DNA that represent units of inheritance.

[0008] A chromosome exists in the nucleus of a cell and consists of a DNA double helix bearing a linear sequence of genes, coiled and recoiled around aggregated proteins, termed histones. The number of chromosomes varies from species to species. Most Human cells carries twenty two pairs of chromosomes plus two sex chromosomes; two 'x' chromosomes in women and one 'x' and one 'y' chromosome in men. Chromosomes carry genetic information in the form of units which are referred to as genes. The entire nuclear genome, forty six chromosomes, is comprised of 3 billion base pairs of nucleotides.

[0009] Mitochondria possess numerous circular DNA. The limited information stored in mitochondrial DNA is thought to assist the mitochondria in producing the enzymes needed to convert glucose to adenosine triphosphate.

[0010] Various standard definitions of a gene exist. Per *Stedman's Medical Dictionary*, 24th edition, copyright 1982: 'The functional unit of heredity. Each gene occupies a specific place or locus on a chromosome, is capable of reproducing itself exactly at cell division, and is capable of directing the formation of an enzyme or other protein. The gene as a functional unit probably consists of a discrete segment of purine (adenine and guanine) and pyrimidine (cytosine and thymine) bases in the correct sequence to code the sequence of amino acids needed to form a specific peptide. Protein synthesis is mediated by molecules of messenger RNA formed on the chromosome with the gene unit of DNA acting as a template, which then pass into the cytoplasm and become oriented on the ribosomes where they in turn act as templates to organize a chain of amino acids to form a peptide. Genes normally occur in pairs in all cells except gametes as a consequence of the fact that all chromosomes are paired except the sex chromosomes (x and y) of the male.'

[0011] Per *Dorland's Pocket Medical Dictionary*, 23rd edition, copyright 1982 the definition of 'gene' is 'the biologic unit of heredity, self-producing, and located at a definite position (locus) on a particular chromosome.'

[0012] Per the text *Understanding Biology*, Second Edition, Peter Raven, George Johnson, Mosby, copyright 1991: 'Gene: The basic unit of heredity. A sequence of DNA nucleotides on a chromosome that encodes a polypeptide or RNA molecule and so determines the nature of an individual's inherited traits.'

[0013] Per *The New Oxford American Dictionary*, Second Edition, copyright 2005: 'Gene: A unit of heredity that is transferred from a parent to offspring and is held to determine some characteristic of the offspring: proteins coded directly by genes. In technical use: a distinct sequence of nucleotides forming part of a chromosome, the order of which determines the order of monomers in a polypeptide or nucleic acid molecule which a cell (or virus) may synthesize.'

[0014] Per MedicineNet.com (Current as of the time of this publication): According to the official Guidelines for Human Gene Nomenclature, a 'gene' is defined as "a DNA segment that contributes to phenotype/function. In the absence of demonstrated function a gene may be characterized by sequence, transcription or homology." DNA: Genes are composed of DNA, a molecule in the memorable shape of a double helix, a spiral ladder. Each rung of the spiral ladder consists of two paired chemicals called bases. There are four types of bases. They are adenine (A), thymine (T), cytosine (C), and guanine (G). As indicated, each base is symbolized by the first letter of its name: A, T, C, and G. Certain bases always pair together (AT and GC). Different sequences of base pairs form coded messages. The gene: A gene is a sequence

319

(a string) of bases. It is made up of combinations of A, T, C, and G. These unique combinations determine the gene's function, much as letters join together to form words. Each person has thousands of genes—billions of base pairs of DNA or bits of information repeated in the nuclei of human cells—which determine individual characteristics (genetic traits).'

[0015] Per Wikipedia.com, referenced to: Group of the Sequence Ontology consortium, coordinated by K. Eilbeck, cited in H. Pearson. (2006). Genetics: what is a gene? *Nature*, 441, 398-401 (Current as of the time of this publication): A modern working definition of a gene is 'a locatable region of genomic sequence, corresponding to a unit of inheritance, which is associated with regulatory regions, transcribed regions, and or other functional sequence regions.'

[0016] The above definitions of a 'gene' are fairly detailed and at present time generally universally accepted in the science and medical communities as representing the definition of a gene. There is a distinct lack of any previous reference in the medical science literature to a unique identifier associated with genetic material.

[0017] Current gene theory is derived from Gregor Mendel (1822-1884), who discovered the basic principles of heredity by breeding garden peas at the abbey where he resided, while teaching at Brunn Modern School. Gregor Mendel built and documented a model of inheritance, often referred to as Mendelian genetics, that has acted as the foundation of modern genetics. Gregor Mendel documented changes in characteristics of the plants he grew and described the physical traits as being related to 'heritable factors'. Over time Mendel's term 'heritable factor' has been replaced by the terms 'gene' and 'allele'. Much of what the current term of a 'gene' describes remains related to and distinctly linked to the physical traits of the live organisms they describe.

[0018] Per J. K. Pal, S.S. Ghaskabi, *Fundamentals of Molecular Biology*, 2009: 'The central dogma of molecular biology . . . states that the genes present in the genome (DNA) are transcribed into mRNAs, which are then translated into polypeptides or proteins, which are phenotypes.' 'Genome, thus, contains the complete set of hereditary information for any organism and is functionally divided into small parts referred to as genes. Each gene is a sequence of nucleotides representing a single protein or RNA. Genome of a living organism may contain as few as 500 genes as in case of Mycoplasma, or as many as 30,000 genes as in case of human beings.'

[0019] Current computer technology utilizes the binary numeric language. Every task a computer performs is related to the language of 'one' and 'zeros'. Transistors that comprise the inside of computer chips are either turned 'on' representing a 'one' or turned 'off' representing a 'zero'. At the core of all computer programs is the machine language of 'ones' and 'zeros'. The most sophisticated central processing unit (CPU) in the world only reads and processes the language of 'ones' and 'zeros'. All text, all pictures, all video, all sound and music is diluted down to the form of one's and zero's, and consequently all of the computing and storage power of a computer is performed by the computer language of 'ones' and 'zeros'.

[0020] The nucleus of a biologically active cell arguably possesses the most sophisticated and well organized processing power in the world. To run such a powerful processing unit, a form of biologic computer language would seem to be a necessary foundation by which to transfer stored information from the DNA to the remainder of the biologically active portions of a cell as needed. Given that the DNA comprising the chromosomes and mitochondrial DNA are both comprised of four different nucleotides including adenosine, cytosine, guanine and thymine, and RNA is comprised of four nucleotides including adenosine, cytosine, guanine and uracil (uracil in place of thymine), it appears evident the biologic computer language used by a cell's genome is an information language derived from base-four mathematics. Instead of current computer technology utilizing binary computer code comprised of 'ones' and 'zeros', the DNA and RNA in a biologically active cell utilize an information language comprised of 'zeros', 'one's', two's' and 'threes' to store and transfer information, which in effect represents a base-four language or quaternary language.

[0021] The above definitions of a 'gene' refer to genes residing in a specific place or locus on a chromosome. Identifying that a gene is present in a particular location is obvious to the human observer, but from a functional standpoint for cell biology this does not necessarily help a cell find or use the information stored in the nucleotide sequence of a particular gene. To rely on location alone, as a means of identifying a gene, would put the function of the entire genome at peril of failure if even a single base pair of nucleotides were added or deleted from the genome. To this point, no discussion regarding genes being organized utilizing a coding system of any form within the genome, other than the mention of physical location in a chromosome, has been made in the medical literature.

[0022] The current understanding of the actual biologic structure of a gene is far more elaborate than the standard definition of a gene leads a casual reader to believe; this knowledge has evolved greatly since Gregor Mendel's work in the 19th century. A gene appears to be comprised of a number of segments loosely strung together along a particular section of DNA. In general there are at least three global segments associated with a gene which include: (1) the Upstream 5' flanking region, (2) the transcriptional unit and (3) the Downstream 3' flanking region.

[0023] The Upstream 5' flanking region is comprised of the 'enhancer region', the 'promoter-proximal region', and 'promoter region'.

[0024] The 'transcriptional unit' begins at a location designated 'transcription start site' (TSS), which is located in a site called the 'initiator region' (inR), which may be described in a general form as Py_2CAPy_5. The transcription unit is comprised of the combination of segments of DNA nucleotides to be transcribed into RNA and spacing units known as 'introns' that are not transcribed or if transcribed are later removed post transcription, such that they do not appear in the final RNA molecule. In the case of a gene coding for a mRNA molecule, the transcription unit will contain all three elements of the mRNA, which includes: (1) the 5' noncoding region, (2) the translational region and (3) the 3' noncoding region. Interspersed between these regions are exons, which will not be transcribed and introns that if transcribed, are removed from the precursor form of mRNA prior to the mRNA reaching its final form. Exons and introns appear to be likened to spacers. The exact role exons and introns play in the transcription process is undetermined.

[0025] The Downstream 3' flanking region contains DNA nucleotides that are not transcribed and may contain what has been termed an 'enhancer region'. An enhancer region in the Downstream 3' flanking region may promote the gene previously transcribed to be transcribed again.

[0026] On either side of the DNA sequencing comprising a gene and its flanking regions, may be inactive DNA which act as boundaries which have been termed 'insulator elements'. The term 'upstream' refers to DNA sequencing that occurs prior to the TSS if viewed from the 5' end to the 3' end of the DNA; where the term 'downstream' refers to DNA sequencing located after the TSS.

[0027] The 'enhancer region' may or may not be present in the Upstream 5' flanking region. If present in the Upstream 5' flanking region, the enhancer region helps facilitate the reading of the gene by encouraging formation of the transcription mechanism. An enhancer may be 50 to 1500 base pairs in length occupying a position upstream from the transcription starting site.

[0028] The 'transcription mechanism', also referred to as the 'transcription machinery' or the 'transcription complex' (TC), in humans, is reported to be comprised of over forty separate proteins that assemble together to ultimately function in a concerted effort to transcribe the nucleotide sequence of the DNA into RNA. The transcription mechanism includes elements such as 'general transcription factor Sp1', 'general transcription factor NF1', 'general transcription factor TATA-binding protein', 'TF$_{II}$D', 'basal transcription complex', and a 'RNA polymerase protein' to name only a few of the forty elements that exist. The elements of the transcription mechanism function as (1) a means to recognize the location of the start of a gene, (2) as proteins to bind the transcription mechanism to the DNA such that transcription may occur or (3) as means of transcribing the DNA nucleotide coding to produce a RNA molecule or a precursor RNA molecule.

[0029] There are at least three RNA polymerase proteins which include: RNA polymerase I, RNA polymerase II, and RNA polymerase III. RNA polymerase I tends to be dedicated to transcribing genetic information that will result in the formation of rRNA molecules. RNA polymerase II tends to be dedicated to transcribing genetic information that will result in the formation of mRNA molecules. RNA polymerase III appears to be dedicated to transcribing genetic information that results in the formation of tRNAs, small cellular RNAs and viral RNAs.

[0030] The 'promoter proximal region' is located upstream from the TSS and upstream from the core promoter region. The 'promoter proximal region' includes two sub-regions termed the GC box and the CAAT box. The 'GC box' appears to be a segment rich in guanine-cytosine nucleotide sequences. The GC box binds to the 'general transcription factor Sp1' of the transcription mechanism. The 'CAAT box' is a segment which contains the nucleotide sequence 'GGCCAATCT' located approximately 75 base pairs (bps) upstream from the transcription start site (TSS). The CAAT box binds to the 'general transcription factor NF1' of the transcription mechanism.

[0031] The 'core promoter' region is considered the shortest sequence within which RNA polymerase II can initiate transcription of a gene The core promoter may include the inR and either a TATA box or a 'downstream promoter element' (DPE). The inR is the region designated Py_2CAPy_5 that surrounds the transcription start site (TSS). The TATA box is located 25 base pairs (bps) upstream from the TSS. The TATA box acts as a site of attachment of the $TF_{II}D$, which is a promoter for binding of the RNA polymerase II molecule. The DPE may appear 28 bps to 32 bps downstream from the TSS. The DPE acts as an alternative site of attachment for the $TF_{II}D$ when the TATA box is not present.

[0032] The transcription mechanism or transcription complex appears to be comprised of different elements depending upon whether rRNA is being transcribed versus mRNA or tRNA or small cellular RNA or viral RNA. The proteins that assemble to assist RNA Polymerase I with transcribing the DNA to produce rRNA appear different the proteins that assemble to assist RNA polymerase II with transcribing the DNA to produce mRNA and from the proteins that assemble to assist RNA polymerase III with transcribing the DNA to produce tRNA, small cellular RNA or viral RNA. A common protein that appears to be present at the initial binding of all three types of RNA polymerase molecules is TATA-binding protein (TBP). TBP appears to be required to attach to the DNA, which then facilitates RNA polymerase to bind to the promoter along the DNA. TBP assembles with TBP-associated factors (TAFs). Together TBF and 11 TAFs comprise the complex referred to as TF$_{II}$D, which has been previously mentioned in the above text.

[0033] Upstream from the TATA box is the 'initiator element', which may be considered as part of the 'core promoter' region. The initiator element is a segment of the nuclear DNA that binds the basal transcription complex. The basal transcription complex is comprised of a number of proteins that make initial contact with the DNA prior to the RNA polymerase binding to the transcription mechanism. The basal transcription complex is associated with an activator.

[0034] An activator is a protein comprised of three components. The three components of the activator include: (1) DNA binding domain, (2) Connecting domain, and (3) Activating domain. When the activator's DNA binding domain attaches to the DNA at a specific point along the DNA, the activator's activating domain then causes the other elements of the transcription mechanism to assemble at this location. Generally the assembly of the other proteins occurs downstream from where the activator's DNA binding domain attached to the DNA. There is evidence that the activator is associated with the activity of small RNAs.

[0035] The design of the cell is so complex, all of its functions so diverse and intricate that some form of practical order is necessitated. The genes must be ordered in some fashion, especially in a human, where there are at least 30,000 different genes used by the cells. Some estimates place the total number of genes present in the human nuclear DNA genome closer to 100,000. If no means of order existed as to how the genes could be identified, then 'random circumstance' would dictate a cell locating a particular portion of genetic information that it requires, at any given time. Randomness tends to favor the occurrence of random events rather than a purposeful order. A 'random circumstance' approach to any living cell would tend to favor failure of the cell rather than survival of the cell.

[0036] To allow a cell to utilize the biologic information stored in a gene a 'unique identifier' (UI) needs to be somehow attached to the gene's specific nucleotide sequence. In the human genome, the cell's transcription mechanisms require an organized means to locate and transcribe any given gene's nucleotide sequence amongst the 3 billion nucleotides that reside in the 46 chromosomes that comprise human DNA. Given how the transcription mechanism assembles upstream from the portion of the gene to be transcribed, the nucleotide sequence acting as a unique identifier associated with a specific gene would be positioned upstream from the transcription start site.

[0037] The transcription complex (TC) engages the DNA upstream from the genetic information segment the TC transcribes. The unique identifier may be attached directly to the RNA coding segment of genetic material, or there may exist one or more base pairs physically separating the unique identifier and the RNA coding portion of genetic material. Regarding some genes, there may be numerous base pairs separating the unique identifier from the transcribing region of the gene.

[0038] For any form of 'gene therapy' to work efficiently, medically therapeutic genetic material inserted into the native DNA of a cell needs to be associated with a unique identification. Attaching a unique identifier to medically therapeutic genetic material is essential in making it possible for the components of a transcription complex to, in a timely organized fashion, locate the exogenous medically therapeutic genetic material, assemble around this exogenous genetic material, and decode the information contained therein. If no such unique identifier is used, then utilization of such exogenous transcribable genetic information occurs based on the occurrence of random events rather than dictated by therapeutic design.

[0039] Naturally occurring unique identifiers in the nuclear genome may occur in numerous forms. Since humans share 47% of their DNA with a banana and 95% of their DNA with a monkey, a portion of the unique identifiers associated with genes in the nuclear DNA may not be specific to a human. Unique identifiers may have a global utility, with a portion of the genome of any organism being shared amongst numerous species. The rational would be that once Nature developed an adequate fundamental design for a particular facet of biologic organisms, this information may be shared amongst numerous species that would benefit from the design. An example might be the basic design of a eukaryote cell; this information would be shared amongst all life that utilized the eukaryote cell design rather than each successive multi-celled species having to repeatedly re-invent the design of a eukaryote cell.

[0040] In order for the knowledge base of cellular genetics to progress forward, the definition of a gene must be expanded to include the presence of a 'unique identifier' associated with each gene present within the DNA. The basis for the presence of this unique identifier (UI) associated with each active gene is so that the cell can locate the biologic information stored in the DNA nucleotide sequencing of the gene. An active gene refers to those genes present in the genome that are utilized by a particular species to support conception, development and maintenance of a species.

[0041] Upon adding a unique identifier to a gene, the current term 'gene' is thus expanded to the term 'quantum gene'. The term 'quantal' in biology generally refers to an 'all or nothing' state or response. The term 'quantal' is a derivative of the word quantum. The term 'quantum means a quantity or amount, and a discrete quantity of energy or a discrete bundle of energy or a discrete quantity of electromagnetic radiation'.

[0042] A 'quantum gene' is comprised of a sequence of nucleotides that represents a 'unique identifier' physically linked to a sequence of nucleotides that represent a discrete quantity of genetic information; these sequences of nucleotides being comprised of some combination of the nucleotides being referred to by their nitrogenous base as adenine (A), thymine (T), cytosine (C), and guanine (G). The genetic information associated with the above-mentioned unique identifier may be comprised of a portion of transcribable genetic information and a portion of nontranscribable genetic information which together define a specific gene, otherwise referred to as a discrete quantity of genetic information.

[0043] Similar to how a gene is described, with regards to a quantum gene, the term 'upstream' refers to DNA sequencing that occurs prior to the transcription start site (TSS) if viewed from the 5' end to the 3' end of the DNA; where the term 'downstream' refers to DNA sequencing located after the TSS.

[0044] Similar to the previously described organization of a standard gene found in nuclear DNA, a quantum gene is structured with at least three global segments which include: (1) the Upstream 5' flanking region, (2) the transcriptional unit and possibly instructional units and (3) the Downstream 3' flanking region. The 'unique identifier' is located in the Upstream 5' flanking region. The current standard definition of a gene strictly encompasses the concept that a gene is comprised of a segment of nuclear DNA that when transcribed produces RNA. Therefore, the differences between the current standard definition of a 'gene' and the definition of a 'quantum gene' is that a quantum gene includes both a unique identifier and a segment of nuclear DNA that when transcribed produces RNA. The segment of nuclear DNA that when transcribed produces RNA is comprised of one or more segments of transcribable genetic information that may be accompanied by one or more segments of nontranscribable genetic information. Nontranscribable segments of genetic information include segments that are removed or ignored during the transcription process or segments that act as commands which includes a START code, STOP code or a REPEAT code. When present, a START code signals initiation of the transcription process. When present, a STOP code signals the discontinuation of the transcription process. When present, a REPEAT code signals that the transcription process should repeat the transcription of the segment of DNA that was just transcribed.

[0045] Similar to the standard description of a 'gene', a quantum gene's Upstream 5' flanking region is comprised of the 'enhancer region', the 'promoter-proximal region', and 'promoter region'.

[0046] Similar to the standard description of a 'gene', a quantum gene's 'transcriptional unit' begins at a location designated 'transcription start site' (TSS), which is located in a site called the 'initiator region' (inR), which may be described in a general form as Py_2CAPy_5. The transcription unit is comprised of the combination of segments of DNA nucleotides to be transcribed into RNA and spacing units known as 'exons' AND 'introns', whereby exons represent segments that are not transcribed and introns represent segments that are transcribed but later removed post transcription, such that they do not appear in the final RNA molecule. In the case of a gene coding for a mRNA molecule, the transcription unit will contain all three elements of the mRNA, which includes: (1) the 5' noncoding region, (2) the translational region and (3) the 3' noncoding region. Interspersed between these regions are exons, which will not be transcribed and introns that if transcribed, are removed from the precursor form of mRNA prior to the mRNA reaching its final form. Exons and introns present in nuclear DNA appear to be likened to spacers interspersed in the nuclear DNA. The exact role exons and introns play in the transcription process is undetermined.

[0047] Similar to the standard description of a 'gene', the quantum gene's Downstream 3' flanking region contains DNA nucleotides that are not transcribed and may contain what has been termed an 'enhancer region'. An enhancer region in the Downstream 3' flanking region may promote the gene previously transcribed to be transcribed again.

[0048] On either side of the DNA sequencing comprising a gene and a quantum gene are flanking regions which represent inactive

DNA, which act as boundaries which have been termed 'insulator elements'. Insulator elements are areas that are not transcribed to produce RNA. The function of insulator elements, other than acting as boundary markers between differing genes, is unknown at this time.

[0049] In nuclear DNA, quantum genes are comprised of a segment of deoxyribonucleic acid where the portion that represents a unique identifier may be separated from the portion that represents transcribable genetic information by a quantity of base pairs of nucleotides that do not represent a unique identifier and do not represent transcribable genetic information. The purpose of the separation of the portion of the unique identifier from the portion of the genetic information by a quantity of base pairs of nucleotides that do not represent a unique identifier and does not represent genetic information may be to act to facilitate a transcription complex attaching to the quantum gene upstream from the portion of the quantum gene that represents genetic information so that transcription of the biologic information associated with the quantum gene may occur at the designated starting point.

[0050] The unique identification or identifier of a quantum gene could be in the form of nucleotide sequence that represents a name assigned to the quantum gene, or a number assigned to a quantum gene or the combination of a name and number assigned to a quantum gene. Irrespective of whether the unique identifier incorporated in a quantum gene is considered a 'name', or a 'number' or a combination of a name or number, the unique identifier is comprised of a sequence of nucleotides linked to the transcribable genetic information for which it acts as a unique identifier. It has been estimated that there are as many as 100,000 separate genes stored in the DNA of the 46 chromosomes comprising the human genome. In a base four language, a string of nine nucleotides is needed to code for 256,144 individual genes. If there were over a million quantum genes, then a string of ten nucleotides could be used since ten nucleotides could represent 1,024,576 unique numbers in a base-four number system.

[0051] Utilizing a base four number system a string of twenty-five nucleotides would represent the number 1,125,899,906,842,624, which could account for 200,000 different quantum genes in 5 billion different species. Therefore 200,000 different quantum genes could be dedicated to producing a biped form of life. In the human genome 5% of the 3 billion base pairs are considered to represent genes by the current definition of a gene. If 5% of the human genome represents the 100,000 quantum genes in the nuclear DNA, then on average 1500 nucleotides can be dedicated to each gene. If 25 nucleotides are dedicated to a unique address or unique identifier, then there remain 1475 nucleotides, on average, to be utilized for coding the biologic information associated with each of the 100,000 quantum genes estimated to exist in the human genome.

[0052] A unique identifier (UI) incorporated in quantum genes could be comprised of a unique number or a unique name or the unique combination of a number and a name. A name might be represented as a single letter or a series of letters. The current convention utilized in science is to apply the four letter alphabet A, C, G, T to represent the four different bases of the nucleotides comprising the DNA, which include adenosine, cytosine, guanine, and thymine respectfully. With regards to RNA, the four letter alphabet A, C, G, U is utilized to represent the bases of the nucleotides which include adenosine, cytosine, guanine, and uracil. Regarding utilizing a unique identifier for DNA, a name could be comprised of a series of letters derived from the four letters A, C, G, and T. Regarding utilizing a unique identifier for purposes of use within an RNA molecule, a unique identifier could be comprised of a series of letters derived from the four letters A, C, G, U. The current scientific convention does not recognize a mathematical base-four nomenclature regarding DNA or RNA. The unique identifier could be represented as a number. Names can be translated into numbers and vice versa.

[0053] In the nuclear DNA, there are several places in the upstream segment of a quantum gene where a segment of twenty-five or more base pairs could exist that acts as the unique identifying code that uniquely identifies the segment of transcribable genetic information. The transcription start site (TSS) is present upstream from a segment of transcribable genetic information. There exists a segment of 25 bps upstream from the TSS that occupies the space along the DNA between the TSS and the TATA box. There exists the downstream promoter element (DPE) 28 bps to 32 bps downstream from the TSS. The DPE acts as an alternative site of attachment for the $TF_{II}D$ when the TATA box is not present. Within the 28 bps to 32 bps of DNA separating the DPE from the TSS may also be a convenient location for a unique identifying code to reside and be associated with the genetic information located just downstream. The cell exists with numerous variability. There exists variation in the arrangement of the elements upstream from the transcribable genetic information, therefore various sites upstream from the transcribable genetic information may function as the unique identifying code for some quantum genes. The unique identifying code may be represented as subsegments of DNA, where subsegments are physically separated from each other, but in combination, the subsegments act in unison to identify a segment of transcribable genetic information.

[0054] By delivering quantum genes containing the genetic information required to produce insulin directly to the cells responsible for the production of insulin, the medical treatment of diabetes mellitus is significantly improved. Diabetes mellitus represents a state of hyperglycemia, a serum blood sugar that is higher than what is considered the normal range for humans. Glucose, a six-carbon molecule, is a form of sugar. Glucose is absorbed by the cells of the body and converted to energy by the processes of glycolysis, the Krebs cycle and phosporylation. Insulin, a protein, facilitates the transfer of glucose from the blood into cells. Normal range for blood glucose in humans is generally defined as a fasting blood plasma glucose level of between 70 to 110 mg/dl. For descriptive purposes, the term 'plasma' refers to the fluid portion of blood.

[0055] Diabetes mellitus is classified as Type One and Type Two. Type One diabetes mellitus is insulin dependent, which refers to the condition where there is a lack of sufficient insulin circulating in the blood stream and insulin must be provided to the body in order to properly regulate the blood glucose level. When insulin is required to regulate the blood glucose level in the body, this condition is often referred to as insulin dependent diabetes mellitus (IDDM). Type Two diabetes mellitus is noninsulin dependent, often referred to as noninsulin dependent diabetes mellitus (NIDDM), meaning the blood glucose level can be managed without insulin, and instead by means of diet, exercise or intervention with oral medications. Type Two diabetes mellitus is considered a progressive disease, the underlying pathogenic mechanisms including pancreatic Beta cell (also often designated as β-Cell) dysfunction and insulin resistance.

[0056] The pancreas serves as an endocrine gland and an exocrine gland. Functioning as an endocrine gland the pancreas produces and secretes hormones including insulin and glucagon. Insulin acts to reduce levels of glucose circulating in the blood. Beta cells secrete insulin into the blood when a higher than normal level of glucose is detected in the serum. For purposes of this description the terms 'blood', 'blood stream' and 'serum' refer to the same substance. Glucagon acts to stimulate an increase in glucose circulating in the blood. Beta cells in the pancreas secrete glucagon when a low level of glucose is detected in the serum.

[0057] Glucose enters the body and then the blood stream as a result of the digestion of food. The Beta cells of the Islets of Langerhans continuously sense the level of glucose in the blood and respond to elevated levels of blood glucose by secreting insulin into the blood. Beta cells produce the protein 'insulin' in their endoplasmic reticulum and store the insulin in vacuoles until it is needed. When Beta cells detect an increase in the glucose level in the blood, Beta cells release insulin into the blood from the described storage vacuoles.

[0058] Insulin is a protein. An insulin protein consists of two chains of amino acids, an alpha chain and a beta chain, linked by two disulfide (S-S) bridges. One chain, the alpha chain consists of 21 amino acids. The second chain the beta chain consists of 30 amino acids.

[0059] Insulin interacts with the cells of the body by means of a cell-surface receptor termed the 'insulin receptor' located on the exterior of a cell's 'outer membrane', otherwise known as the 'plasma membrane'. Insulin interacts with muscle and liver cells by means of the insulin receptor to rapidly remove excess blood sugar when the glucose level in the blood is higher than the upper limit of the normal physiologic range. Recognized functions of insulin include stimulating cells to take up glucose from the blood and convert it to glycogen to facilitate the cells in the body to utilize glucose to generate biochemically usable energy, and to stimulate fat cells to take up glucose and synthesize fat.

[0060] Diabetes Mellitus may be the result of one or more factors. Causes of diabetes mellitus may include: (1) mutation of the insulin gene itself causing miscoding, which results in the production of ineffective insulin molecules; (2) mutations to genes that code for the 'transcription factors' needed for transcription of the insulin gene in the deoxyribonucleic acid (DNA) to create messenger ribonucleic acid (mRNA) molecules, which facilitate the manufacture of the insulin molecule; (3) mutations of the gene encoding for the insulin receptor, which produces inactive or an insufficient number of insulin receptors; (4) mutation to the gene encoding for glucokinase, the enzyme that phosphorylates glucose in the first step of glycolysis; (5) mutations to the genes encoding portions of the potassium channels in the plasma membrane of the Beta cells, preventing proper closure of the channel, thus blocking insulin release; (6) mutations to mitochondrial genes that as a result, decreases the energy available to be used facilitate the release of insulin, therefore reducing insulin secretion; (7) failure of glucose transporters to properly permit the facilitated diffusion of glucose from plasma into the cells of the body.

[0061] A 'eukaryote' refers to a nucleated cell. Eukaryotes comprise nearly all animal and plant cells. A human eukaryote or nucleated cell is comprised of an exterior lipid bilayer plasma membrane, cytoplasm, a nucleus, and organelles. The exterior plasma membrane defines the perimeter of the cell, regulates the flow of nutrients, water and regulating molecules in and out of the cell, and has embedded into its structure receptors that the cell uses to detect properties of the environment surrounding the cell membrane. The cytoplasm acts as a filling medium inside the boundaries of the plasma cell membrane and is comprised mainly of water and nutrients such as amino acids, oxygen, and glucose. The nucleus, organelles, and ribosomes are suspended in the cytoplasm. The nucleus contains the majority of the cell's genetic information in the form of double stranded deoxyribonucleic acid (DNA). Organelles generally carry out specialized functions for the cell and include such structures as the mitochondria, the endoplasmic reticulum, storage vacuoles, lysosomes and Golgi complex (sometimes referred to as a Golgi apparatus). Floating in the cytoplasm, but also located in the endoplasmic reticulum and mitochondria are ribosomes. Ribosomes are complex macromolecule structures comprised of ribosomal ribonucleic acid (rRNA) molecules and ribosomal proteins that combine and couple to a messenger ribonucleic acid (mRNA) molecule. The rRNAs and the ribosomal proteins congregate to form a macromolecule structure that surrounds a mRNA molecule. Ribosomes decode genetic information in a mRNA molecule and manufacture proteins to the specifications of the instruction code physically present in the mRNA molecule. More than one ribosome may be attached to a single mRNA at a time.

[0062] Proteins are comprised of a series of amino acids bonded together in a linear strand, sometimes referred to as a chain; a protein may be further modified to be a structure comprised of one or more similar or differing strands of amino acids bonded together. Insulin is a protein structure comprised of two strands of amino acids; one strand comprised of 21 amino acids long and the second strand comprised of 30 amino acids, the two strands attached by two disulfide bridges. There are an estimated 30,000 different proteins the cells of the human body may manufacture. The human body is comprised of a wide variety of cells, many with specialized functions requiring unique combinations of proteins and protein structures such as glycoproteins (a protein combined with a carbohydrate) to accomplish the required task or tasks a specialized cell is designed to perform. Forms of glycoproteins are known to be utilized as cell-surface receptors. Messenger RNAs (mRNA) are created by transcription of DNA, they generally migrate to other locations inside the cell and are utilized by ribosomes as protein manufacturing templates. A ribosome is a protein complex that manufactures proteins by deciphering the instruction code located in a mRNA molecule. When a specific protein is needed, pieces of the ribosome complex, which include rRNA molecules and ribosomal proteins, bind around the strand of a mRNA that carries the specific instruction code that will generate the required protein. The ribosome traverses the mRNA strand and deciphers the genetic information coded into the sequence of nucleotides that comprise the mRNA molecule to produce a protein molecule and this process is referred to as translation.

[0063] The insulin molecule is a protein produced by Beta cells located in the pancreas. The 'insulin messenger RNA' is created in a Beta cell by a polymerase complex transcribing the insulin gene from nuclear DNA in the nucleus of the cell. The native messenger RNA (mRNA) for insulin then travels to the endoplasmic reticulum, where numerous ribosomes, comprised of rRNA and ribosomal proteins, engage these mRNA molecules. Many ribosomes may be attached to a single strand of mRNA simultaneously, each generating an identical copy of the protein as dictated by the information encoded in the mRNA. Insulin is produced by ribosomes translating the information in a mRNA molecule coded for the insulin protein, which produce strands of amino acids that are coded for an immature form of the biologically active insulin molecule referred to as 'pro-insulin'. Once the pro-insulin molecule is generated it then undergoes modification by several enzymes including prohormone convertase one (PC1), prohormone convertase two (PC2) and carboxypeptidase E, which results in the production of a biologically active insulin molecule. Once the biologically active insulin protein is generated it is stored in a vacuole in the Beta cell to await being released into the blood stream.

[0064] Insulin receptors, which appear on the surface of cells, offer binding sites for insulin circulating in the blood. When insulin binds to an insulin receptor, the biologic response inside the cell causes glucose to enter the cell and undergo processing in the cytoplasm. Processed glucose molecules then enter the mitochondria. The mitochondria further process the modified glucose molecules to produce usable energy in the form of adenosine triphosphate molecules (ATP). Thirty-eight ATP molecules may be generated from one molecule of glucose during the process of aerobic respiration. ATP molecules are utilized as an energy source by biologic processes throughout the cell.

[0065] The current medical therapeutic approach to the management of diabetes mellitus has produced limited results. Patients with diabetes generally struggle with an inadequate production of insulin, or an ineffective release of biologically active insulin molecules, or a release of an insufficient number of biologically active insulin molecules, or an insufficient production of cell-surface receptors, or a production of ineffective cell-surface receptors, or a production of ineffective insulin molecules that are unable to interact properly with insulin receptors to produce the required biologic effect. Type One diabetes requires administration of exogenous insulin. The traditional approach to Type Two diabetes has generally first been to adjust the diet to limit the caloric intake the individual consumes. Exercise is used as an initial approach to both Type One and Type Two diabetes as a means of up-regulating the utilization of fats and sugar so as to reduce the amount of circulating plasma glucose. When diet and exercise are inadequate in properly managing Type Two diabetes, oral medications are often introduced. The action of sulfonylureas, a commonly prescribed class of oral medication, is to stimulate the Beta cells to produce additional insulin receptors and enhance the insulin receptors' response to insulin. Biguanides, another form of oral treatment, inhibit gluconeogenesis, the production of glucose in the liver, thereby attempting to reduce plasma glucose levels. Thiazolidinediones (TZDs) lower blood sugar levels by activating peroxisome proliferator-activated receptor gamma (PPAR-γ), a transcription factor, which when activated regulates the activity of various target genes, particularly ones involved in glucose and lipid metabolism. If diet, exercise and oral medications do not produce a satisfactory control of the level of blood glucose in a diabetic patient, exogenous insulin is injected into the body in an effort to normalize the amount of glucose present in the serum. Insulin, a protein, has not successfully been made available as an oral medication to date due to the fact that proteins in general become degraded when they encounter the acid environment present in the stomach.

337

[0066] Despite strict monitoring of blood glucose and potentially multiple doses of insulin injected throughout the day, many patients with diabetes mellitus still experience devastating adverse effects from elevated blood glucose levels. Microvascular damage and elevated tissue sugar levels contribute to such complications as renal failure, retinopathy involving the eyes, neuropathy, and accelerated heart disease despite aggressive efforts to maintain the blood sugar within the physiologic normal range using exogenous insulin by itself or a combination of exogenous insulin and one or more oral medications. Diabetes remains the number one cause of renal failure in the United States. Especially in diabetic patients that are dependent upon administering exogenous insulin into their body, though dosing of the insulin may be four or more times a day and even though this may produce adequate control of the blood glucose level to prevent the clinical symptoms of hyperglycemia; this does not unerringly supplement the body's natural capacity to monitor the blood sugar level minute to minute, twenty-four hours a day, and deliver an immediate response to a rise in blood glucose by the release of insulin from Beta cells as required. The deleterious effects of diabetes may still evolve despite strict and persistent control of the glucose level in the blood stream.

[0067] The current treatment of diabetes may be augmented by the unique approach to utilizing modified viruses as vehicles to transport quantum genes into cells in order to increase the production of biologically active insulin. By utilizing modified viruses to transport quantum genes to facilitate and enhance the production of mRNAs, which would then facilitate the assembly of proteins would offer a new treatment option for patients with diabetes.

[0068] Viruses are obligate parasites. Viruses simply represent a carrier of genetic material and by themselves viruses are unable to replicate or carry out any form of biologic function outside their host cell. Viruses are generally comprised of one or more nested shells constructed of one or more layers of protein or lipid material, a genetic payload that represents the instruction code necessary to replicate the virus, and protein enzymes to help facilitate the genetic payload in the function of replicating copies of the virus once the genetic payload has been delivered to a host cell. Located on the outer shell or envelope of a virus are probes. The function of a virus's probes is to locate and engage a host cell's receptors. The virus's surface probes are designed to detect, make contact with and functionally engage one or more receptors located on the exterior of a cell type that will offer the virus the proper environment in which to construct copies of itself. A host cell provides the virus the proper biochemical machinery for the virus to successfully replicate itself.

[0069] Protected by an outer protein coat or lipid envelope, viruses carry a genetic payload in the form of deoxyribonucleic acid (DNA) or ribonucleic acid (RNA). Once a virus's exterior probes locate and functionally engage the surface receptor or receptors on a host cell, the virus inserts its genetic payload into the interior of the host cell. In the event a virus is carrying a DNA payload, the virus's DNA travels to the host cell's nucleus and is known to become inserted into the host cell's own native DNA. In the case where a virus is carrying its genetic payload as RNA, the virus inserts the RNA payload into the host cell and may also insert one or more enzymes to facilitate the RNA being utilized properly to replicate copies of the virus. Once inside the host cell, some species of virus facilitate use of their RNA by having the RNA converted to DNA. Once the viral RNA has been converted to DNA, the virus's DNA travels to the host cell's nucleus and is known to become inserted into the host cell's native DNA. Once a virus's genetic material has been inserted into the host cell's native DNA, the virus's genetic material takes command of certain cell functions and redirects the resources of the host cell to generate copies of the virus. Other forms of RNA viruses bypass the need to use the nuclear DNA and simply utilize portions of the viral genome to act as messenger RNA (mRNA). RNA viruses that bypass the host cell's DNA, cause the cell to in general generate copies of the necessary parts of the virus directly from the virus's RNA genome.

[0070] Present medical care is attempting to utilize viruses to deliver genetic information into cells. Research in the field of gene therapy has involved certain naturally occurring viruses. Some of the common viral vectors that have been investigated include: Adeno-associated virus, Adenovirus, Alphavirus, Epstein-Barr virus, Gammaretrovirus, Herpes simplex virus, Letivirus, Poliovirus, Rhabdovirus, Vaccinia virus. Naturally occurring virus vectors are limited to the naturally occurring external probes that are affixed to the outer wall of the virus. The external probes fixed to the outside wall of a virus virion dictate which type of cell the virus can engage and infect. Therefore, as an example, the function of the adenovirus, a respiratory virus, is strictly limited to engaging and infecting specific lung cells. Used as a medical treatment device, the adenovirus can only deliver gene therapy to specific lung cells, which severely limits this vector's usefulness as a deliver device. The therapeutic function of all naturally occurring viral vectors is limited to delivering a DNA or RNA payload to the cell type the viral vector naturally targets as its host cell.

[0071] Naturally occurring viruses also have the disadvantage of being susceptible to detection and elimination by a body's immune system. Viruses have been infecting humans for hundreds of thousands of years. A human's innate immune system is very efficient at detecting the presence of most naturally occurring viruses when such a virus is inside the body. The human immune system is quite capable of generating a vigorous response to most intruding viruses, attacking and neutralizing virus virions whenever a virus virion physically exists are outside the exterior wall of the virus's host cell. If gene therapy in its current state were to become a clinical therapeutic tool, the naturally occurring viruses selected for gene therapy research will have limited effectiveness due the fact that once the viral vector is introduced into the body, the body's the immune system will quickly engage and eliminate the viral vectors, possibly before the vector is able to deliver its payload to its host cell or target cell.

[0072] Cichutek, K., 2001 (US Patent No. 6,323,031 B1) teaches preparation and use of novel lentiviral SiVagm-derived vectors for gene transfer into selected cell types, specifically into proliferatively active and resting human cells.

[0073] Cichutek teaches that it is indeed plausible to re-configure an existing virus and use it as a transport vehicle, though Cichutek's specification and claims are too limited to describe a method that will work for all cell types, if indeed if it will work for any cell type.

[0074] Cichutek describes vectors for 'gene transfer'; in the claims the language that is used is 'genetic information'. Cichutek's Claim 1 of the cited patent states 'A propagation-incompetent SIVagm vector comprising a viral core and a viral envelope, wherein the viral core comprises a simian immunodeficiency virus (SIVagm) viral core of the African vervet monkey Chlorocebus.' Cichutek's does not describe in his claims any further details of the intended payload other than the stating 'SIVagm viral core' in claim 1; in claims 5 & 6 Cichutek describes only 'genetic information'. Transfer of 'genetic information' dramatically limits the useful application of Cichutek's patent in the treatment of medical diseases.

[0075] Cichutek does not claim the use of specific glycogen probes to target specific types of cells. Cichutek's approach is dependent upon the probes naturally present on the viral vectors reported in the patent, which will direct the viral vectors to only those cells the viruses naturally use as their host cell. Cichutek's approach is very restrictive, limited to gene transfer to only cells the viruses use as their natural host cell.

[0076] Cichutek's claim 4, states 'The SIVagm vector of claim 1, wherein the viral envelope further comprises a single chain antibody (scFv) or a ligand of a cell surface molecule.' By use of the words 'a' and 'or' in the claim, the claim is limited in the singular, meaning Cichutek claims a single chain antibody or a singular ligand. Singular type antibodies or ligands can be used for cell to cell communication, but to open an access portal into a cell and insert a payload into the cell requires two different types antibodies or ligands. As an example human immunodeficiency virus requires the use of both the gp120 and gp41 probes to open a portal into a T-Helper cell and insert its viral genome into the T-Helper cell. The gp120 probe engages the CD4+ cell-surface receptor on the T-cell. Once the gp120 probe has successfully engaged a CD4+ cell-surface receptor on the

341

target T-Helper cell, then the HIV virion's gp41 probe can engage either a CXCR4 or a CCR5 cell-surface receptor on the T-Helper cell in order to open up an access portal for HIV to insert its viral genome into a T-Helper cell. It is well documented in the medical literature that a genetic defect leading to an abnormality in the CXCR4 cell-surface receptor prevents HIV virions from opening an access portal and inserting its genetic payload into such T-Helper cells. This genetic defect in the CXCR4 cell-surface receptor offers the subset of people carrying the genetic defect resistance to HIV infection. This example demonstrates the need for at least two types of glycoprotein probes to be present on the surface of a viral vector in order for a viral vector to be capable of opening an access portal and delivering the payload the vector carries into its host cell or target cell.

[0077] A delivery system that offered a defined means of targeting specific types of cells would invoke minimal or no response by the innate immune system and the adaptable immune system when present in the body, and a delivery system that would be capable of inserting into cells a wide variety of quantum gene molecules would significantly improve the current medical treatment options available to clinicians treating patients.

[0078] The solution to arriving at a versatile, workable delivery system that will meet the needs of a number of medical treatments involves three important elements. These elements include:

(1) configurable external probes whereby more than one type of protein structure probe or more than one type of glycoprotein probe is to be used to engage and access specific target cell types in order to successfully deliver a payload into a specific type of cell,

(2) an external envelope comprised of a protein shell or lipid layer expressing the least number of cell-surface markers, such as the use of a stem cell to act as the host cell to manufacture the delivery devices,

(3) configuring the core of the vector to enable it to carry and deliver quantum genes.

For purposes of this text, the use of the terms 'specific target cell type', 'target cell', 'specific type of cell', 'specific cell', 'specific type of cell' are equivalent and interchangeable; the configuration of cell-surface receptors that a specific type of cell has located on and protruding from its outer cell membrane determines the cell type.

[0079] Viruses are obligate parasites. Viruses simply represent a carrier of genetic material and by themselves viruses are unable to replicate or carry out any form of biologic function outside their host cell. A 'virion' refers to the physical structure of a single complete virus as it exists outside of the host cell; a more archaic term for 'viral virion' was 'viral particle'. Viruses are generally comprised of one or more nested shells constructed of one or more layers of protein, some with a lipid outer envelope, a genetic payload that represents the instruction code necessary to replicate the virus, and protein enzymes to help facilitate the genetic payload in the function of replicating copies of the virus once the genetic payload has been delivered to a host cell. Located on the outer shell or envelope of a virus are probes. The function of a virus's external probes is to locate and engage a host cell's receptors. The virus's surface probes are designed to detect, make contact with and functionally engage one or more receptors located on the exterior of the type of cell that will offer the virus the proper environment in which to construct copies of itself. A host cell provides the virus the proper biologic machinery for the virus to successfully replicate itself. Once the virus's genome is inside the host cell, the viral genome takes command of the cell's production machinery and causes the host cell to generate copies of the virus. As the viral copies exit the host cell, these virions set off in search of other host cells to infect.

[0080] Naturally occurring viruses exist in a number of differing shapes. The shape of a virus may be rod or filament like, icosahedral, or complex structures combining filament and polygonal shapes. Viruses generally have their outer wall comprised of a protein coat or an envelope comprised of lipids.

[0081] An outer envelope comprised of lipids may be in the form of one or two phospholipid layers. When the outer envelope is comprised of two phospholipid layers this is termed a lipid bilayer. For purposes of this text the term 'lipid' includes 'phospholipid' molecules. A phospholipid is a composite molecule comprised of a polar or hydrophilic region on one end and a nonpolar or hydrophobic region on the opposite end. A lipid bilayer covering a virus, like the membrane of a cell, is constructed with the hydrophilic region of one of the phospholipid layers pointed toward the exterior of the virion and the hydrophilic region of the second phospholipid layer pointed inward toward the center of the virus virion; with the hydrophobic regions of each of the two lipid layers pointed toward each other. The outer envelope of some forms of virus may be comprised of an outer lipid layer or lipid bilayer affixed to a protein matrix for support, the protein matrix being located closer to the center of the virus virion than the lipid layer or lipid bilayer.

[0082] Spherical viruses are generally spherical in shape and may be comprised of an outer envelope and one inner shell or alternatively an outer envelope and multiple inner shells. Inner shells are approximately spherical in shape; this is because the proteins comprising the protein matrix shell have an irregular shape to their structure, but when constructed together for a shape that resembles a sphere. In the case of a spherical virus with an outer envelope and one inner shell, the inner shell is often referred to as a nucleocapsid shell comprised of numerous capsid proteins attached to each other. In the case of a spherical virus being comprised of an outer envelope and multiple inner shells, the outermost inner viral shells may be referred to as comprised of a quantity of matrix proteins, where the innermost shell is referred to as a nucleocapsid and is comprised of a quantity of capsid proteins. The inner protein shells are nested inside each other. The cavity created by the innermost shell or nucleocapsid is referred to as the 'core' or 'center of the virus'. Any payload carried by the virus virion is generally carried in the core or center of the virion.

[0083] Viruses carry genetic material in the form of deoxyribonucleic acid (DNA) or ribonucleic acid (RNA) as their payload. DNA or RNA genome payloads are carried in the cavity of the nucleocapsid referred to as the core. A virus is therefore generally considered to be a DNA virus if its genome is comprised of DNA or the virus is considered a RNA virus if its genome is comprised of RNA that acts as genetic instructions to generate copies of the virus. Viruses may also carry enzymes as part of their payload. An enzyme such as 'reverse transcriptase' transforms a RNA viral genome into DNA. Protease enzymes modify the viral genome once it has entered a host cell. An integrase enzyme assists a DNA viral genome with insertion into the host cell's nuclear DNA. The entire genetic payload is carried inside the cavity created by the virus's nucleocapsid shell.

[0084] The probes attached to the exterior of a virus are constructed to engage specific cell-surface receptors on specific type of cells in the body. Only a cell that expresses cell-surface receptors that are capable of being engaged by the probes of a specific virus can act as a host for the virus. Viruses generally use two probes to access a host cell. The first probe makes an initial attachment to the host cell, while the action of the virus's second probe often in conjunction with the action of the first probe cause an access portal to be created in the host cell's exterior plasma membrane. Once an access portal is formed, the virus inserts the contents of its payload into the host cell utilizing the open access portal. Certain types of virus may be engulfed whole by a target cell. Once the virus's genome is inside the cytoplasm of the host cell, any enzymes that accompanied the viral genome into the cell, may begin to modify or assist the virus's genome with infecting and taking control of the host cell's biologic functions.

[0085] Probes are attached to the external envelope of a virus virion. Probes may be in the form of a protein structure or may be in the form of a glycoprotein molecule. For viruses constructed with a protein matrix as its outer envelope, the probes tend to be protein structures. A portion of the protein structure probe is fixed or anchored in the protein matrix, while a portion of the protein structure probe extends out and away from the protein matrix. The portion of the protein structure probe extending out away from the virus virion is referred to as the 'exterior domain', the portion anchored in the protein matrix is the 'transcending domain'. Some protein probes have a third segment that extends through the envelope and exists inside the virus virion, which is referred to as the 'interior domain'. The exterior domain of a protein structure probe is intended to engage a specific cell-surface receptor on a biologically active cell the virus is targeting as its host cell.

[0086] Viruses that utilize a lipid layer as the outer envelope, are constructed with probes that tend to be glycoproteins. A glycoprotein is comprised of a protein segment and a carbohydrate segment. The carbohydrate segment of the glycoprotein molecule is fixed or anchored in the lipid layer of the outer envelope, while the protein segment extends outward and away from the outer envelope. The protein portion of a glycoprotein probe that extends outward and away from the outer envelope of a virus virion is intended to engage a cell-surface receptor on a biologically active cell the virus is targeting as its host cell.

[0087] Some forms of viruses that utilize a lipid layer as its envelope use protein structure probes. In this case, the portion of the protein structure probe that extends outward and away from the outer envelope is the 'exterior domain', the portion that is anchored in the lipid layer is the 'transcending domain' and again some protein structure probes have an 'interior domain' that exist inside the virion, which may also help anchor the protein structure probe to the virion. The exterior domain of a protein structure probe that extends outward and away from the outer envelope of a virus virion is intended to engage a cell-surface receptor on a biologically active cell the virus is targeting as its host cell.

[0088] When a virus carries a DNA payload and the viral DNA is inserted into the host cell, the virus's DNA travels to the host cell's nucleus and is known to become inserted into the host cell's own native DNA. In the case where a virus is carrying its genetic payload as RNA, the virus inserts the RNA payload into the host cell and may also insert one or more enzymes to facilitate the RNA being utilized properly to replicate copies of the virus. Once inside the host cell, some species of virus facilitate use of the viral RNA by having the RNA converted to DNA. Once the viral RNA has been converted to

DNA, the virus's DNA travels to the host cell's nucleus and is known to become inserted into the host cell's native DNA. Once a virus's genetic material has been inserted into the host cell's native DNA, the virus's genetic material takes command of certain cell functions and redirects the resources of the host cell to generate copies of the virus. Other forms of RNA viruses bypass the need to use the nuclear DNA and simply utilize portions of the viral genome to act as messenger RNA. RNA viruses that bypass the host cell's DNA, cause the cell in general to generate copies of the necessary parts of the virus directly from the virus's RNA genome.

[0089] The human immunodeficiency virus (HIV) is a RNA virus and has an outer envelope comprised of a lipid bilayer. The lipid bilayer covers a protein matrix consisting of p17^{gag} proteins. Inside the p17^{gag} protein is nested a nucleocapsid comprised of p24^{gag} proteins. Inside the nucleocapsid HIV carries its payload. HIV's genetic payload consists of two single strands of RNA and several enzymes. The enzymes that accompany HIV's genome include 'reverse transcriptase', 'integrase' and 'protease' molecules.

[0090] The T-Helper cell acts as HIV's host cell. The HIV virion utilizes two types of glycoprotein probes affixed to its external envelope to locate and engage a T-Helper cell. HIV utilizes a glycoprotein probe 120 to locate a CD4 cell-surface receptor on a T-Helper cell. Once an HIV glycoprotein 120 probe has successfully engaged a CD4 cell surface-receptor on a T-Helper cell a conformational change occurs in the glycoprotein 120 probe and a glycoprotein 41 probe is exposed. The glycoprotein 41 probe's intent is to engage a CXCR4 or CCR5 cell-surface receptor on the same T-Helper cell. Once a glycoprotein 41 probe on the HIV virion successfully engages a CXCR4 or CCR5 cell-surface receptor, the HIV virion opens an access portal through the T-Helper cell's outer membrane.

[0091] Once the HIV virion has opened an access portal through the T-Helper cell's outer plasma membrane, the HIV virion inserts two positive strand RNA molecules and the associated enzymes it carries into the T-Helper cell. Each RNA strand is approximately 9500 nucleotides in length. Inserted along with the RNA strands are the enzymes reverse transcriptase, protease and integrase. Once the virus's genome gains access to the interior of the T-Helper cell, in the cytoplasm the pair of RNA molecules are transformed to deoxyribonucleic acid by the reverse transcriptase enzyme. Following modification of the virus's genome to DNA, the virus's genetic information migrates to the host cell's nucleus. In the nucleus, with the assistance of the integrase protein, the HIV's DNA becomes inserted into the T-Helper cell's native nuclear DNA. When the timing is appropriate, the now integrated viral DNA is decoded by the host cell's polymerase molecules and the virus's genetic information commands certain cell functions to carry out the replication process to construct copies of the human immunodeficiency virus.

[0092] The outer layer of the HIV virion is comprised of a portion of the T-Helper cell's outer cell membrane. In the final stage of the replication process, as a copy of the HIV virion, carrying the HIV genome, buds through the host cell's cell membrane the outer protein shell acquires as its external envelope, a wrapping of lipid bilayer from the host cell's cell membrane. In the case of HIV, since the surface of the pathogen is covered by an envelope comprised of lipid bilayer taken from the host T-Helper cells, this feature allows the HIV virion the capacity to elude the two immune systems, since the detectors comprising the innate immune system and the adaptable immune system may find it difficult to distinguish between the surface of an infectious HIV virion and the surface characteristics of a noninfected T-Helper cell.

[0093] The Hepatitis C virus (HCV) is a positive sense RNA virus, meaning a type of RNA that is capable of bypassing the need for involving the host cell's nucleus by having its RNA genome function as messenger RNA. Hepatitis C infects liver cells. The Hepatitis C viral genome becomes divided once it gains access to the interior of a liver host cell. Portions of the subdivisions of the Hepatitis C genome directly interact with ribosomes to produce proteins necessary to construct copies of the virus.

[0094] HCV belongs to the Flaviviridae family and is the only member of the Hepacivirus genus. There are considered to be at least 100 different strains of Hepatitis C virus based on genome sequencing variability.

[0095] HCV is comprised of an outer lipoprotein envelope and an internal nucleocapsid. The genetic payload is carried within the nucleocapsid. In its natural state, present on the surface of the outer envelope of the Hepatitis C virus are probes that detect receptors present on the surface of liver cells. The glycoprotein E1 probe and the glycoprotein E2 probe have been identified to be affixed to the surface of HCV. The E2 probe binds with high affinity to the large external loop of a CD81 cell-surface receptor. CD81 is found on the surface of many cell types including liver cells. Once the E2 probe has engaged the CD81 cell-surface receptor, cofactors on the surface of HCV's external envelope engage either or both the low density lipoprotein receptor (LDLR) or the scavenger receptor class B type I (SR-BI) present on the liver cell in order to effect the mechanism to facilitate HCV breaching the cell membrane and inserting its RNA genome payload through the plasma cell membrane of the liver cell into the liver cell. Upon successful engagement of the HCV surface probes with a liver cell's cell-surface receptors, HCV inserts the single strand of RNA and other payload elements it carries into the liver cell targeted to be a host cell. The HCV RNA genome then interacts with enzymes and ribosomes inside the liver cell in a translational process to produce the proteins required to construct copies of the protein components of HCV. The HCV genome undergoes a method of transcription to replicate copies of the virus's RNA genome. Inside the host, pieces of the HCV virus are assembled together and ultimately loaded with a copy of the HCV genome. Replicas of the original HCV then escape the host cell and migrate the environment in search of additional host liver cells to infect and continue the replication process.

[0096] The HCV's naturally occurring genetic payload consists of a single molecule of linear positive sense, single stranded RNA approximately 9600 nucleotides in length. By means of a translational process a polyprotein of approximately 3000 amino

acids is generated. This polyprotein is cleaved post translation by host and viral proteases into individual viral proteins which include: the structural proteins of C, E1, E2, the nonstructural proteins NS1, NS2, NS3, NS4A, NS4B, NS5A, NS5B, p7 and ARFP/F protein. Hepatitis C virus's proteins direct the host liver cell to construction copies of the Hepatitis C virus. A membrane associated replicase complex consisting of the virus's nonstructural proteins NS3 and NS5B facilitate the replication of the viral genome. The membrane of the endoplasmic reticulum appears to be the site of protein maturation and viral assembly. Once copies of the Hepatitis C Virus are generated, they exit the host cell and each copy of HCV migrates in search of another appropriate liver cell that will act as a host to continue the replication process.

[0097] Hepatitis C virus life-cycle demonstrates that copies of a virus virion can be generated by inserting RNA into a host cell that functions as messenger RNA in the host cell. The Hepatitis C viral RNA genome functions as messenger RNA, acting as the template in conjunction with the biologic machinery of a host cell to produce the components that comprise copies of the Hepatitis C virion and the Hepatitis C viral RNA provides the biologic instructions to assemble the components into complete copies of the Hepatitis C virions. The Hepatitis C virus life-cycle clearly demonstrates that viral virions can be manufactured by a host cell without involving the nucleus of the cell.

[0098] Deciphering the existence, replication and behavior of viruses provides clear examples of several fundamental concepts, which include: (1) Viruses target specific cells in the body by means of identifying and engaging such target cells utilizing the probes projecting outward from the virus's exterior shell to make contact with cell-surface receptors located on the surface of the target cells, and (2) Viruses are capable of carrying a variety of different types of payloads including DNA, RNA and a variety of proteins.

[0099] Current gene therapy approach to attempting to deliver a payload to cells in the body use modified forms of existing viruses to act as transport devices to deliver genetic information. This approach is severely limited by restricting the virus virion to the target only cells the viral vector naturally seeks out and infects. Current gene therapy approach is further limited by using the pre-existing size of naturally occurring viruses, rather than being able to modify the size of the structure to be able to tailor the volumetric carrying capacity of the payload portion of the modified virus. Further, gene therapy is restricted to utilizing naturally occurring viruses to deliver only genetic information; it has not previously been appreciated by those skilled in the art that virus-like transport devices might deliver to a variety of specific type of cells a wide variety of differing payloads such as quantum genes.

[0100] A dramatic, not previously recognized by those expert in the art is the need to develop a transport vehicle that can be fashioned to seek out specific types of cells and deliver to these cells DNA genetic material. The external envelope of a transport should be constructed so as not to alert the immune system of its presence to prevent rejection of the vehicles. Transport vehicles should be capable of being configured to target any specific type of cell and engage and deliver their payload only to that specific type of cell.

[0101] An equally dramatic, not previously recognized is the need for strict organization of the genes that comprise the human genome. The individual genes must each be labeled with some form of unique identifier to facilitate the nuclear transcription mechanisms in easily finding the transcribable genetic information when needed.

[0102] Merging these two concepts together suggests a transport device that would be capable of inserting quantum genes into specifically targeted cells; a constellation of concepts not previously before recognized by those skilled in the art.

[0103] For purposes of this text, the term 'exogenous' refers to an item which originates outside the boundaries of a particular cell or cell type and becomes a part of a particular cell or cell type. The term 'endogenous' refers to an item which originates as a part of a particular cell or cell type and remains a part of that particular cell or cell type.

BRIEF SUMMARY OF THE INVENTION

[0104] Utilization of configurable microscopic medical payload delivery devices to deliver quantum genes to specific type of cells facilitates a dramatic new approach to medical care. By selecting the type of probes that are present on the surface of the configurable microscopic medical payload delivery devices, specific types of cells can be targeted. By delivering quantum genes to specific type of cells, genetic instructions delivered to cell can be located and transcribed in an efficient manner, and thus utilized in the specific type of cells in a timely fashion. A wide variety of medical conditions are manageable by utilizing this new and unique approach.

DETAILED DESCRIPTION

[0105] The future of medical treatment will be the widespread utilization of configurable microscopic medical payload delivery devices (CMMPDD) to deliver quantum genes directly to targeted cell types in the body.

[0106] Introduced herein are the concepts: (1) configurable microscopic medical payload delivery devices can carry quantum gene molecules as the payload, and (2) glycoprotein probes present on the exterior of the configurable microscopic medical payload delivery devices include specific glycoprotein probes or protein structure probes affixed to the exterior, these glycoprotein probes or protein structure probes intended to seek out and engage cell-surface receptors attached to the exterior of whichever cell the configurable microscopic medical payload delivery devices is intended to deliver its payload of quantum gene molecules in order to produce a predetermined medically beneficial effect.

[0107] For the purposes of this text a 'quantum gene' is comprised of a sequence of nucleotides that represents a 'unique identifier' physically linked to a sequence of nucleotides that represent a discrete quantity of genetic information; these sequences of nucleotides being comprised of some combination of the nucleotides being referred to by their nitrogenous base as <u>adenine</u>

(A), thymine (T), cytosine (C), and guanine (G). The genetic information associated with the above-mentioned unique identifier may be comprised of a portion of transcribable genetic information and a portion of nontranscribable genetic information which together define a specific gene, otherwise referred to as a discrete quantity of genetic information. The nontranscribable segments of a quantum gene may represent segments that act as instructions such as a START code, STOP code and REPEAT code or may help facilitated the attachment of a transcription complex or be simply ignored during the transcription process. Quantum gene molecules can be comprised of a segment of nucleotides where the portion that represents a unique identifier is separated from the portion that represents genetic information by a quantity of base pairs of nucleotides that do not represent a unique identifier and do not represent genetic information. The purpose of the separation of the portion of the unique identifier from the portion of the genetic information by a quantity of base pairs of nucleotides that do not represent a unique identifier and does not represent genetic information is to facilitate a transcription complex attaching to the quantum gene upstream from the portion of the quantum gene that represents genetic information so that transcription of the biologic information associated with the quantum gene may occur.

[0108] The genetic information in a quantum gene codes for some combination of protein coding RNA (pcRNA), non-coding RNAs (ncRNA) and spacers. Spacers represent segments of the DNA that do not code for a RNA molecule. The genetic information in a quantum gene, when transcribed, produces protein coding RNA and non-coding RNA. Protein coding RNAs, usually referred to as messenger RNAs, undergo the process of translation in the cytoplasm of the cell and produce proteins. Non-coding RNAs are highly abundant and functionally important for the cell's operation. Non-coding RNAs have also been referred by such terms as non-protein-coding RNAs (npcRNA) or non-messenger RNA (nmRNA) or small non-messenger RNA (snmRNA) or functional RNAs (fRNA). The non-coding RNAs include: transfer RNAs (tRNA), ribosomal RNAs (rRNA), small nuclear RNAs (snRNA), small nucleolar RNAs (snoRNA), signal recognition particle RNA

(SRP RNA), antisense RNA (aRNA), micro RNA (miRNA), small interfering RNA (siRNA), Y RNA, telomerase RNA.

[0109] Transfer RNAs (tRNA), are RNAs that carries amino acids and deliver them to a ribosome. Ribosomal RNAs (rRNA), are RNAs that couple with ribosomal proteins and participate in translation of mRNA to produce protein molecules. Small nuclear RNAs (snRNA) are RNAs involved in splicing and other nuclear functions. Small nucleolar RNAs (snoRNA) are RNAs involved in nucleotide modification. Signal recognition particle RNA (SRP RNA) are RNAs are involved in membrane integration. Antisense RNA (aRNA) are RNAs involved in transcription attenuation, mRNA degradation, mRNA stabilization, and translation blockage. Micro RNA (miRNA) are RNAs involved in gene regulation and have been implicated in a wide range of cell functions including cell growth, apoptosis, neuronal plasticity, and insulin secretion. Small interfering RNA (siRNA) are RNAs involved in gene regulation, often interfering with the expression of a single gene. Y RNA are RNAs involved in RNA processing and DNA replication. Telomerase RNA are RNAs involved in telomere synthesis.

[0110] In addition to the unique identifier, a quantum gene is comprised of the biologic instruction code, which when transcribed produces one or more of the same RNA molecules or different RNA molecules. A quantum gene must be comprised of a unique identifier and the genetic material to code for at least one RNA molecule. The definition of a 'quantum gene' differs from all previous definitions of a 'gene' due to the requirement that the quantum gene must have a unique identifier that accompanies a segment of genetic information. From a medical treatment perspective, the quantum gene's unique identifier allows the genetic information present in the quantum gene to be located by a cell's transcription machinery, once the quantum gene is inserted into a cell's nuclear DNA.

[0111] Ribonucleic acid molecules directly transcribed from the DNA or quantum gene, may be precursor ribonucleic acid molecules that require modification by nuclear enzymes prior to being translatable or may be ribonucleic acid molecules which are directly translatable without further modification.

[0112] In the DNA there are a number of nucleotides physically existing along the deoxyribonucleic acid between the unique identifier and the transcribable genetic information; or in other terms a number of nucleotides that are not a part of the identification code and are not transcribable, exist downstream from the unique identifier and upstream from the transcribable genetic information.

[0113] It is well recognized that within the transcribable genetic information there exist subsegments of nucleotides that are not transcribable and there are subsegments of nucleotides that are transcribed but are not found in the final version of the RNA molecule. Subsegments of transcribable genetic information that are not transcribed are subsegments such as 'STOP' codes, which indicate to the transcription complex a potential point at which to cease transcribing the genetic information. Certain factors may influence whether a transcription complex actually ceases transcription at that point or whether the transcription complex continues transcribing when the transcription complex reaches a 'STOP' code. Subsegments of nucleotides that are transcribed and appear in the final active form of a RNA are referred to as exons. Subsegments of nucleotides that are transcribed, but do not appear in the final active form of a RNA are referred to as introns. Precursor RNA molecules include both exons and introns. Introns are removed by modification of the initial RNA segment directly transcribed from the transcribable genetic information.

[0114] Utilization of the sigma summation symbol to show summation over a series of indexed variables or expression can be represented as:

$$\sum_{j=1}^{n} [K]_j = [K]_1 + [K]_2 + \ldots + [K]_n$$

[0115] An equation to represent a quantum gene would be:

Quantum gene = [unique identifier] +

$$\sum_{a=0}^{n}[nontranscribable\ connector\ nucleotide]_a\ +$$

$$\sum_{b=1}^{n}[nucleotide\ segment\ transcribable\ for\ RNA]_b\ +$$

$$\sum_{c=0}^{n}[nontranscribable\ spacer\ nucleotide]_c\ +$$

$$\sum_{d=0}^{n}[nontranscribable\ nucleotide\ commands]_d$$

Where 'unique identifier' represents a number, a name or the combination of a number and a name that the transcription complex utilizes to locate a specific quantum gene amongst the DNA material present in a biologically active cell.

Where 'nontranscribable connector nucleotide' represents one or more nucleotides that physically exists between the 'unique identifier' and the segment of 'transcribable genetic information'.

Where a 'nontranscribable spacer nucleotide' represents one or more nucleotides comprising the transcribable genetic information that is not transcribed when the transcription complex transcribes the genetic information of the quantum gene.

Where a 'nontranscribable nucleotide command' represents one or more nucleotides comprising the transcribable genetic information that is not transcribed when the transcription complex transcribes the genetic information of the quantum gene, but acts as an instruction to the transcription complex to cause the transcription complex to function in a certain manner; examples include a STOP code that causes the transcription complex to cease transcription and a REPEAT code that causes the transcription complex to repeat its transcription of a segment of genetic material.

Where 'a' represents the range of 'zero to any positive whole number. Where 'b' represents the range of 'one to any positive whole number'.

Where 'c' represents the range of 'zero to any positive whole number'.
Where 'd' represents the range of 'zero to any positive whole number'.

Where the DNA segment that is transcribable for RNA may transcribe RNAs that may exist in a precursor form; such a precursor form may include elements such as introns that are removed following transcription by modifying proteins.

[0116] For purposes of this text an 'external envelope' refers to the outermost covering of a virus or a virus-like transport device or a configurable microscopic medical payload delivery device. The external envelope may be comprised of a lipid layer, a lipid bilayer, the combination of a lipid layer affixed to a protein matrix or the combination of a lipid bilayer affixed to a protein matrix. A protein matrix is equivalent to a protein shell and may be referred to as a protein matrix shell. The terms protein matrix, protein shell, protein matrix shell are equivalent to the term capsid, where the term capsid is meant to represent 'a protein coat or shell of a virus particle, surrounding the nucleic acid or nucleoprotein core'. For purposes of this text, the term 'particle' is equivalent to the term 'virion'; further the term 'virus particle' is equivalent to 'viral virion'.

[0117] For purposes of this text an 'internal shell' refers to a protein matrix shell nested inside the external envelope. Multiple inner shells may exist, with those of smaller diameter concentrically nested inside those of a larger diameter. The inner most protein matrix shell is termed the nucleocapsid. The proteins that comprise the nucleocapsid are termed capsid proteins. In the cavity created by the nucleocapsid, referred to as the center or core of the nucleocapsid, is where the payload of quantum gene molecules is carried.

[0118] For purposes of this text 'external probes' are molecular structures that are utilized to locate and engage cell-surface receptors on biologically active cells. External probes are generally comprised of a portion which is anchored or fixed in the external envelope and a second portion that extends out and away from the external envelope. The portion of the external probe that extends out and away from the external envelope is intended to make contact and engage a specific cell-surface receptor located on a biologically active cell. External probes may be comprised solely of a protein structure or an external probe may be a glycoprotein molecule.

[0119] For purposes of this text 'glycoprotein molecule' refers to a molecule comprised of a carbohydrate region and a protein region. Glycoprotein molecules that act as probes are generally anchored or fixed to a lipid layer utilizing the carbohydrate portion of the molecule as an anchor. The protein portion of the glycoprotein molecule which extends outward and away from the external envelope the glycoprotein has been affixed such that the protein region may function as a probe to locate and attach to the cell-surface receptor it was created to engage.

[0120] The concept of configurable microscopic medical payload delivery devices is modeled after naturally existing viruses. Configurable microscopic medical payload delivery devices in general are spherical in shape; though other shapes may be used as function might warrant the use of a particular shape. The spherical configurable microscopic medical payload delivery devices are comprised of an external envelope and one or more inner nested protein shells. A quantity of exterior protein structure probes and/or glycoprotein probes are anchored in the external envelope and a portion extend out and away from the exterior lipid envelope. Nesting of protein shells refers to progressively smaller diameter shells fitting snugly inside protein shells of a larger diameter. Inside the inner most protein shell, referred to as the nucleocapsid, is a cavity referred to as the core of the device. The core of the device is the space where the medically therapeutic payload the device carries is located. The payload of the device is comprised of ribonucleic acid molecules.

[0121] Configurable microscopic medical payload delivery devices (CMMPDD) target specific types of cells in the body. Configurable microscopic medical payload delivery devices engage specific types of cells by the configuration of probes affixed to the external envelope of the CMMPDD. By fixing specific probes to the external envelope of the CMMPDD, these probes intended to engage and attach only to specific cell-surface receptors located on certain cell types in the body, the CMMPDD will deliver its payload only to those cell types that express compatible and engagable specific cell-surface receptors. In a similar fashion where the exterior probes of a naturally occurring virus engage specific cell-surface receptors present on the surface of the virus's host cell and only the designated host cell, the CMMPDD's exterior probes are configured to engage cell-surface receptors on a specific type of target cell and only those cells. In this manner, the payload of quantum gene molecules carried by CMMPDD will be delivered only to specific types of cells in the body. The configuration of exterior probes on the surface of a CMMPDD varies as needed so as to effect the CMMPDD delivery of specific quantum gene payloads to specific type of cells as needed to effect a particular predetermined medical treatment.

[0122] The size of the configurable microscopic medical payload delivery devices is dependent upon the diameter of the inner protein matrix shells and this is dictated by the volume size of the payload the CMMPDD is required to carry and deliver to a target cell. The diameter of the each inner protein matrix shell is governed by the number of protein molecules utilized to construct the protein matrix shell at the time the protein matrix shell is generated. Increasing the number of proteins that comprise a protein matrix shell increases the diameter of the protein matrix shell. When applicable, as dictated by the capacity the CMMPDD is to be utilized to function as, an external lipid envelope wraps around and covers the outer protein matrix shell. The larger the volume of the core of the CMMPDD, the greater the physical size of the payload the CMMPDD is able to carry. The size of the configurable microscopic medical payload delivery device is to be generally the size of cell (approximately 10^{-4} m in diameter) or less, generally detectable by a light microscope or, as needed, an electron microscope. The size of the CMMPDD is not to be too large such that it would generate a burden to the body by damaging organ tissues through clogging blood vessels or the glomeruli in the kidneys. The dimensions of each type of

CMMPDD are to be tailored to the mission of the CMMPDD, which takes into account factors such as the type of target cell, the size of the payload that is to be delivered to the target cells and the length of time the CMMPDD may engage the target cell.

[0123] Being enveloped in an external lipid layer, configurable microscopic medical payload delivery devices possess the advantage of having their exterior appear similar to the plasma membrane that acts as an outside covering for the cells that comprise the body. By appearing similar to existing plasma membranes, the CMMPDDs appear similar to naturally occurring structures found in the body. CMMPDD are afforded the capability to avoid detection by a body's immune system because the exterior of the CMMPDD mimics the cells comprising the body and the surveillance elements of the immune system find it difficult to discern between the CMMPDD and naturally occurring cells comprising the body.

[0124] To carry out the process of manufacturing a configurable microscopic medical payload delivery device, a primitive cell such as a stem cell is selected. The reason for utilizing primitive cells such as stems cells as the host cell, is that the CMMPDD acquires its outer envelope from the host cell and the more primitive the host cell, the fewer in number the identifying protein markers are present on the surface of the CMMPDD. The fewer the identifying surface proteins present on the outer envelope of the CMMPDD, the less likely a body's immune system will identify the CMMPDD as an invader and therefore less likely the body's immune system will react to the presence of the CMMPDD and reject the CMMPDD by attacking and neutralizing the CMMPDD.

[0125] Stem cells used as host cells to manufacture quantities of CMMPDD product are selected per histocompatibility markers present on their surface. Certain histocompatibility markers present on the surface of the final CMMPDD product will be less likely to cause a reaction in a specific patient based on the genetic profile of the patient's histocompatibility markers. A similar histocompatibility match is done when donor organs are selected to be given to recipients to avoid rejection of the donor organ by the recipient's immune system.

[0126] The selected stem cell used to manufacture configurable microscopic medical payload delivery devices goes through several steps of maturation before it is capable of generating therapeutic CMMPDD product. RNA inserted into the host stem cell code for the general physical outer structures of the CMMPDD. RNA inserted into the host generate surface probes that target the cell-surface receptors on a specific target cell type. RNA would be inserted into the host that would be used to generate the payload of quantum genes. Similar to how copies of a naturally occurring virus, such as the Hepatitis C virus or HIV, are produced, assembled and released from a host cell, copies of the CMMPDD would be produced, assembled and released from a stem cell functioning as a de facto host cell. Once released from the host cell, the copies of the CMMPDD would be collected, then pooled together to produce a therapeutic dose that would result in a medically beneficial effect.

[0127] The stem cells used as host cells are suspended in a broth of nutrients and are kept at an optimum temperature to govern the rate of production of the CMMPDD product. Similar to the natural production of the Hepatitis C virus, the configurable microscopic medical payload delivery devices 'production genome' is introduced into the host stem cells. The configurable microscopic medical payload delivery devices production genome carries genetic instructions to cause the host cells to manufacture the configurable microscopic medical payload delivery devices' outer protein wall, the inner protein matrixes, the surface probes the configurable microscopic medical payload delivery device is to have affixed to its outer envelope and the quantity of quantum gene molecules the configurable microscopic medical payload delivery devices are to carry; and the instructions to assemble the various pieces into the final form of the configurable microscopic medical payload delivery devices and the instructions to activate the budding process. The resultant configurable microscopic medical payload delivery devices are collected from the nutrient broth surrounding the host cells and placed together into doses to be used as a treatment for a medical disease.

[0128] The 'production genome' are an array of RNAs, which include messenger RNAs that are directly translated by the host cell's ribosomes. The production genome dictates the characteristics of the final version of the CMMPDD that buds from the host stem cell and is released and is to be utilized as a medical treatment. The production genome is specifically tailored to code for the surface probes that will seek and engage a specific type of target cell. The production genome also carries the instructions to code for the production of the type of quantum genes to be delivered to the specific type of target cell. The 'production genome' varies depending upon the configuration of the CMMPDD and the specific type of quantum genes the CMMPDD will transport to effect a specific medical treatment on a specific type of cell.

[0129] The configurable microscopic medical payload delivery device transporting quantum gene molecules represents a very versatile medical treatment delivery device. CMMPDD is used to deliver a number of different quantum gene molecules to a wide variety of cells in the body.

[0130] The construction of a naturally occurring virus can be likened to the act of following a programmed script to produce a specific result. It is known that the genetic code that a virus carries dictates the production of copies of the virus. It is known that specific segments of the viral genetic code represent instructions that dictate the construction of different parts of the virus so that copies of the virus can be made inside the host cell. It is well documented that there exist different subtypes of most viruses, based off of mutations that have occurred to the viral genome over time; these mutations to the viral genome producing variants in the construction of the virus. Configurable microscopic medical payload delivery devices which carry quantum genes are constructed much like a naturally occurring virus virions would be constructed in a host cell. Altering the production RNA alters the configuration of the external probes or alters the configuration of the size of the inner shells or alters the type of quantum gene the CMMPDD will carry or alters any combination of the three.

[0131] As an example of the method to produce a device to treat diabetes mellitus utilizing configurable microscopic medical payload delivery devices to deliver to Beta cells quantum genes, which when transcribed produce messenger RNA coded to produce insulin, the following production process is followed in the lab: (1) human stem cells are selected. (2) Into the selected stem cells is placed the RNA production genome constructed, in this case, specifically as a means to treat diabetes mellitus. The RNA production genome contains genetic instructions to cause the host stem cells to manufacture the CMMPDDs' outer protein wall, the inner protein matrix, surface probes to include a quantity of glycoprotein probes that engage the GPR40 cell-surface receptor present on the surface of Beta cells located in the Islets of Langerhans in the pancreas, and the payload of quantum genes, in this case the quantum genes to facilitate the production of the insulin molecules in Beta cells; and the biologic instructions to assemble the components into the final form of the CMMPDD; and the biologic instructions to activate the budding process. (3) Upon insertion of the RNA production genome into the host stem cells, host stem cells' production cellular machinery responds by simultaneously translating the different segments of the RNA production genome to produce the proteins that comprise the exterior protein wall, the inner protein matrix molecules, the surface probes, the quantum gene payload to produce the messenger RNA that will produce insulin, and decode the instructions to assemble the components into the CMMPDDs. (4) Upon assembly, the CMMPDDs bud through the cell membrane of the host stem cell. (5) At the time of the budding process, the CMMPDDs acquire an outside envelope wrapped over the outer protein shell, this outer envelope comprised of a portion of the plasma membrane from the host stem cell as the CMMPDDs exit the host cell. (6) The resultant CMMPDDs are collected from the nutrient broth surrounding the host stem cells. (7) The CMMPDD product is washed in sterile solution to separate the CMMPDD product from any unwanted elements of the nutrient broth. (8) The configurable microscopic medical payload delivery devices are removed from the sterile solvent and suspended in a hypoallergenic liquid medium. (9) The configurable microscopic medical payload delivery devices are separated into individual quantities to facilitate storage and delivery to physicians and patients. (10) The configurable microscopic medical payload delivery devices transported in the hypoallergenic liquid medium is administered to a diabetic patient per injection in a dose that is tailored to receiving patient's requirement to produce sufficient amount of insulin to control the blood sugar. (11) Upon being injected into the body, the configurable microscopic medical payload delivery devices migrate to the Beta cells located in the Islets of Langerhans by means of the patient's blood stream. (12) Upon the configurable microscopic medical payload delivery devices reaching the Beta cells, the configurable microscopic medical payload delivery devices engage the cell-surface receptors located on the Beta cells and insert the payload of quantum genes they carry into the Beta cells. The payload of quantum genes migrate to the nucleus of the Beta cells. The quantum genes inserts into the nuclear DNA of the Beta cells. Transcription machinery present in the nucleus transcribes the quantum genes. Messenger RNAs generated by transcribing the exogenous quantum genes enhances the Beta cells' production of insulin molecules. The increase in insulin production by Beta cells successfully manages diabetes mellitus.

[0132] In a similar fashion, configurable microscopic medical payload delivery devices can be fashioned to deliver a payload of a specific type of quantum gene molecule to any type of cell in the body. Different cell types express different cell-surface markers on the exterior of their plasma membrane. The differing configurations of cell-surface markers on differing types of cells distinguish one cell type from another cell type. By configuring the exterior probes that extend from the surface of the configurable microscopic medical payload delivery device to seek out and engage specific cell-surface receptors present on a specific type of cell, payloads of any quantum gene molecule can be delivered to specific cells in the body.

[0133] The transcribable genetic information linked to the unique identifier may occur in the form of naturally found transcribable genetic information or may occur as artificially created transcribable genetic information, referred to as 'artificial transcribable genetic information'. Naturally found transcribable genetic information would be a segment of transcribable genetic information that would be found in a cell's genome otherwise referred to as a gene.

Artificial transcribable genetic information would be transcribable genetic information that would represent either (i) a modified form of a naturally occurring gene or (ii) a segment of nucleotides that represents transcribable genetic information that is artificially created to produce a medically beneficial result.

[0134] A quantum gene, as it exists as a functional part of the deoxyribonucleic acid of a cell, is a segment of deoxyribonucleic acid, comprised of both a unique identifier and a segment of transcribable biologic information, that is capable of being inserted into a cell's nuclear DNA. DNA is comprised of two parallel strands of nucleotides. Each strand of DNA is a mirror image of each other since adenine must combine with thymine and cytosine must combine with guanine. Therefore, since each strand of DNA is a mirror image of each other, one strand of DNA possesses the nucleotide sequence that codes for both strands; one strand represents the DNA code, while the second strand represents the mirror image of the first strand. In this manner, a quantum gene can be defined in its most elemental form as a sequence of nucleotides comprising a single strand of nucleotides.

[0135] A quantum gene could thus be represented as a single strand of nucleotides comprised of the nucleotides adenine, cytosine, guanine and thymine. The double stranded form of a quantum gene would be the single strand of nucleotides attached in parallel to a second strand of nucleotides that represents the mirror image of the single strand of nucleotides. Double stranded deoxyribonucleic acid segments is the form quantum genes take when a quantum gene is inserted into a cell's nuclear genome.

Conclusions, Ramification, and Scope

[0136] Accordingly, the reader will see that the configurable microscopic medical payload delivery device to deliver quantum genes to specific targeted cell types provides advantages over existing art by (1) being a delivery device that seeks out specific types of cells, (2) by being a delivery device that is versatile enough to deliver a variety of quantum genes to accomplish various medical treatments and (3) by being a delivery device constructed with a surface envelope that will avoid detection by the innate as well as the adaptable immune systems so as not to activate the immune system to its presence; for these reasons this represents a new and unique medical delivery device that has never before been recognized nor appreciated by those skilled in the art.

[0137] The reader will also see that the concept and utilization of the quantum gene as described in this text has never before been recognized nor appreciated by those skilled in the art.

[0138] Although the description above contains specificities, these should not be construed as limiting the scope of the invention but as merely providing illustrations of some of the presently preferred embodiments of the invention.

[0139] Thus the scope of the invention should be determined by the appended claims and their legal equivalents, rather than by the examples given.

CLAIMS: Reserved.

PATENT APPLICATION
SPECIFICATION NUMBER 2

TITLE OF THE INVENTION:

QUANTUM UNIT OF INHERITANCE VECTOR THERAPY METHOD

BACKGROUND OF THE INVENTION

1. Field of the Invention

This invention relates to any medical method intended to correct a protein deficiency or genetic deficiency in the body by utilizing a configurable microscopic medical payload delivery device to insert one or more quantum genes into one or more specific type of cells in the body to improve cell function.

2. Description of Background Art

[0001] The Central Dogma of Microbiology dictates that in the nucleus of a cell, genes are transcribed to produce messenger ribonucleic acid molecules (mRNAs), these mRNAs migrate to the cytoplasm where they are translated to produce proteins. One of the great unknowns that has challenged the study of microbiology is the subject of understanding of how the genes, comprising the genome of a species, are organized such that the nuclear transcription machinery can efficiently locate specific transcribable genetic information and instructions that the cell requires to maintain itself, grow and conduct cell replication. Decoding the means as to how the genetic information contained in the nuclear deoxyribonucleic acid (DNA) of a cell is organized, helps to further the efforts to produce an effective gene therapy treatment strategy. Understanding the basis of genetic instruction code information stored in a cell's DNA and utilizing such knowledge of labeling and cataloging of genetic information, makes inserting biologic instruction into the DNA of cells a practical and effective means of treating a wide scope of medical conditions.

[0002] The human genome is comprised of deoxyribonucleic acid (DNA) separated into 46 chromosomes. The chromosomes are further subdivided into genes. Genes represent units of transcribable DNA. Transcription of the DNA refers to generating one or more of a variety of RNA molecules. Regarding the human genome, currently it is estimated that 5% of the total nuclear DNA is thought to represent genes and 95% is thought to represent redundant non-gene genetic material. The DNA genome in a cell is therefore comprised of transcribable genetic information and nontranscribable genetic information. Transcribable genetic information represent the segments of DNA that when transcribed by transcription machinery yield RNA molecules, usually in a precursor form that require modification before the RNA molecules are capable of being translated. The nontranscribable genetic information represent segments that act as either points of attachment for the transcription machinery or act as commands to direct the transcription machinery or act as spacers between transcribable segments of genetic information or have no known function at this time. A segment of nontranslatable DNA that is coded as a STOP command, under the proper circumstances, will cause the transcription machinery to cease transcribing the DNA at that point. A segment of DNA coded to signal a REPEAT command, will cause the transcription machinery to repeat its transcription of a segment of genetic information. The term 'genetic information' refers to a sequence of nucleotides that comprise transcribable portions of DNA and nontranscribable portions of DNA. In the DNA, four different nucleotides comprise the nucleotide sequences. The four different nucleotides that comprise the DNA include adenine, cytosine, guanine, and thymine.

[0003] Computer programs, commonly utilized in desk top computers, laptop computers, mainframe computers are comprised of a series of software instructions and data. In order for a computer program to run its digital programming in an orderly fashion, each software instruction and each element of data is assigned or associated with a unique identifier such that the software instructions can be carried out in an orderly fashion and each element of data can be efficiently located when there is a need to process the data elements. Similarly, each unit of genetic information, often referred to as a gene, comprising the nuclear DNA of a species genome, must have a unique identifier assigned to it such that the genetic information can be readily located by the transcription machinery and utilized when needed by a cell.

[0004] When a gene is to be transcribed, approximately forty proteins assemble together into what is referred to as a transcription complex, which acts as the transcription machinery. The transcription complex forms along a segment of DNA, upstream from the start of the transcribable genetic information. The transcription complex transcribes the genetic information to produce RNA. It is vital to the cell that the transcription complex is able to locate a specific gene amongst the 3 billion base pairs comprising the human genome in an orderly and efficient fashion to enable it to perform functions the cell requires to operate, survive, grow and replicate.

[0005] For purposes of this text there are several general definitions. A 'ribose' is a five carbon or pentose sugar ($C_5H_{10}O_5$) present in the structural components of ribonucleic acid, riboflavin, and other nucleotides and nucleosides. A 'deoxyribose' is a deoxypentose ($C_5H_{10}O_4$) found in deoxyribonucleic acid. A 'nucleoside' is a compound of a sugar usually ribose or deoxyribose with a nitrogenous base by way of an N-glycosyl link. A 'nucleotide' is a single unit of a nucleic acid, composed of a five carbon sugar (either a ribose or a deoxyribose), a nitrogenous base and a phosphate group. There are two families of 'nitrogenous bases', which include: pyrimidine and purine. A 'pyrimidine' is a six member ring made up of carbon and nitrogen atoms; the members of the pyrimidine family include: cytosine (C), thymine (T) and uracil (U). A 'purine' is a five-member ring fused to a pyrimidine type ring; the members of the purine family include: adenine (A) and guanine (G). A 'nucleic acid' is a polynucleotide which is a biologic molecule such as ribonucleic acid or deoxyribonucleic acid that allow organisms to reproduce. A 'ribonucleic acid' (RNA) is a linear polymer of nucleotides formed by repeated riboses linked by phosphodiester bonds between the 3-hydroxyl group of one and the 5-hydroxyl group of the next; RNAs are a single strand macromolecule comprised of a sequence of nucleotides, these nucleotides are generally referred to by their nitrogenous bases, which include: adenine, cytosine, guanine or uracil. The term macromolecule refers to any very large molecule. RNAs are subset into different types which include messenger RNA (mRNA), transport RNA (tRNA), ribosomal RNA (rRNA) and a variety of small RNAs. Messenger RNAs act as templates to produce proteins. A ribosome is a complex comprised of rRNAs and proteins and is responsible for the correct positioning of mRNA and charged tRNA to facilitate the proper alignment and bonding of amino acids into a strand to produce a protein. A 'charged' tRNA is a tRNA that is carrying an amino acid. Ribosomal RNA (rRNA) represents a subset of RNAs that form part of the physical structure of a ribosome. Small RNAs include snoRNA, U snRNA, and miRNA. The snoRNAs modify precursor rRNA molecules. U snRNAs modify precursor mRNA molecules. The miRNA molecules modify the function of mRNA molecules.

[0006] A 'deoxyribose' is a deoxypentose ($C_5H_{10}O_4$) sugar. Deoxyribonucleic acid (DNA) is comprised of three basic elements: a deoxyribose sugar, a phosphate group and nitrogen containing bases. DNA is a macromolecule made up of two chains of repeating deoxyribose sugars linked by phosphodiester bonds between the 3-hydroxyl group of one and the 5-hydroxyl group of the next; the two chains are held antiparallel to each other by weak hydrogen bonds. DNA strands contain a sequence of nucleotides, which include: adenine, cytosine, guanine and thymine. Adenine is always paired with thymine of the opposite strand, and guanine is always paired with cytosine of the opposite strand; one side or strand of a DNA macromolecule is the mirror image of the opposite strand. Nuclear DNA is regarded as the medium for storing the master plan of hereditary information.

[0007] Genes are considered segments of the DNA that represent units of inheritance.

[0008] A chromosome exists in the nucleus of a cell and consists of a DNA double helix bearing a linear sequence of genes, coiled and recoiled around aggregated proteins, termed histones. The number of chromosomes varies from species to species. Most Human cells carries twenty two pairs of chromosomes plus two sex chromosomes; two 'x' chromosomes in women and one 'x' and one 'y' chromosome in men. Chromosomes carry genetic information in the form of units which are referred to as genes. The entire nuclear genome, forty six chromosomes, is comprised of 3 billion base pairs of nucleotides.

[0009] Mitochondria possess numerous circular DNA. The limited information stored in mitochondrial DNA is thought to assist the mitochondria in producing the enzymes needed to convert glucose to adenosine triphosphate.

[0010] Various standard definitions of a gene exist. Per *Stedman's Medical Dictionary*, 24th edition, copyright 1982: 'The functional unit of heredity. Each gene occupies a specific place or locus on a chromosome, is capable of reproducing itself exactly at cell division, and is capable of directing the formation of an enzyme or other protein. The gene as a functional unit probably consists of a discrete segment of purine (adenine and guanine) and pyrimidine (cytosine and thymine) bases in the correct sequence to code the sequence of amino acids needed to form a specific peptide. Protein synthesis is mediated by molecules of messenger RNA formed on the chromosome with the gene unit of DNA acting as a template, which then pass into the cytoplasm and become oriented on the ribosomes where they in turn act as templates to organize a chain of amino acids to form a peptide. Genes normally occur in pairs in all cells except gametes as a consequence of the fact that all chromosomes are paired except the sex chromosomes (x and y) of the male.'

[0011] Per *Dorland's Pocket Medical Dictionary*, 23rd edition, copyright 1982 the definition of 'gene' is 'the biologic unit of heredity, self-producing, and located at a definite position (locus) on a particular chromosome.'

[0012] Per the text *Understanding Biology*, Second Edition, Peter Raven, George Johnson, Mosby, copyright 1991: 'Gene: The basic unit of heredity. A sequence of DNA nucleotides on a chromosome that encodes a polypeptide or RNA molecule and so determines the nature of an individual's inherited traits.'

[0013] Per *The New Oxford American Dictionary*, Second Edition, copyright 2005: 'Gene: A unit of heredity that is transferred from a parent to offspring and is held to determine some characteristic of the offspring: proteins coded directly by genes. In technical use: a distinct sequence of nucleotides forming part of a chromosome, the order of which determines the order of monomers in a polypeptide or nucleic acid molecule which a cell (or virus) may synthesize.'

[0014] Per MedicineNet.com (Current as of the time of this publication): According to the official Guidelines for Human Gene Nomenclature, a 'gene' is defined as "a DNA segment that contributes to phenotype/function. In the absence of demonstrated function a gene may be characterized by sequence, transcription or homology." DNA: Genes are composed of DNA, a molecule in the memorable shape of a double helix, a spiral ladder. Each rung of the spiral ladder consists of two paired chemicals called bases. There are four types of bases. They are adenine (A), thymine (T), cytosine (C), and guanine (G). As indicated, each base is symbolized by the first letter of its name: A, T, C, and G. Certain bases always pair together (AT and GC). Different sequences of base pairs form coded messages. The gene: A gene is a sequence (a string) of bases. It is made up of combinations of A, T, C, and G. These unique combinations determine the gene's function, much as letters join together to form words. Each person has thousands of genes—billions of base pairs of DNA or bits of information repeated in the nuclei of human cells—which determine individual characteristics (genetic traits).'

[0015] Per Wikipedia.com, referenced to: Group of the Sequence Ontology consortium, coordinated by K. Eilbeck, cited in H. Pearson. (2006). Genetics: what is a gene? *Nature*, 441, 398-401 (Current as of the time of this publication): A modern working definition of a gene is 'a locatable region of genomic sequence, corresponding to a unit of inheritance, which is associated with regulatory regions, transcribed regions, and or other functional sequence regions.'

[0016] The above definitions of a 'gene' are fairly detailed and at present time generally universally accepted in the science and medical communities as representing the definition of a gene. There is a distinct lack of any previous reference in the medical science literature to a unique identifier associated with genetic material.

[0017] Current gene theory is derived from Gregor Mendel (1822-1884), who discovered the basic principles of heredity by breeding garden peas at the abbey where he resided, while teaching at Brunn Modern School. Gregor Mendel built and documented a model of inheritance, often referred to as Mendelian genetics, that has acted as the foundation of modern genetics. Gregor Mendel documented changes in characteristics of the plants he grew and described the physical traits as being related to 'heritable factors'. Over time Mendel's term 'heritable factor' has been replaced by the terms 'gene' and 'allele'. Much of what the current term of a 'gene' describes remains related to and distinctly linked to the physical traits of the live organisms they describe.

[0018] Per J. K. Pal, S.S. Ghaskabi, *Fundamentals of Molecular Biology*, 2009: 'The central dogma of molecular biology . . . states that the genes present in the genome (DNA) are transcribed into mRNAs, which are then translated into polypeptides or proteins, which are phenotypes.' 'Genome, thus, contains the complete set of hereditary information for any organism and is functionally divided into small parts referred to as genes. Each gene is a sequence of nucleotides representing a single protein or RNA. Genome of a living organism may contain as few as 500 genes as in case of Mycoplasma, or as many as 30,000 genes as in case of human beings.'

[0019] Current computer technology utilizes the binary numeric language. Every task a computer performs is related to the language of 'one' and 'zeros'. Transistors that comprise the inside of computer chips are either turned 'on' representing a 'one' or turned 'off' representing a 'zero'. At the core of all computer programs is the machine language of 'ones' and 'zeros'. The most sophisticated central processing unit (CPU) in the world only reads and processes the language of 'ones' and 'zeros'. All text, all pictures, all video, all sound and music is diluted down to the form of one's and zero's, and consequently all of the computing and storage power of a computer is performed by the computer language of 'ones' and 'zeros'.

[0020] The nucleus of a biologically active cell arguably possesses the most sophisticated and well organized processing power in the world. To run such a powerful processing unit, a form of biologic computer language would seem to be a necessary foundation by which to transfer stored information from the DNA to the remainder of the biologically active portions of a cell as needed. Given that the DNA comprising the chromosomes and mitochondrial DNA are both comprised of four different nucleotides including adenosine, cytosine, guanine and thymine, and RNA is comprised of four nucleotides including adenosine, cytosine, guanine and uracil (uracil in place of thymine), it appears evident the biologic computer language used by a cell's genome is an information language derived from base-four mathematics. Instead of current computer technology utilizing binary computer code comprised of 'ones' and 'zeros', the DNA and RNA in a biologically active cell utilize an information language comprised of 'zeros', 'one's', two's' and 'threes' to store and transfer information, which in effect represents a base-four language or quaternary language.

[0021] The above definitions of a 'gene' refer to genes residing in a specific place or locus on a chromosome. Identifying that a gene is present in a particular location is obvious to the human observer, but from a functional standpoint for cell biology this does not necessarily help a cell find or use the information stored in the nucleotide sequence of a particular gene. To rely on location alone, as a means of identifying a gene, would put the function of the entire genome at peril of failure if even a single base pair of nucleotides were added or deleted from the genome. To this point, no discussion regarding genes being organized utilizing a coding system of any form within the genome, other than the mention of physical location in a chromosome, has been made in the medical literature.

[0022] The current understanding of the actual biologic structure of a gene is far more elaborate than the standard definition of a gene leads a casual reader to believe; this knowledge has evolved greatly since Gregor Mendel's work in the 19th century. A gene appears to be comprised of a number of segments loosely strung together along a particular section of DNA. In general there are at least three global segments associated with a gene which include: (1) the Upstream 5' flanking region, (2) the transcriptional unit and (3) the Downstream 3' flanking region.

[0023] The Upstream 5' flanking region is comprised of the 'enhancer region', the 'promoter-proximal region', and 'promoter region'.

[0024] The 'transcriptional unit' begins at a location designated 'transcription start site' (TSS), which is located in a site called the 'initiator region' (inR), which may be described in a general form as Py_2CAPy_5. The transcription unit is comprised of the combination of segments of DNA nucleotides to be transcribed into RNA and spacing units known as 'introns' that are not transcribed or if transcribed are later removed post transcription, such that they do not appear in the final RNA molecule. In the case of a gene coding for a mRNA molecule, the transcription unit will contain all three elements of the mRNA, which includes: (1) the 5' noncoding region, (2) the translational region and (3) the 3' noncoding region. Interspersed between these regions are exons, which will not be transcribed and introns that if transcribed, are removed from the precursor form of mRNA prior to the mRNA reaching its final form. Exons and introns appear to be likened to spacers. The exact role exons and introns play in the transcription process is undetermined.

[0025] The Downstream 3' flanking region contains DNA nucleotides that are not transcribed and may contain what has been termed an 'enhancer region'. An enhancer region in the Downstream 3' flanking region may promote the gene previously transcribed to be transcribed again.

[0026] On either side of the DNA sequencing comprising a gene and its flanking regions, may be inactive DNA which act as boundaries which have been termed 'insulator elements'. The term 'upstream' refers to DNA sequencing that occurs prior to the TSS if viewed from the 5' end to the 3' end of the DNA; where the term 'downstream' refers to DNA sequencing located after the TSS.

[0027] The 'enhancer region' may or may not be present in the Upstream 5' flanking region. If present in the Upstream 5' flanking region, the enhancer region helps facilitate the reading of the gene by encouraging formation of the transcription mechanism. An enhancer may be 50 to 1500 base pairs in length occupying a position upstream from the transcription starting site.

[0028] The 'transcription mechanism', also referred to as the 'transcription machinery' or the 'transcription complex' (TC), in humans, is reported to be comprised of over forty separate proteins that assemble together to ultimately function in a concerted effort to transcribe the nucleotide sequence of the DNA into RNA. The transcription mechanism includes elements such as 'general transcription factor Sp1', 'general transcription factor NF1', 'general transcription factor TATA-binding protein', 'TF$_{II}$D', 'basal transcription complex', and a 'RNA polymerase protein' to name only a few of the forty elements that exist. The elements of the transcription mechanism function as (1) a means to recognize the location of the start of a gene, (2) as proteins to bind the transcription mechanism to the DNA such that transcription may occur or (3) as means of transcribing the DNA nucleotide coding to produce a RNA molecule or a precursor RNA molecule.

[0029] There are at least three RNA polymerase proteins which include: RNA polymerase I, RNA polymerase II, and RNA polymerase III. RNA polymerase I tends to be dedicated to transcribing genetic information that will result in the formation of rRNA molecules. RNA polymerase II tends to be dedicated to transcribing genetic information that will result in the formation of mRNA molecules. RNA polymerase III appears to be dedicated to transcribing genetic information that results in the formation of tRNAs, small cellular RNAs and viral RNAs.

[0030] The 'promoter proximal region' is located upstream from the TSS and upstream from the core promoter region. The 'promoter proximal region' includes two sub-regions termed the GC box and the CAAT box. The 'GC box' appears to be a segment rich in guanine-cytosine nucleotide sequences. The GC box binds to the 'general transcription factor Sp1' of the transcription mechanism. The 'CAAT box' is a segment which contains the nucleotide sequence 'GGCCAATCT' located approximately 75 base pairs (bps) upstream from the transcription start site (TSS). The CAAT box binds to the 'general transcription factor NF1' of the transcription mechanism.

[0031] The 'core promoter' region is considered the shortest sequence within which RNA polymerase II can initiate transcription of a gene The core promoter may include the inR and either a TATA box or a 'downstream promoter element' (DPE). The inR is the region designated Py2CAPy5 that surrounds the transcription start site (TSS). The TATA box is located 25 base pairs (bps) upstream from the TSS. The TATA box acts as a site of attachment of the TFIID, which is a promoter for binding of the RNA polymerase II molecule. The DPE may appear 28 bps to 32 bps downstream from the TSS. The DPE acts as an alternative site of attachment for the TFIID when the TATA box is not present.

[0032] The transcription mechanism or transcription complex appears to be comprised of different elements depending upon

377

whether rRNA is being transcribed versus mRNA or tRNA or small cellular RNA or viral RNA. The proteins that assemble to assist RNA Polymerase I with transcribing the DNA to produce rRNA appear different the proteins that assemble to assist RNA polymerase II with transcribing the DNA to produce mRNA and from the proteins that assemble to assist RNA polymerase III with transcribing the DNA to produce tRNA, small cellular RNA or viral RNA. A common protein that appears to be present at the initial binding of all three types of RNA polymerase molecules is TATA-binding protein (TBP). TBP appears to be required to attach to the DNA, which then facilitates RNA polymerase to bind to the promoter along the DNA. TBP assembles with TBP-associated factors (TAFs). Together TBF and 11 TAFs comprise the complex referred to as TFIID, which has been previously mentioned in the above text.

[0033] Upstream from the TATA box is the 'initiator element', which may be considered as part of the 'core promoter' region. The initiator element is a segment of the nuclear DNA that binds the basal transcription complex. The basal transcription complex is comprised of a number of proteins that make initial contact with the DNA prior to the RNA polymerase binding to the transcription mechanism. The basal transcription complex is associated with an activator.

[0034] An activator is a protein comprised of three components. The three components of the activator include: (1) DNA binding domain, (2) Connecting domain, and (3) Activating domain. When the activator's DNA binding domain attaches to the DNA at a specific point along the DNA, the activator's activating domain then causes the other elements of the transcription mechanism to assemble at this location. Generally the assembly of the other proteins occurs downstream from where the activator's DNA binding domain attached to the DNA. There is evidence that the activator is associated with the activity of small RNAs.

[0035] The design of the cell is so complex, all of its functions so diverse and intricate that some form of practical order is necessitated. The genes must be ordered in some fashion, especially in a human, where there are at least 30,000 different genes used by the cells.

Some estimates place the total number of genes present in the human nuclear DNA genome closer to 100,000. If no means of order existed as to how the genes could be identified, then 'random circumstance' would dictate a cell locating a particular portion of genetic information that it requires, at any given time. Randomness tends to favor the occurrence of random events rather than a purposeful order. A 'random circumstance' approach to any living cell would tend to favor failure of the cell rather than survival of the cell.

[0036] To allow a cell to utilize the biologic information stored in a gene a 'unique identifier' (UI) needs to be somehow attached to the gene's specific nucleotide sequence. In the human genome, the cell's transcription mechanisms require an organized means to locate and transcribe any given gene's nucleotide sequence amongst the 3 billion nucleotides that reside in the 46 chromosomes that comprise human DNA. Given how the transcription mechanism assembles upstream from the portion of the gene to be transcribed, the nucleotide sequence acting as a unique identifier associated with a specific gene would be positioned upstream from the transcription start site.

[0037] The transcription complex (TC) engages the DNA upstream from the genetic information segment the TC transcribes. The unique identifier may be attached directly to the RNA coding segment of genetic material, or there may exist one or more base pairs physically separating the unique identifier and the RNA coding portion of genetic material. Regarding some genes, there may be numerous base pairs separating the unique identifier from the transcribing region of the gene.

[0038] For any form of 'gene therapy' to work efficiently, medically therapeutic genetic material inserted into the native DNA of a cell needs to be associated with a unique identification. Attaching a unique identifier to medically therapeutic genetic material is essential in making it possible for the components of a transcription complex to, in a timely organized fashion, locate the exogenous medically therapeutic genetic material, assemble around this exogenous genetic material, and decode the information contained therein. If no such unique identifier is used, then utilization of such exogenous transcribable genetic information occurs based on the occurrence of random events rather than dictated by therapeutic design.

[0039] Naturally occurring unique identifiers in the nuclear genome may occur in numerous forms. Since humans share 47% of their DNA with a banana and 95% of their DNA with a monkey, a portion of the unique identifiers associated with genes in the nuclear DNA may not be specific to a human. Unique identifiers may have a global utility, with a portion of the genome of any organism being shared amongst numerous species. The rational would be that once Nature developed an adequate fundamental design for a particular facet of biologic organisms, this information may be shared amongst numerous species that would benefit from the design. An example might be the basic design of a eukaryote cell; this information would be shared amongst all life that utilized the eukaryote cell design rather than each successive multi-celled species having to repeatedly re-invent the design of a eukaryote cell.

[0040] In order for the knowledge base of cellular genetics to progress forward, the definition of a gene must be expanded to include the presence of a 'unique identifier' associated with each gene present within the DNA. The basis for the presence of this unique identifier (UI) associated with each active gene is so that the cell can locate the biologic information stored in the DNA nucleotide sequencing of the gene. An active gene refers to those genes present in the genome that are utilized by a particular species to support conception, development and maintenance of a species.

[0041] Upon adding a unique identifier to a gene, the current term 'gene' is thus expanded to the term 'quantum gene'. The term 'quantal' in biology generally refers to an 'all or nothing' state or response. The term 'quantal' is a derivative of the word quantum. The term 'quantum means a quantity or amount, and a discrete quantity of energy or a discrete bundle of energy or a discrete quantity of electromagnetic radiation'.

[0042] A 'quantum gene' is comprised of a sequence of nucleotides that represents a 'unique identifier' physically linked to a sequence of nucleotides that represent a discrete quantity of genetic information; these sequences of nucleotides being comprised of some combination of the nucleotides being referred to by their nitrogenous base as <u>adenine</u> (A), <u>thymine</u> (T), <u>cytosine</u> (C), and <u>guanine</u> (G). The genetic information associated with the above-mentioned unique identifier may be comprised of a portion of transcribable genetic information and a portion of nontranscribable genetic information which together define a specific gene, otherwise referred to as a discrete quantity of genetic information.

[0043] Similar to how a gene is described, with regards to a quantum gene, the term 'upstream' refers to DNA sequencing that occurs prior to the transcription start site (TSS) if viewed from the 5' end to the 3' end of the DNA; where the term 'downstream' refers to DNA sequencing located after the TSS.

[0044] Similar to the previously described organization of a standard gene found in nuclear DNA, a quantum gene is structured with at least three global segments which include: (1) the Upstream 5' flanking region, (2) the transcriptional unit and possibly instructional units and (3) the Downstream 3' flanking region. The 'unique identifier' is located in the Upstream 5' flanking region. The current standard definition of a gene strictly encompasses the concept that a gene is comprised of a segment of nuclear DNA that when transcribed produces RNA. Therefore, the differences between the current standard definition of a 'gene' and the definition of a 'quantum gene' is that a quantum gene includes both a unique identifier and a segment of nuclear DNA that when transcribed produces RNA. The segment of nuclear DNA that when transcribed produces RNA is comprised of one or more segments of transcribable genetic information that may be accompanied by one or more segments of nontranscribable genetic information. Nontranscribable segments of genetic information include segments that are removed or ignored during the transcription process or segments that act as commands which includes a START code, STOP code or a REPEAT code. When present, a START code signals initiation of the transcription process. When present, a STOP code signals the discontinuation of the transcription process. When present, a REPEAT code signals that the transcription process should repeat the transcription of the segment of DNA that was just transcribed.

[0045] Similar to the standard description of a 'gene', a quantum gene's Upstream 5' flanking region is comprised of the 'enhancer region', the 'promoter-proximal region', and 'promoter region'.

[0046] Similar to the standard description of a 'gene', a quantum gene's 'transcriptional unit' begins at a location designated 'transcription start site' (TSS), which is located in a site called the 'initiator region' (inR), which may be described in a general form as Py2CAPy5. The transcription unit is comprised of the combination of segments of DNA nucleotides to be transcribed into RNA and spacing units known as 'exons' AND 'introns', whereby exons represent segments that are not transcribed and introns represent segments that are transcribed but later removed post transcription, such that they do not appear in the final RNA molecule. In the case of a gene coding for a mRNA molecule, the transcription unit will contain all three elements of the mRNA, which includes: (1) the 5' noncoding region, (2) the translational region and (3) the 3' noncoding region. Interspersed between these regions are exons, which will not be transcribed and introns that if transcribed, are removed from the precursor form of mRNA prior to the mRNA reaching its final form. Exons and introns present in nuclear DNA appear to be likened to spacers interspersed in the nuclear DNA. The exact role exons and introns play in the transcription process is undetermined.

[0047] Similar to the standard description of a 'gene', the quantum gene's Downstream 3' flanking region contains DNA nucleotides that are not transcribed and may contain what has been termed an 'enhancer region'. An enhancer region in the Downstream 3' flanking region may promote the gene previously transcribed to be transcribed again.

[0048] On either side of the DNA sequencing comprising a gene and a quantum gene are flanking regions which represent inactive

DNA, which act as boundaries which have been termed 'insulator elements'. Insulator elements are areas that are not transcribed to produce RNA. The function of insulator elements, other than acting as boundary markers between differing genes, is unknown at this time.

[0049] In nuclear DNA, quantum genes are comprised of a segment of deoxyribonucleic acid where the portion that represents a unique identifier may be separated from the portion that represents transcribable genetic information by a quantity of base pairs of nucleotides that do not represent a unique identifier and do not represent transcribable genetic information. The purpose of the separation of the portion of the unique identifier from the portion of the genetic information by a quantity of base pairs of nucleotides that do not represent a unique identifier and does not represent genetic information may be to act to facilitate a transcription complex attaching to the quantum gene upstream from the portion of the quantum gene that represents genetic information so that transcription of the biologic information associated with the quantum gene may occur at the designated starting point.

[0050] The unique identification or identifier of a quantum gene could be in the form of nucleotide sequence that represents a name assigned to the quantum gene, or a number assigned to a quantum gene or the combination of a name and number assigned to a quantum gene. Irrespective of whether the unique identifier incorporated in a quantum gene is considered a 'name', or a 'number' or a combination of a name or number, the unique identifier is comprised of a sequence of nucleotides linked to the transcribable genetic information for which it acts as a unique identifier. It has been estimated that there are as many as 100,000 separate genes stored in the DNA of the 46 chromosomes comprising the human genome. In a base four language, a string of nine nucleotides is needed to code for 256,144 individual genes. If there were over a million quantum genes, then a string of ten nucleotides could be used since ten nucleotides could represent 1,024,576 unique numbers in a base-four number system.

[0051] Utilizing a base four number system a string of twenty-five nucleotides would represent the number 1,125,899,906,842,624, which could account for 200,000 different quantum genes in 5 billion different species. Therefore 200,000 different quantum genes could be dedicated to producing a biped form of life. In the human genome 5% of the 3 billion base pairs are considered to represent genes by the current definition of a gene. If 5% of the human genome represents the 100,000 quantum genes in the nuclear DNA, then on average 1500 nucleotides can be dedicated to each gene. If 25 nucleotides are dedicated to a unique address or unique identifier, then there remain 1475 nucleotides, on average, to be utilized for coding the biologic information associated with each of the 100,000 quantum genes estimated to exist in the human genome.

[0052] A unique identifier (UI) incorporated in quantum genes could be comprised of a unique number or a unique name or the unique combination of a number and a name. A name might be represented as a single letter or a series of letters. The current convention utilized in science is to apply the four letter alphabet A, C, G, T to represent the four different bases of the nucleotides comprising the DNA, which include adenosine, cytosine, guanine, and thymine respectfully. With regards to RNA, the four letter alphabet A, C, G, U is utilized to represent the bases of the nucleotides which include adenosine, cytosine, guanine, and uracil. Regarding utilizing a unique identifier for DNA, a name could be comprised of a series of letters derived from the four letters A, C, G, and T. Regarding utilizing a unique identifier for purposes of use within an RNA molecule, a unique identifier could be comprised of a series of letters derived from the four letters A, C, G, U. The current scientific convention does not recognize a mathematical base-four nomenclature regarding DNA or RNA. The unique identifier could be represented as a number. Names can be translated into numbers and vice versa.

[0053] In the nuclear DNA, there are several places in the upstream segment of a quantum gene where a segment of twenty-five or more base pairs could exist that acts as the unique identifying code that uniquely identifies the segment of transcribable genetic information. The transcription start site (TSS) is present upstream from a segment of transcribable genetic information. There exists a segment of 25 bps upstream from the TSS that occupies the space along the DNA between the TSS and the TATA box. There exists the downstream promoter element (DPE) 28 bps to 32 bps downstream from the TSS. The DPE acts as an alternative site of attachment for the TFIID when the TATA box is not present. Within the 28 bps to 32 bps of DNA separating the DPE from the TSS may also be a convenient location for a unique identifying code to reside and be associated with the genetic information located just downstream. The cell exists with numerous variability. There exists variation in the arrangement of the elements upstream from the transcribable genetic information, therefore various sites upstream from the transcribable genetic information may function as the unique identifying code for some quantum genes. The unique identifying code may be represented as subsegments of DNA, where subsegments are physically separated from each other, but in combination, the subsegments act in unison to identify a segment of transcribable genetic information.

[0054] By delivering quantum genes containing the genetic information required to produce insulin directly to the cells responsible for the production of insulin, the medical treatment of diabetes mellitus is significantly improved. Diabetes mellitus represents a state of hyperglycemia, a serum blood sugar that is higher than what is considered the normal range for humans. Glucose, a six-carbon molecule, is a form of sugar. Glucose is absorbed by the cells of the body and converted to energy by the processes of glycolysis, the Krebs cycle and phosporylation. Insulin, a protein, facilitates the transfer of glucose from the blood into cells. Normal range for blood glucose in humans is generally defined as a fasting blood plasma glucose level of between 70 to 110 mg/dl. For descriptive purposes, the term 'plasma' refers to the fluid portion of blood.

[0055] Diabetes mellitus is classified as Type One and Type Two. Type One diabetes mellitus is insulin dependent, which refers to the condition where there is a lack of sufficient insulin circulating in the blood stream and insulin must be provided to the body in order to properly regulate the blood glucose level. When insulin is required to regulate the blood glucose level in the body, this condition is often referred to as insulin dependent diabetes mellitus (IDDM). Type Two diabetes mellitus is noninsulin dependent, often referred to as noninsulin dependent diabetes mellitus (NIDDM), meaning the blood glucose level can be managed without insulin, and instead by means of diet, exercise or intervention with oral medications. Type Two diabetes mellitus is considered a progressive disease, the underlying pathogenic mechanisms including pancreatic Beta cell (also often designated as β-Cell) dysfunction and insulin resistance.

[0056] The pancreas serves as an endocrine gland and an exocrine gland. Functioning as an endocrine gland the pancreas produces and secretes hormones including insulin and glucagon. Insulin acts to reduce levels of glucose circulating in the blood. Beta cells secrete insulin into the blood when a higher than normal level of glucose is detected in the serum. For purposes of this description the terms 'blood', 'blood stream' and 'serum' refer to the same substance. Glucagon acts to stimulate an increase in glucose circulating in the blood. Beta cells in the pancreas secrete glucagon when a low level of glucose is detected in the serum.

[0057] Glucose enters the body and then the blood stream as a result of the digestion of food. The Beta cells of the Islets of Langerhans continuously sense the level of glucose in the blood and respond to elevated levels of blood glucose by secreting insulin into the blood. Beta cells produce the protein 'insulin' in their endoplasmic reticulum and store the insulin in vacuoles until it is needed. When Beta cells detect an increase in the glucose level in the blood, Beta cells release insulin into the blood from the described storage vacuoles.

[0058] Insulin is a protein. An insulin protein consists of two chains of amino acids, an alpha chain and a beta chain, linked by two disulfide (S-S) bridges. One chain, the alpha chain consists of 21 amino acids. The second chain the beta chain consists of 30 amino acids.

[0059] Insulin interacts with the cells of the body by means of a cell-surface receptor termed the 'insulin receptor' located on the exterior of a cell's 'outer membrane', otherwise known as the 'plasma membrane'. Insulin interacts with muscle and liver cells by means of the insulin receptor to rapidly remove excess blood sugar when the glucose level in the blood is higher than the upper limit of the normal physiologic range. Recognized functions of insulin include stimulating cells to take up glucose from the blood and convert it to glycogen to facilitate the cells in the body to utilize glucose to generate biochemically usable energy, and to stimulate fat cells to take up glucose and synthesize fat.

[0060] Diabetes Mellitus may be the result of one or more factors. Causes of diabetes mellitus may include: (1) mutation of the insulin gene itself causing miscoding, which results in the production of ineffective insulin molecules; (2) mutations to genes that code for the 'transcription factors' needed for transcription of the insulin gene in the deoxyribonucleic acid (DNA) to create messenger ribonucleic acid (mRNA) molecules, which facilitate the manufacture of the insulin molecule; (3) mutations of the gene encoding for the insulin receptor, which produces inactive or an insufficient number of insulin receptors; (4) mutation to the gene encoding for glucokinase, the enzyme that phosphorylates glucose in the first step of glycolysis; (5) mutations to the genes encoding portions of the potassium channels in the plasma membrane of the Beta cells, preventing proper closure of the channel, thus blocking insulin release; (6) mutations to mitochondrial genes that as a result, decreases the energy available to be used facilitate the release of insulin, therefore reducing insulin secretion; (7) failure of glucose transporters to properly permit the facilitated diffusion of glucose from plasma into the cells of the body.

[0061] A 'eukaryote' refers to a nucleated cell. Eukaryotes comprise nearly all animal and plant cells. A human eukaryote or nucleated cell is comprised of an exterior lipid bilayer plasma membrane, cytoplasm, a nucleus, and organelles. The exterior plasma membrane defines the perimeter of the cell, regulates the flow of nutrients, water and regulating molecules in and out of the cell, and has embedded into its structure receptors that the cell uses to detect properties of the environment surrounding the cell membrane.

The cytoplasm acts as a filling medium inside the boundaries of the plasma cell membrane and is comprised mainly of water and nutrients such as amino acids, oxygen, and glucose. The nucleus, organelles, and ribosomes are suspended in the cytoplasm. The nucleus contains the majority of the cell's genetic information in the form of double stranded deoxyribonucleic acid (DNA). Organelles generally carry out specialized functions for the cell and include such structures as the mitochondria, the endoplasmic reticulum, storage vacuoles, lysosomes and Golgi complex (sometimes referred to as a Golgi apparatus). Floating in the cytoplasm, but also located in the endoplasmic reticulum and mitochondria are ribosomes. Ribosomes are complex macromolecule structures comprised of ribosomal ribonucleic acid (rRNA) molecules and ribosomal proteins that combine and couple to a messenger ribonucleic acid (mRNA) molecule. The rRNAs and the ribosomal proteins congregate to form a macromolecule structure that surrounds a mRNA molecule. Ribosomes decode genetic information in a mRNA molecule and manufacture proteins to the specifications of the instruction code physically present in the mRNA molecule. More than one ribosome may be attached to a single mRNA at a time.

[0062] Proteins are comprised of a series of amino acids bonded together in a linear strand, sometimes referred to as a chain; a protein may be further modified to be a structure comprised of one or more similar or differing strands of amino acids bonded together. Insulin is a protein structure comprised of two strands of amino acids; one strand comprised of 21 amino acids long and the second strand comprised of 30 amino acids, the two strands attached by two disulfide bridges. There are an estimated 30,000 different proteins the cells of the human body may manufacture. The human body is comprised of a wide variety of cells, many with specialized functions requiring unique combinations of proteins and protein structures such as glycoproteins (a protein combined with a carbohydrate) to accomplish the required task or tasks a specialized cell is designed to perform. Forms of glycoproteins are known to be utilized as cell-surface receptors. Messenger RNAs (mRNA) are created by transcription of DNA, they generally migrate to other locations inside the cell and are utilized by ribosomes as protein manufacturing templates. A ribosome is a protein complex that manufactures proteins by deciphering the instruction code located in a mRNA molecule. When a specific protein is needed, pieces of the ribosome complex, which include rRNA molecules and ribosomal proteins, bind around the strand of a mRNA that carries the specific instruction code that will generate the required protein. The ribosome traverses the mRNA strand and deciphers the genetic information coded into the sequence of nucleotides that comprise the mRNA molecule to produce a protein molecule and this process is referred to as translation.

[0063] The insulin molecule is a protein produced by Beta cells located in the pancreas. The 'insulin messenger RNA' is created in a Beta cell by a polymerase complex transcribing the insulin gene from nuclear DNA in the nucleus of the cell. The native messenger RNA (mRNA) for insulin then travels to the endoplasmic reticulum, where numerous ribosomes, comprised of rRNA and ribosomal proteins, engage these mRNA molecules. Many ribosomes may be attached to a single strand of mRNA simultaneously, each generating an identical copy of the protein as dictated by the information encoded in the mRNA. Insulin is produced by ribosomes translating the information in a mRNA molecule coded for the insulin protein, which produce strands of amino acids that are coded for an immature form of the biologically active insulin molecule referred to as 'pro-insulin'. Once the pro-insulin molecule is generated it then undergoes modification by several enzymes including prohormone convertase one (PC1), prohormone convertase two (PC2) and carboxypeptidase E, which results in the production of a biologically active insulin molecule. Once the biologically active insulin protein is generated it is stored in a vacuole in the Beta cell to await being released into the blood stream.

[0064] Insulin receptors, which appear on the surface of cells, offer binding sites for insulin circulating in the blood. When insulin binds to an insulin receptor, the biologic response inside the cell causes glucose to enter the cell and undergo processing in the cytoplasm. Processed glucose molecules then enter the mitochondria. The mitochondria further process the modified glucose molecules to produce usable energy in the form of adenosine triphosphate molecules (ATP). Thirty-eight ATP molecules may be generated from one molecule of glucose during the process of aerobic respiration. ATP molecules are utilized as an energy source by biologic processes throughout the cell.

[0065] The current medical therapeutic approach to the management of diabetes mellitus has produced limited results. Patients with diabetes generally struggle with an inadequate production of insulin, or an ineffective release of biologically active insulin molecules, or a release of an insufficient number of biologically active insulin molecules, or an insufficient production of cell-surface receptors, or a production of ineffective cell-surface receptors, or a production of ineffective insulin molecules that are unable to interact properly with insulin receptors to produce the required biologic effect. Type One diabetes requires administration of exogenous insulin. The traditional approach to Type Two diabetes has generally first been to adjust the diet to limit the caloric intake the individual consumes. Exercise is used as an initial approach to both Type One and Type Two diabetes as a means of up-regulating the utilization of fats and sugar so as to reduce the amount of circulating plasma glucose. When diet and exercise are inadequate in properly managing Type Two diabetes, oral medications are often introduced. The action of sulfonylureas, a commonly prescribed class of oral medication, is to stimulate the Beta cells to produce additional insulin receptors and enhance the insulin receptors' response to insulin. Biguanides, another form of oral treatment, inhibit gluconeogenesis, the production of glucose in the liver, thereby attempting to reduce plasma glucose levels. Thiazolidinediones (TZDs) lower blood sugar levels by activating peroxisome proliferator-activated receptor gamma (PPAR-γ), a transcription factor, which when activated regulates the activity of various target genes, particularly ones involved in glucose and lipid metabolism. If diet, exercise and oral medications do not produce a satisfactory control of the level of blood glucose in a diabetic patient, exogenous insulin is injected into the body in an effort to normalize the amount of glucose present in the serum. Insulin, a protein, has not successfully been made available as an oral medication to date due to the fact that proteins in general become degraded when they encounter the acid environment present in the stomach.

[0066] Despite strict monitoring of blood glucose and potentially multiple doses of insulin injected throughout the day, many patients with diabetes mellitus still experience devastating adverse effects from elevated blood glucose levels. Microvascular damage and elevated tissue sugar levels contribute to such complications as renal failure, retinopathy involving the eyes, neuropathy, and accelerated heart disease despite aggressive efforts to maintain the blood sugar within the physiologic normal range using exogenous insulin by itself or a combination of exogenous insulin and one or more oral medications. Diabetes remains the number one cause of renal failure in the United States. Especially in diabetic patients that are dependent upon administering exogenous insulin into their body, though dosing of the insulin may be four or more times a day and even though this may produce adequate control of the blood glucose level to prevent the clinical symptoms of hyperglycemia; this does not unerringly supplement the body's natural capacity to monitor the blood sugar level minute to minute, twenty-four hours a day, and deliver an immediate response to a rise in blood glucose by the release of insulin from Beta cells as required. The deleterious effects of diabetes may still evolve despite strict and persistent control of the glucose level in the blood stream.

[0067] The current treatment of diabetes may be augmented by the unique approach to utilizing modified viruses as vehicles to transport quantum genes into cells in order to increase the production of biologically active insulin. By utilizing modified viruses to transport quantum genes to facilitate and enhance the production of mRNAs, which would then facilitate the assembly of proteins would offer a new treatment option for patients with diabetes.

[0068] Viruses are obligate parasites. Viruses simply represent a carrier of genetic material and by themselves viruses are unable to replicate or carry out any form of biologic function outside their host cell. Viruses are generally comprised of one or more nested shells constructed of one or more layers of protein or lipid material,

391

a genetic payload that represents the instruction code necessary to replicate the virus, and protein enzymes to help facilitate the genetic payload in the function of replicating copies of the virus once the genetic payload has been delivered to a host cell. Located on the outer shell or envelope of a virus are probes. The function of a virus's probes is to locate and engage a host cell's receptors. The virus's surface probes are designed to detect, make contact with and functionally engage one or more receptors located on the exterior of a cell type that will offer the virus the proper environment in which to construct copies of itself. A host cell provides the virus the proper biochemical machinery for the virus to successfully replicate itself.

[0069] Protected by an outer protein coat or lipid envelope, viruses carry a genetic payload in the form of deoxyribonucleic acid (DNA) or ribonucleic acid (RNA). Once a virus's exterior probes locate and functionally engage the surface receptor or receptors on a host cell, the virus inserts its genetic payload into the interior of the host cell. In the event a virus is carrying a DNA payload, the virus's DNA travels to the host cell's nucleus and is known to become inserted into the host cell's own native DNA. In the case where a virus is carrying its genetic payload as RNA, the virus inserts the RNA payload into the host cell and may also insert one or more enzymes to facilitate the RNA being utilized properly to replicate copies of the virus. Once inside the host cell, some species of virus facilitate use of their RNA by having the RNA converted to DNA. Once the viral RNA has been converted to DNA, the virus's DNA travels to the host cell's nucleus and is known to become inserted into the host cell's native DNA. Once a virus's genetic material has been inserted into the host cell's native DNA, the virus's genetic material takes command of certain cell functions and redirects the resources of the host cell to generate copies of the virus. Other forms of RNA viruses bypass the need to use the nuclear DNA and simply utilize portions of the viral genome to act as messenger RNA (mRNA). RNA viruses that bypass the host cell's DNA, cause the cell to in general generate copies of the necessary parts of the virus directly from the virus's RNA genome.

[0070] Present medical care is attempting to utilize viruses to deliver genetic information into cells. Research in the field of gene therapy has involved certain naturally occurring viruses. Some of the common viral vectors that have been investigated include: Adeno-associated virus, Adenovirus, Alphavirus, Epstein-Barr virus, Gammaretrovirus, Herpes simplex virus, Letivirus, Poliovirus, Rhabdovirus, Vaccinia virus. Naturally occurring virus vectors are limited to the naturally occurring external probes that are affixed to the outer wall of the virus. The external probes fixed to the outside wall of a virus virion dictate which type of cell the virus can engage and infect. Therefore, as an example, the function of the adenovirus, a respiratory virus, is strictly limited to engaging and infecting specific lung cells. Used as a medical treatment device, the adenovirus can only deliver gene therapy to specific lung cells, which severely limits this vector's usefulness as a deliver device. The therapeutic function of all naturally occurring viral vectors is limited to delivering a DNA or RNA payload to the cell type the viral vector naturally targets as its host cell.

[0071] Naturally occurring viruses also have the disadvantage of being susceptible to detection and elimination by a body's immune system. Viruses have been infecting humans for hundreds of thousands of years. A human's innate immune system is very efficient at detecting the presence of most naturally occurring viruses when such a virus is inside the body. The human immune system is quite capable of generating a vigorous response to most intruding viruses, attacking and neutralizing virus virions whenever a virus virion physically exists are outside the exterior wall of the virus's host cell. If gene therapy in its current state were to become a clinical therapeutic tool, the naturally occurring viruses selected for gene therapy research will have limited effectiveness due the fact that once the viral vector is introduced into the body, the body's the immune system will quickly engage and eliminate the viral vectors, possibly before the vector is able to deliver its payload to its host cell or target cell.

[0072] Cichutek, K., 2001 (US Patent No. 6,323,031 B1) teaches preparation and use of novel lentiviral SiVagm-derived vectors for gene transfer into selected cell types, specifically into proliferatively active and resting human cells.

[0073] Cichutek teaches that it is indeed plausible to re-configure an existing virus and use it as a transport vehicle, though Cichutek's specification and claims are too limited to describe a method that will work for all cell types, if indeed if it will work for any cell type.

[0074] Cichutek describes vectors for 'gene transfer'; in the claims the language that is used is 'genetic information'. Cichutek's Claim 1 of the cited patent states 'A propagation-incompetent SIVagm vector comprising a viral core and a viral envelope, wherein the viral core comprises a simian immunodeficiency virus (SIVagm) viral core of the African vervet monkey Chlorocebus.' Cichutek's does not describe in his claims any further details of the intended payload other than the stating 'SIVagm viral core' in claim 1; in claims 5 & 6 Cichutek describes only 'genetic information'. Transfer of 'genetic information' dramatically limits the useful application of Cichutek's patent in the treatment of medical diseases.

[0075] Cichutek does not claim the use of specific glycogen probes to target specific types of cells. Cichutek's approach is dependent upon the probes naturally present on the viral vectors reported in the patent, which will direct the viral vectors to only those cells the viruses naturally use as their host cell. Cichutek's approach is very restrictive, limited to gene transfer to only cells the viruses use as their natural host cell.

[0076] Cichutek's claim 4, states 'The SIVagm vector of claim 1, wherein the viral envelope further comprises a single chain antibody (scFv) or a ligand of a cell surface molecule.' By use of the words 'a' and 'or' in the claim, the claim is limited in the singular, meaning Cichutek claims a single chain antibody or a singular ligand. Singular type antibodies or ligands can be used for cell to cell communication, but to open an access portal into a cell and insert a payload into the cell requires two different types antibodies or ligands. As an example human immunodeficiency virus requires the use of both the gp120 and gp41 probes to open a portal into a T-Helper cell and insert its viral genome into the T-Helper cell. The gp120 probe engages the CD4+ cell-surface receptor on the T-cell. Once the gp120 probe has successfully engaged a CD4+ cell-surface receptor on the target T-Helper cell, then the HIV virion's gp41 probe can engage either a CXCR4 or a CCR5 cell-surface receptor on the T-Helper cell in order to open up an access portal for HIV to insert its viral genome into a T-Helper cell. It is well documented in the medical literature that a genetic defect leading to an abnormality in the CXCR4 cell-surface receptor prevents HIV virions from opening an access portal and inserting its genetic payload into such T-Helper cells. This genetic defect in the CXCR4 cell-surface receptor offers the subset of people carrying the genetic defect resistance to HIV infection. This example demonstrates the need for at least two types of glycoprotein probes to be present on the surface of a viral vector in order for a viral vector to be capable of opening an access portal and delivering the payload the vector carries into its host cell or target cell.

[0077] A delivery system that offered a defined means of targeting specific types of cells would invoke minimal or no response by the innate immune system and the adaptable immune system when present in the body, and a delivery system that would be capable of inserting into cells a wide variety of quantum gene molecules would significantly improve the current medical treatment options available to clinicians treating patients.

[0078] The solution to arriving at a versatile, workable delivery system that will meet the needs of a number of medical treatments involves three important elements. These elements include:

   (1) configurable external probes whereby more than one type of protein structure probe or more than one type of glycoprotein probe is to be used to engage and access specific target cell types in order to successfully deliver a payload into a specific type of cell,

   (2) an external envelope comprised of a protein shell or lipid layer expressing the least number of cell-surface markers,

such as the use of a stem cell to act as the host cell to manufacture the delivery devices,

(3) configuring the core of the vector to enable it to carry and deliver quantum genes.

For purposes of this text, the use of the terms 'specific target cell type', 'target cell', 'specific type of cell', 'specific cell', 'specific type of cell' are equivalent and interchangeable; the configuration of cell-surface receptors that a specific type of cell has located on and protruding from its outer cell membrane determines the cell type.

[0079] Viruses are obligate parasites. Viruses simply represent a carrier of genetic material and by themselves viruses are unable to replicate or carry out any form of biologic function outside their host cell. A 'virion' refers to the physical structure of a single complete virus as it exists outside of the host cell; a more archaic term for 'viral virion' was 'viral particle'. Viruses are generally comprised of one or more nested shells constructed of one or more layers of protein, some with a lipid outer envelope, a genetic payload that represents the instruction code necessary to replicate the virus, and protein enzymes to help facilitate the genetic payload in the function of replicating copies of the virus once the genetic payload has been delivered to a host cell. Located on the outer shell or envelope of a virus are probes. The function of a virus's external probes is to locate and engage a host cell's receptors. The virus's surface probes are designed to detect, make contact with and functionally engage one or more receptors located on the exterior of the type of cell that will offer the virus the proper environment in which to construct copies of itself. A host cell provides the virus the proper biologic machinery for the virus to successfully replicate itself. Once the virus's genome is inside the host cell, the viral genome takes command of the cell's production machinery and causes the host cell to generate copies of the virus. As the viral copies exit the host cell, these virions set off in search of other host cells to infect.

[0080] Naturally occurring viruses exist in a number of differing shapes. The shape of a virus may be rod or filament like, icosahedral, or complex structures combining filament and polygonal shapes.

Viruses generally have their outer wall comprised of a protein coat or an envelope comprised of lipids.

[0081] An outer envelope comprised of lipids may be in the form of one or two phospholipid layers. When the outer envelope is comprised of two phospholipid layers this is termed a lipid bilayer. For purposes of this text the term 'lipid' includes 'phospholipid' molecules. A phospholipid is a composite molecule comprised of a polar or hydrophilic region on one end and a nonpolar or hydrophobic region on the opposite end. A lipid bilayer covering a virus, like the membrane of a cell, is constructed with the hydrophilic region of one of the phospholipid layers pointed toward the exterior of the virion and the hydrophilic region of the second phospholipid layer pointed inward toward the center of the virus virion; with the hydrophobic regions of each of the two lipid layers pointed toward each other. The outer envelope of some forms of virus may be comprised of an outer lipid layer or lipid bilayer affixed to a protein matrix for support, the protein matrix being located closer to the center of the virus virion than the lipid layer or lipid bilayer.

[0082] Spherical viruses are generally spherical in shape and may be comprised of an outer envelope and one inner shell or alternatively an outer envelope and multiple inner shells. Inner shells are approximately spherical in shape; this is because the proteins comprising the protein matrix shell have an irregular shape to their structure, but when constructed together for a shape that resembles a sphere. In the case of a spherical virus with an outer envelope and one inner shell, the inner shell is often referred to as a nucleocapsid shell comprised of numerous capsid proteins attached to each other. In the case of a spherical virus being comprised of an outer envelope and multiple inner shells, the outermost inner viral shells may be referred to as comprised of a quantity of matrix proteins, where the innermost shell is referred to as a nucleocapsid and is comprised of a quantity of capsid proteins. The inner protein shells are nested inside each other. The cavity created by the innermost shell or nucleocapsid is referred to as the 'core' or 'center of the virus'. Any payload carried by the virus virion is generally carried in the core or center of the virion.

[0083] Viruses carry genetic material in the form of deoxyribonucleic acid (DNA) or ribonucleic acid (RNA) as their payload. DNA or RNA genome payloads are carried in the cavity of the nucleocapsid referred to as the core. A virus is therefore generally considered to be a DNA virus if its genome is comprised of DNA or the virus is considered a RNA virus if its genome is comprised of RNA that acts as genetic instructions to generate copies of the virus. Viruses may also carry enzymes as part of their payload. An enzyme such as 'reverse transcriptase' transforms a RNA viral genome into DNA. Protease enzymes modify the viral genome once it has entered a host cell. An integrase enzyme assists a DNA viral genome with insertion into the host cell's nuclear DNA. The entire genetic payload is carried inside the cavity created by the virus's nucleocapsid shell.

[0084] The probes attached to the exterior of a virus are constructed to engage specific cell-surface receptors on specific type of cells in the body. Only a cell that expresses cell-surface receptors that are capable of being engaged by the probes of a specific virus can act as a host for the virus. Viruses generally use two probes to access a host cell. The first probe makes an initial attachment to the host cell, while the action of the virus's second probe often in conjunction with the action of the first probe cause an access portal to be created in the host cell's exterior plasma membrane. Once an access portal is formed, the virus inserts the contents of its payload into the host cell utilizing the open access portal. Certain types of virus may be engulfed whole by a target cell. Once the virus's genome is inside the cytoplasm of the host cell, any enzymes that accompanied the viral genome into the cell, may begin to modify or assist the virus's genome with infecting and taking control of the host cell's biologic functions.

[0085] Probes are attached to the external envelope of a virus virion. Probes may be in the form of a protein structure or may be in the form of a glycoprotein molecule. For viruses constructed with a protein matrix as its outer envelope, the probes tend to be protein structures. A portion of the protein structure probe is fixed or anchored in the protein matrix, while a portion of the protein structure probe extends out and away from the protein matrix. The portion of the protein structure probe extending out away from the virus virion is referred to as the 'exterior domain', the portion anchored in the protein matrix is the 'transcending domain'. Some protein probes have a third segment that extends through the envelope and exists inside the virus virion, which is referred to as the 'interior domain'. The exterior domain of a protein structure probe is intended to engage a specific cell-surface receptor on a biologically active cell the virus is targeting as its host cell.

[0086] Viruses that utilize a lipid layer as the outer envelope, are constructed with probes that tend to be glycoproteins. A glycoprotein is comprised of a protein segment and a carbohydrate segment. The carbohydrate segment of the glycoprotein molecule is fixed or anchored in the lipid layer of the outer envelope, while the protein segment extends outward and away from the outer envelope. The protein portion of a glycoprotein probe that extends outward and away from the outer envelope of a virus virion is intended to engage a cell-surface receptor on a biologically active cell the virus is targeting as its host cell.

[0087] Some forms of viruses that utilize a lipid layer as its envelope use protein structure probes. In this case, the portion of the protein structure probe that extends outward and away from the outer envelope is the 'exterior domain', the portion that is anchored in the lipid layer is the 'transcending domain' and again some protein structure probes have an 'interior domain' that exist inside the virion, which may also help anchor the protein structure probe to the virion. The exterior domain of a protein structure probe that extends outward and away from the outer envelope of a virus virion is intended to engage a cell-surface receptor on a biologically active cell the virus is targeting as its host cell.

[0088] When a virus carries a DNA payload and the viral DNA is inserted into the host cell, the virus's DNA travels to the host cell's nucleus and is known to become inserted into the host cell's own native DNA. In the case where a virus is carrying its genetic payload as RNA, the virus inserts the RNA payload into the host cell and may also insert one or more enzymes to facilitate the RNA being utilized properly to replicate copies of the virus. Once inside the host cell, some species of virus facilitate use of the viral RNA by having the RNA converted to DNA. Once the viral RNA has been converted to DNA, the virus's DNA travels to the host cell's nucleus and is known to become inserted into the host cell's native DNA. Once a virus's genetic material has been inserted into the host cell's native DNA, the virus's genetic material takes command of certain cell functions and redirects the resources of the host cell to generate copies of the virus. Other forms of RNA viruses bypass the need to use the nuclear DNA and simply utilize portions of the viral genome to act as messenger RNA. RNA viruses that bypass the host cell's DNA, cause the cell in general to generate copies of the necessary parts of the virus directly from the virus's RNA genome.

[0089] The human immunodeficiency virus (HIV) is a RNA virus and has an outer envelope comprised of a lipid bilayer. The lipid bilayer covers a protein matrix consisting of $p17^{gag}$ proteins. Inside the $p17^{gag}$ protein is nested a nucleocapsid comprised of $p24^{gag}$ proteins. Inside the nucleocapsid HIV carries its payload. HIV's genetic payload consists of two single strands of RNA and several enzymes. The enzymes that accompany HIV's genome include 'reverse transcriptase', 'integrase' and 'protease' molecules.

[0090] The T-Helper cell acts as HIV's host cell. The HIV virion utilizes two types of glycoprotein probes affixed to its external envelope to locate and engage a T-Helper cell. HIV utilizes a glycoprotein probe 120 to locate a CD4 cell-surface receptor on a T-Helper cell. Once an HIV glycoprotein 120 probe has successfully engaged a CD4 cell surface-receptor on a T-Helper cell a conformational change occurs in the glycoprotein 120 probe and a glycoprotein 41 probe is exposed. The glycoprotein 41 probe's intent is to engage a CXCR4 or CCR5 cell-surface receptor on the same T-Helper cell. Once a glycoprotein 41 probe on the HIV virion successfully engages a CXCR4 or CCR5 cell-surface receptor, the HIV virion opens an access portal through the T-Helper cell's outer membrane.

[0091] Once the HIV virion has opened an access portal through the T-Helper cell's outer plasma membrane, the HIV virion inserts two positive strand RNA molecules and the associated enzymes it carries into the T-Helper cell. Each RNA strand is approximately 9500 nucleotides in length. Inserted along with the RNA strands are the enzymes reverse transcriptase, protease and integrase. Once the virus's genome gains access to the interior of the T-Helper cell, in the cytoplasm the pair of RNA molecules are transformed to deoxyribonucleic acid by the reverse transcriptase enzyme. Following modification of the virus's genome to DNA, the virus's genetic information migrates to the host cell's nucleus. In the nucleus, with the assistance of the integrase protein, the HIV's DNA becomes inserted into the T-Helper cell's native nuclear DNA. When the timing is appropriate, the now integrated viral DNA is decoded by the host cell's polymerase molecules and the virus's genetic information commands certain cell functions to carry out the replication process to construct copies of the human immunodeficiency virus.

[0092] The outer layer of the HIV virion is comprised of a portion of the T-Helper cell's outer cell membrane. In the final stage of the replication process, as a copy of the HIV virion, carrying the HIV genome, buds through the host cell's cell membrane the outer protein shell acquires as its external envelope, a wrapping of lipid bilayer from the host cell's cell membrane. In the case of HIV, since the surface of the pathogen is covered by an envelope comprised of lipid bilayer taken from the host T-Helper cells, this feature allows the HIV virion the capacity to elude the two immune systems, since the detectors comprising the innate immune system and the adaptable immune system may find it difficult to distinguish between the surface of an infectious HIV virion and the surface characteristics of a noninfected T-Helper cell.

[0093] The Hepatitis C virus (HCV) is a positive sense RNA virus, meaning a type of RNA that is capable of bypassing the need for involving the host cell's nucleus by having its RNA genome function as messenger RNA. Hepatitis C infects liver cells. The Hepatitis C viral genome becomes divided once it gains access to the interior of a liver host cell. Portions of the subdivisions of the Hepatitis C genome directly interact with ribosomes to produce proteins necessary to construct copies of the virus.

[0094] HCV belongs to the Flaviviridae family and is the only member of the Hepacivirus genus. There are considered to be at least 100 different strains of Hepatitis C virus based on genome sequencing variability.

[0095] HCV is comprised of an outer lipoprotein envelope and an internal nucleocapsid. The genetic payload is carried within the nucleocapsid. In its natural state, present on the surface of the outer envelope of the Hepatitis C virus are probes that detect receptors present on the surface of liver cells. The glycoprotein E1 probe and the glycoprotein E2 probe have been identified to be affixed to the surface of HCV. The E2 probe binds with high affinity to the large external loop of a CD81 cell-surface receptor. CD81 is found on the surface of many cell types including liver cells. Once the E2 probe has engaged the CD81 cell-surface receptor, cofactors on the surface of HCV's external envelope engage either or both the low density lipoprotein receptor (LDLR) or the scavenger receptor class B type I (SR-BI) present on the liver cell in order to effect the mechanism to facilitate HCV breaching the cell membrane and inserting its RNA genome payload through the plasma cell membrane of the liver cell into the liver cell. Upon successful engagement of the HCV surface probes with a liver cell's cell-surface receptors, HCV inserts the single strand of RNA and other payload elements it carries into the liver cell targeted to be a host cell. The HCV RNA genome then interacts with enzymes and ribosomes inside the liver cell in a translational process to produce the proteins required to construct copies of the protein components of HCV. The HCV genome undergoes a method of transcription to replicate copies of the virus's RNA genome. Inside the host, pieces of the HCV virus are assembled together and ultimately loaded with a copy of the HCV genome. Replicas of the original HCV then escape the host cell and migrate the environment in search of additional host liver cells to infect and continue the replication process.

[0096] The HCV's naturally occurring genetic payload consists of a single molecule of linear positive sense, single stranded RNA approximately 9600 nucleotides in length. By means of a translational process a polyprotein of approximately 3000 amino

acids is generated. This polyprotein is cleaved post translation by host and viral proteases into individual viral proteins which include: the structural proteins of C, E1, E2, the nonstructural proteins NS1, NS2, NS3, NS4A, NS4B, NS5A, NS5B, p7 and ARFP/F protein. Hepatitis C virus's proteins direct the host liver cell to construction copies of the Hepatitis C virus. A membrane associated replicase complex consisting of the virus's nonstructural proteins NS3 and NS5B facilitate the replication of the viral genome. The membrane of the endoplasmic reticulum appears to be the site of protein maturation and viral assembly. Once copies of the Hepatitis C Virus are generated, they exit the host cell and each copy of HCV migrates in search of another appropriate liver cell that will act as a host to continue the replication process.

[0097] Hepatitis C virus life-cycle demonstrates that copies of a virus virion can be generated by inserting RNA into a host cell that functions as messenger RNA in the host cell. The Hepatitis C viral RNA genome functions as messenger RNA, acting as the template in conjunction with the biologic machinery of a host cell to produce the components that comprise copies of the Hepatitis C virion and the Hepatitis C viral RNA provides the biologic instructions to assemble the components into complete copies of the Hepatitis C virions. The Hepatitis C virus life-cycle clearly demonstrates that viral virions can be manufactured by a host cell without involving the nucleus of the cell.

[0098] Deciphering the existence, replication and behavior of viruses provides clear examples of several fundamental concepts, which include: (1) Viruses target specific cells in the body by means of identifying and engaging such target cells utilizing the probes projecting outward from the virus's exterior shell to make contact with cell-surface receptors located on the surface of the target cells, and (2) Viruses are capable of carrying a variety of different types of payloads including DNA, RNA and a variety of proteins.

[0099] Current gene therapy approach to attempting to deliver a payload to cells in the body use modified forms of existing viruses to act as transport devices to deliver genetic information. This approach is severely limited by restricting the virus virion to the target only cells the viral vector naturally seeks out and infects. Current gene therapy approach is further limited by using the pre-existing size of naturally occurring viruses, rather than being able to modify the size of the structure to be able to tailor the volumetric carrying capacity of the payload portion of the modified virus. Further, gene therapy is restricted to utilizing naturally occurring viruses to deliver only genetic information; it has not previously been appreciated by those skilled in the art that virus-like transport devices might deliver to a variety of specific type of cells a wide variety of differing payloads such as quantum genes.

[0100] A dramatic, not previously recognized by those expert in the art is the need to develop a transport vehicle that can be fashioned to seek out specific types of cells and deliver to these cells DNA genetic material. The external envelope of a transport should be constructed so as not to alert the immune system of its presence to prevent rejection of the vehicles. Transport vehicles should be capable of being configured to target any specific type of cell and engage and deliver their payload only to that specific type of cell.

[0101] An equally dramatic, not previously recognized is the need for strict organization of the genes that comprise the human genome. The individual genes must each be labeled with some form of unique identifier to facilitate the nuclear transcription mechanisms in easily finding the transcribable genetic information when needed.

[0102] Merging these two concepts together suggests a transport device that would be capable of inserting quantum genes into specifically targeted cells; a constellation of concepts not previously before recognized by those skilled in the art.

[0103] For purposes of this text, the term 'exogenous' refers to an item which originates outside the boundaries of a particular cell or cell type and becomes a part of a particular cell or cell type. The term 'endogenous' refers to an item which originates as a part of a particular cell or cell type and remains a part of that particular cell or cell type.

BRIEF SUMMARY OF THE INVENTION

[0104] Utilization of configurable microscopic medical payload delivery devices to deliver quantum genes to specific type of cells facilitates a dramatic new approach to medical care. By selecting the type of probes that are present on the surface of the configurable microscopic medical payload delivery devices, specific types of cells can be targeted. By delivering quantum genes to specific type of cells, genetic instructions delivered to cell can be located and transcribed in an efficient manner, and thus utilized in the specific type of cells in a timely fashion. A wide variety of medical conditions are manageable by utilizing this new and unique approach.

DETAILED DESCRIPTION

[0105] The future of medical treatment will be the widespread utilization of a medical treatment delivery method the incorporates configurable microscopic medical payload delivery devices (CMMPDD) to deliver quantum genes directly to targeted cell types in the body.

[0106] Introduced herein is a delivery method that includes the concepts: (1) configurable microscopic medical payload delivery devices can carry quantum gene molecules as the payload, and (2) glycoprotein probes present on the exterior of the configurable microscopic medical payload delivery devices include specific glycoprotein probes or protein structure probes affixed to the exterior, these glycoprotein probes or protein structure probes intended to seek out and engage cell-surface receptors attached to the exterior of whichever cell the configurable microscopic medical payload delivery devices is intended to deliver its payload of quantum gene molecules in order to produce a predetermined medically beneficial effect.

[0107] For the purposes of this text a 'quantum gene' is comprised of a sequence of nucleotides that represents a 'unique identifier' physically linked to a sequence of nucleotides that represent a discrete quantity of genetic information; these sequences of nucleotides being comprised of some combination of the nucleotides being referred to by their nitrogenous base as <u>adenine</u> (A), <u>thymine</u> (T), <u>cytosine</u> (C), and <u>guanine</u> (G). The genetic information associated with the above-mentioned unique identifier may be comprised of a portion of transcribable genetic information and a portion of nontranscribable genetic information which together define a specific gene, otherwise referred to as a discrete quantity of genetic information. The nontranscribable segments of a quantum gene may represent segments that act as instructions such as a START code, STOP code and REPEAT code or may help facilitated the attachment of a transcription complex or be simply ignored during the transcription process. Quantum gene molecules can be comprised of a segment of nucleotides where the portion that represents a unique identifier is separated from the portion that represents genetic information by a quantity of base pairs of nucleotides that do not represent a unique identifier and do not represent genetic information. The purpose of the separation of the portion of the unique identifier from the portion of the genetic information by a quantity of base pairs of nucleotides that do not represent a unique identifier and does not represent genetic information is to facilitate a transcription complex attaching to the quantum gene upstream from the portion of the quantum gene that represents genetic information so that transcription of the biologic information associated with the quantum gene may occur.

[0108] The genetic information in a quantum gene codes for some combination of protein coding RNA (pcRNA), non-coding RNAs (ncRNA) and spacers. Spacers represent segments of the DNA that do not code for a RNA molecule. The genetic information in a quantum gene, when transcribed, produces protein coding RNA and non-coding RNA. Protein coding RNAs, usually referred to as messenger RNAs, undergo the process of translation in the cytoplasm of the cell and produce proteins. Non-coding RNAs are highly abundant and functionally important for the cell's operation. Non-coding RNAs have also been referred by such terms as non-protein-coding RNAs (npcRNA) or non-messenger RNA (nmRNA) or small non-messenger RNA (snmRNA) or functional RNAs (fRNA). The non-coding RNAs include: transfer RNAs (tRNA), ribosomal RNAs (rRNA), small nuclear RNAs (snRNA), small nucleolar RNAs (snoRNA), signal recognition particle RNA

(SRP RNA), antisense RNA (aRNA), micro RNA (miRNA), small interfering RNA (siRNA), Y RNA, telomerase RNA.

[0109] Transfer RNAs (tRNA), are RNAs that carries amino acids and deliver them to a ribosome. Ribosomal RNAs (rRNA), are RNAs that couple with ribosomal proteins and participate in translation of mRNA to produce protein molecules. Small nuclear RNAs (snRNA) are RNAs involved in splicing and other nuclear functions. Small nucleolar RNAs (snoRNA) are RNAs involved in nucleotide modification. Signal recognition particle RNA (SRP RNA) are RNAs are involved in membrane integration. Antisense RNA (aRNA) are RNAs involved in transcription attenuation, mRNA degradation, mRNA stabilization, and translation blockage. Micro RNA (miRNA) are RNAs involved in gene regulation and have been implicated in a wide range of cell functions including cell growth, apoptosis, neuronal plasticity, and insulin secretion. Small interfering RNA (siRNA) are RNAs involved in gene regulation, often interfering with the expression of a single gene. Y RNA are RNAs involved in RNA processing and DNA replication. Telomerase RNA are RNAs involved in telomere synthesis.

[0110] In addition to the unique identifier, a quantum gene is comprised of the biologic instruction code, which when transcribed produces one or more of the same RNA molecules or different RNA molecules. A quantum gene must be comprised of a unique identifier and the genetic material to code for at least one RNA molecule. The definition of a 'quantum gene' differs from all previous definitions of a 'gene' due to the requirement that the quantum gene must have a unique identifier that accompanies a segment of genetic information. From a medical treatment perspective, the quantum gene's unique identifier allows the genetic information present in the quantum gene to be located by a cell's transcription machinery, once the quantum gene is inserted into a cell's nuclear DNA.

[0111] Ribonucleic acid molecules directly transcribed from the DNA or quantum gene, may be precursor ribonucleic acid molecules that require modification by nuclear enzymes prior to being translatable or may be ribonucleic acid molecules which are directly translatable without further modification.

[0112] In the DNA there are a number of nucleotides physically existing along the deoxyribonucleic acid between the unique identifier and the transcribable genetic information; or in other terms a number of nucleotides that are not a part of the identification code and are not transcribable, exist downstream from the unique identifier and upstream from the transcribable genetic information.

[0113] It is well recognized that within the transcribable genetic information there exist subsegments of nucleotides that are not transcribable and there are subsegments of nucleotides that are transcribed but are not found in the final version of the RNA molecule. Subsegments of transcribable genetic information that are not transcribed are subsegments such as 'STOP' codes, which indicate to the transcription complex a potential point at which to cease transcribing the genetic information. Certain factors may influence whether a transcription complex actually ceases transcription at that point or whether the transcription complex continues transcribing when the transcription complex reaches a 'STOP' code. Subsegments of nucleotides that are transcribed and appear in the final active form of a RNA are referred to as exons. Subsegments of nucleotides that are transcribed, but do not appear in the final active form of a RNA are referred to as introns. Precursor RNA molecules include both exons and introns. Introns are removed by modification of the initial RNA segment directly transcribed from the transcribable genetic information.

[0114] Utilization of the sigma summation symbol to show summation over a series of indexed variables or expression can be represented as:

$$\sum_{j=1}^{n} [K]_j = [K]_1 + [K]_2 + \ldots\ldots + [K]_n$$

[0115] An equation to represent a quantum gene would be:

Quantum gene = [unique identifier] +

$$\sum_{a=0}^{n}[nontranscribable\ connector\ nucleotide]_{a}\ +$$

$$\sum_{b=1}^{n}[nucleotide\ segment\ transcribable\ for\ RNA]_{b}\ +$$

$$\sum_{c=0}^{n}[nontranscribable\ spacer\ nucleotide]_{c}\ +$$

$$\sum_{d=0}^{n}[nontranscribable\ nucleotide\ commands]_{d}$$

Where 'unique identifier' represents a number, a name or the combination of a number and a name that the transcription complex utilizes to locate a specific quantum gene amongst the DNA material present in a biologically active cell.

Where 'nontranscribable connector nucleotide' represents one or more nucleotides that physically exists between the 'unique identifier' and the segment of 'transcribable genetic information'.

Where a 'nontranscribable spacer nucleotide' represents one or more nucleotides comprising the transcribable genetic information that is not transcribed when the transcription complex transcribes the genetic information of the quantum gene.

Where a 'nontranscribable nucleotide command' represents one or more nucleotides comprising the transcribable genetic information that is not transcribed when the transcription complex transcribes the genetic information of the quantum gene, but acts as an instruction to the transcription complex to cause the transcription complex to function in a certain manner; examples include a STOP code that causes the transcription complex to cease transcription and a REPEAT code that causes the transcription complex to repeat its transcription of a segment of genetic material.

Where 'a' represents the range of 'zero to any positive whole number. Where 'b' represents the range of 'one to any positive whole number'.

Where 'c' represents the range of 'zero to any positive whole number'.
Where 'd' represents the range of 'zero to any positive whole number'.

Where the DNA segment that is transcribable for RNA may transcribe RNAs that may exist in a precursor form; such a precursor form may include elements such as introns that are removed following transcription by modifying proteins.

[0116] For purposes of this text an 'external envelope' refers to the outermost covering of a virus or a virus-like transport device or a configurable microscopic medical payload delivery device. The external envelope may be comprised of a lipid layer, a lipid bilayer, the combination of a lipid layer affixed to a protein matrix or the combination of a lipid bilayer affixed to a protein matrix. A protein matrix is equivalent to a protein shell and may be referred to as a protein matrix shell. The terms protein matrix, protein shell, protein matrix shell are equivalent to the term capsid, where the term capsid is meant to represent 'a protein coat or shell of a virus particle, surrounding the nucleic acid or nucleoprotein core'. For purposes of this text, the term 'particle' is equivalent to the term 'virion'; further the term 'virus particle' is equivalent to 'viral virion'.

[0117] For purposes of this text an 'internal shell' refers to a protein matrix shell nested inside the external envelope. Multiple inner shells may exist, with those of smaller diameter concentrically nested inside those of a larger diameter. The inner most protein matrix shell is termed the nucleocapsid. The proteins that comprise the nucleocapsid are termed capsid proteins. In the cavity created by the nucleocapsid, referred to as the center or core of the nucleocapsid, is where the payload of quantum gene molecules is carried.

[0118] For purposes of this text 'external probes' are molecular structures that are utilized to locate and engage cell-surface receptors on biologically active cells. External probes are generally comprised of a portion which is anchored or fixed in the external envelope and a second portion that extends out and away from the external envelope. The portion of the external probe that extends out and away from the external envelope is intended to make contact and engage a specific cell-surface receptor located on a biologically active cell. External probes may be comprised solely of a protein structure or an external probe may be a glycoprotein molecule.

[0119] For purposes of this text 'glycoprotein molecule' refers to a molecule comprised of a carbohydrate region and a protein region. Glycoprotein molecules that act as probes are generally anchored or fixed to a lipid layer utilizing the carbohydrate portion of the molecule as an anchor. The protein portion of the glycoprotein molecule which extends outward and away from the external envelope the glycoprotein has been affixed such that the protein region may function as a probe to locate and attach to the cell-surface receptor it was created to engage.

[0120] The concept of configurable microscopic medical payload delivery devices is modeled after naturally existing viruses. Configurable microscopic medical payload delivery devices in general are spherical in shape; though other shapes may be used as function might warrant the use of a particular shape. The spherical configurable microscopic medical payload delivery devices are comprised of an external envelope and one or more inner nested protein shells. A quantity of exterior protein structure probes and/or glycoprotein probes are anchored in the external envelope and a portion extend out and away from the exterior lipid envelope. Nesting of protein shells refers to progressively smaller diameter shells fitting snugly inside protein shells of a larger diameter. Inside the inner most protein shell, referred to as the nucleocapsid, is a cavity referred to as the core of the device. The core of the device is the space where the medically therapeutic payload the device carries is located. The payload of the device is comprised of ribonucleic acid molecules.

[0121] Configurable microscopic medical payload delivery devices (CMMPDD) target specific types of cells in the body. Configurable microscopic medical payload delivery devices engage specific types of cells by the configuration of probes affixed to the external envelope of the CMMPDD. By fixing specific probes to the external envelope of the CMMPDD, these probes intended to engage and attach only to specific cell-surface receptors located on certain cell types in the body, the CMMPDD will deliver its payload only to those cell types that express compatible and engagable specific cell-surface receptors. In a similar fashion where the exterior probes of a naturally occurring virus engage specific cell-surface receptors present on the surface of the virus's host cell and only the designated host cell, the CMMPDD's exterior probes are configured to engage cell-surface receptors on a specific type of target cell and only those cells. In this manner, the payload of quantum gene molecules carried by CMMPDD will be delivered only to specific types of cells in the body. The configuration of exterior probes on the surface of a CMMPDD varies as needed so as to effect the CMMPDD delivery of specific quantum gene payloads to specific type of cells as needed to effect a particular predetermined medical treatment.

[0122] The size of the configurable microscopic medical payload delivery devices is dependent upon the diameter of the inner protein matrix shells and this is dictated by the volume size of the payload the CMMPDD is required to carry and deliver to a target cell. The diameter of the each inner protein matrix shell is governed by the number of protein molecules utilized to construct the protein matrix shell at the time the protein matrix shell is generated. Increasing the number of proteins that comprise a protein matrix shell increases the diameter of the protein matrix shell. When applicable, as dictated by the capacity the CMMPDD is to be utilized to function as, an external lipid envelope wraps around and covers the outer protein matrix shell. The larger the volume of the core of the CMMPDD, the greater the physical size of the payload the CMMPDD is able to carry. The size of the configurable microscopic medical payload delivery device is to be generally the size of cell (approximately 10^{-4} m in diameter) or less, generally detectable by a light microscope or, as needed, an electron microscope. The size of the CMMPDD is not to be too large such that it would generate a burden to the body by damaging organ tissues through clogging blood vessels or the glomeruli in the kidneys. The dimensions of each type of CMMPDD are to be tailored to the mission of the CMMPDD, which takes into account factors such as the type of target cell, the size of the payload that is to be delivered to the target cells and the length of time the CMMPDD may engage the target cell.

[0123] Being enveloped in an external lipid layer, configurable microscopic medical payload delivery devices possess the advantage of having their exterior appear similar to the plasma membrane that acts as an outside covering for the cells that comprise the body. By appearing similar to existing plasma membranes, the CMMPDDs appear similar to naturally occurring structures found in the body. CMMPDD are afforded the capability to avoid detection by a body's immune system because the exterior of the CMMPDD mimics the cells comprising the body and the surveillance elements of the immune system find it difficult to discern between the CMMPDD and naturally occurring cells comprising the body.

[0124] To carry out the process of manufacturing a configurable microscopic medical payload delivery device, a primitive cell such as a stem cell is selected. The reason for utilizing primitive cells such as stems cells as the host cell, is that the CMMPDD acquires its outer envelope from the host cell and the more primitive the host cell, the fewer in number the identifying protein markers are present on the surface of the CMMPDD. The fewer the identifying surface proteins present on the outer envelope of the CMMPDD, the less likely a body's immune system will identify the CMMPDD as an invader and therefore less likely the body's immune system will react to the presence of the CMMPDD and reject the CMMPDD by attacking and neutralizing the CMMPDD.

[0125] Stem cells used as host cells to manufacture quantities of CMMPDD product are selected per histocompatibility markers present on their surface. Certain histocompatibility markers present on the surface of the final CMMPDD product will be less likely to cause a reaction in a specific patient based on the genetic profile of the patient's histocompatibility markers. A similar histocompatibility match is done when donor organs are selected to be given to recipients to avoid rejection of the donor organ by the recipient's immune system.

413

[0126] The selected stem cell used to manufacture configurable microscopic medical payload delivery devices goes through several steps of maturation before it is capable of generating therapeutic CMMPDD product. RNA inserted into the host stem cell code for the general physical outer structures of the CMMPDD. RNA inserted into the host generate surface probes that target the cell-surface receptors on a specific target cell type. RNA would be inserted into the host that would be used to generate the payload of quantum genes. Similar to how copies of a naturally occurring virus, such as the Hepatitis C virus or HIV, are produced, assembled and released from a host cell, copies of the CMMPDD would be produced, assembled and released from a stem cell functioning as a de facto host cell. Once released from the host cell, the copies of the CMMPDD would be collected, then pooled together to produce a therapeutic dose that would result in a medically beneficial effect.

[0127] The stem cells used as host cells are suspended in a broth of nutrients and are kept at an optimum temperature to govern the rate of production of the CMMPDD product. Similar to the natural production of the Hepatitis C virus, the configurable microscopic medical payload delivery devices 'production genome' is introduced into the host stem cells. The configurable microscopic medical payload delivery devices production genome carries genetic instructions to cause the host cells to manufacture the configurable microscopic medical payload delivery devices' outer protein wall, the inner protein matrixes, the surface probes the configurable microscopic medical payload delivery device is to have affixed to its outer envelope and the quantity of quantum gene molecules the configurable microscopic medical payload delivery devices are to carry; and the instructions to assemble the various pieces into the final form of the configurable microscopic medical payload delivery devices and the instructions to activate the budding process. The resultant configurable microscopic medical payload delivery devices are collected from the nutrient broth surrounding the host cells and placed together into doses to be used as a treatment for a medical disease.

[0128] The 'production genome' are an array of RNAs, which include messenger RNAs that are directly translated by the host cell's ribosomes. The production genome dictates the characteristics of the final version of the CMMPDD that buds from the host stem cell and is released and is to be utilized as a medical treatment. The production genome is specifically tailored to code for the surface probes that will seek and engage a specific type of target cell. The production genome also carries the instructions to code for the production of the type of quantum genes to be delivered to the specific type of target cell. The 'production genome' varies depending upon the configuration of the CMMPDD and the specific type of quantum genes the CMMPDD will transport to effect a specific medical treatment on a specific type of cell.

[0129] The configurable microscopic medical payload delivery device transporting quantum gene molecules represents a very versatile medical treatment delivery device. CMMPDD is used to deliver a number of different quantum gene molecules to a wide variety of cells in the body.

[0130] The construction of a naturally occurring virus can be likened to the act of following a programmed script to produce a specific result. It is known that the genetic code that a virus carries dictates the production of copies of the virus. It is known that specific segments of the viral genetic code represent instructions that dictate the construction of different parts of the virus so that copies of the virus can be made inside the host cell. It is well documented that there exist different subtypes of most viruses, based off of mutations that have occurred to the viral genome over time; these mutations to the viral genome producing variants in the construction of the virus. Configurable microscopic medical payload delivery devices which carry quantum genes are constructed much like a naturally occurring virus virions would be constructed in a host cell. Altering the production RNA alters the configuration of the external probes or alters the configuration of the size of the inner shells or alters the type of quantum gene the CMMPDD will carry or alters any combination of the three.

[0131] As an example of the method to produce a device to treat diabetes mellitus utilizing configurable microscopic medical payload delivery devices to deliver to Beta cells quantum genes, which when transcribed produce messenger RNA coded to produce insulin, the following production process is followed in the lab: (1) human stem cells are selected. (2) Into the selected stem cells is placed the RNA production genome constructed, in this case, specifically as a means to treat diabetes mellitus. The RNA production genome contains genetic instructions to cause the host stem cells to manufacture the CMMPDDs' outer protein wall, the inner protein matrix, surface probes to include a quantity of glycoprotein probes that engage the GPR40 cell-surface receptor present on the surface of Beta cells located in the Islets of Langerhans in the pancreas, and the payload of quantum genes, in this case the quantum genes to facilitate the production of the insulin molecules in Beta cells; and the biologic instructions to assemble the components into the final form of the CMMPDD; and the biologic instructions to activate the budding process. (3) Upon insertion of the RNA production genome into the host stem cells, host stem cells' production cellular machinery responds by simultaneously translating the different segments of the RNA production genome to produce the proteins that comprise the exterior protein wall, the inner protein matrix molecules, the surface probes, the quantum gene payload to produce the messenger RNA that will produce insulin, and decode the instructions to assemble the components into the CMMPDDs. (4) Upon assembly, the CMMPDDs bud through the cell membrane of the host stem cell. (5) At the time of the budding process, the CMMPDDs acquire an outside envelope wrapped over the outer protein shell, this outer envelope comprised of a portion of the plasma membrane from the host stem cell as the CMMPDDs exit the host cell. (6) The resultant CMMPDDs are collected from the nutrient broth surrounding the host stem cells. (7) The CMMPDD product is washed in sterile solution to separate the CMMPDD product from any unwanted elements of the nutrient broth. (8) The configurable microscopic medical payload delivery devices are removed from the sterile solvent and suspended in a hypoallergenic liquid medium. (9) The configurable microscopic medical payload delivery devices are separated into individual quantities to facilitate storage and delivery to physicians and patients. (10) The configurable microscopic medical payload delivery devices transported in the hypoallergenic liquid medium is administered to a diabetic patient per injection in a dose that is tailored to receiving patient's requirement to produce sufficient amount of insulin to control the blood sugar. (11) Upon being injected into the body, the configurable microscopic medical payload delivery devices migrate to the Beta cells located in the Islets of Langerhans by means of the patient's blood stream. (12) Upon the configurable microscopic medical payload delivery devices reaching the Beta cells, the configurable microscopic medical payload delivery devices engage the cell-surface receptors located on the Beta cells and insert the payload of quantum genes they carry into the Beta cells. The payload of quantum genes migrate to the nucleus of the Beta cells. The quantum genes inserts into the nuclear DNA of the Beta cells. Transcription machinery present in the nucleus transcribes the quantum genes. Messenger RNAs generated by transcribing the exogenous quantum genes enhances the Beta cells' production of insulin molecules. The increase in insulin production by Beta cells successfully manages diabetes mellitus.

[0132] In a similar fashion, configurable microscopic medical payload delivery devices can be fashioned to deliver a payload of a specific type of quantum gene molecule to any type of cell in the body. Different cell types express different cell-surface markers on the exterior of their plasma membrane. The differing configurations of cell-surface markers on differing types of cells distinguish one cell type from another cell type. By configuring the exterior probes that extend from the surface of the configurable microscopic medical payload delivery device to seek out and engage specific cell-surface receptors present on a specific type of cell, payloads of any quantum gene molecule can be delivered to specific cells in the body.

[0133] The transcribable genetic information linked to the unique identifier may occur in the form of naturally found transcribable genetic information or may occur as artificially created transcribable genetic information, referred to as 'artificial transcribable genetic information'. Naturally found transcribable genetic information would be a segment of transcribable genetic information that would be found in a cell's genome otherwise referred to as a gene.

Artificial transcribable genetic information would be transcribable genetic information that would represent either (i) a modified form of a naturally occurring gene or (ii) a segment of nucleotides that represents transcribable genetic information that is artificially created to produce a medically beneficial result.

[0134] A quantum gene, as it exists as a functional part of the deoxyribonucleic acid of a cell, is a segment of deoxyribonucleic acid, comprised of both a unique identifier and a segment of transcribable biologic information, that is capable of being inserted into a cell's nuclear DNA. DNA is comprised of two parallel strands of nucleotides. Each strand of DNA is a mirror image of each other since adenine must combine with thymine and cytosine must combine with guanine. Therefore, since each strand of DNA is a mirror image of each other, one strand of DNA possesses the nucleotide sequence that codes for both strands; one strand represents the DNA code, while the second strand represents the mirror image of the first strand. In this manner, a quantum gene can be defined in its most elemental form as a sequence of nucleotides comprising a single strand of nucleotides.

[0135] A quantum gene could thus be represented as a single strand of nucleotides comprised of the nucleotides adenine, cytosine, guanine and thymine. The double stranded form of a quantum gene would be the single strand of nucleotides attached in parallel to a second strand of nucleotides that represents the mirror image of the single strand of nucleotides. Double stranded deoxyribonucleic acid segments is the form quantum genes take when a quantum gene is inserted into a cell's nuclear genome.

Conclusions, Ramification, and Scope

[0136] Accordingly, the reader will see that the method to utilize configurable microscopic medical payload delivery device to deliver quantum genes to specific targeted cell types provides advantages over existing art by (1) being a method to use delivery devices that seeks out specific types of cells, (2) by being method that uses delivery devices that are versatile enough to deliver a variety of quantum genes to accomplish various medical treatments and (3) by being a method to use delivery devices constructed with a surface envelope that will avoid detection by the innate as well as the adaptable immune systems so as not to activate the immune system to its presence; for these reasons this represents a new and unique medical delivery device that has never before been recognized nor appreciated by those skilled in the art.

[0137] The reader will also see that the concept and utilization of a method that incorporates the use of the quantum gene as described in this text has never before been recognized nor appreciated by those skilled in the art.

[0138] Although the description above contains specificities, these should not be construed as limiting the scope of the invention but as merely providing illustrations of some of the presently preferred embodiments of the invention.

[0139] Thus the scope of the invention should be determined by the appended claims and their legal equivalents, rather than by the examples given.

CLAIMS: Reserved.

PATENT APPLICATION
SPECIFICATION NUMBER 3

TITLE OF THE INVENTION:

CONFIGURABLE MICROSCOPIC MEDICAL PAYLOAD DELIVERY DEVICE TO DELIVER NUCLEAR SIGNALING PROTEINS TO SPECIFIC CELLS TO MANAGE DIABETES MELLITUS AND GENETIC DEFICIENCY DISORDERS

BACKGROUND OF THE INVENTION

Field of the Invention

This invention relates to any medical device intended to correct a protein deficiency or genetic deficiency in the body by utilizing a configurable microscopic medical payload delivery device to insert one or more nuclear signaling proteins into one or more specific cell types in the body to improve cell function.

Description of Background Art

[0001] For purposes of this text a 'nuclear signaling protein' molecule (NSP) is a protein molecule intended to attach to nuclear deoxyribonucleic acid, by means of zinc fingers, for the purpose of initiating or inhibiting the process of transcription of a segment of the deoxyribonucleic acid. Nuclear signaling protein molecules include nuclear receptors (NR), nuclear binding proteins (NBP), and artificial transcription factors (ATF).

[0002] Proteins are comprised of one or more linear strings of amino acids. Particular segments of a protein may be termed a 'domain'. Zinc fingers refer to small protein domains that are folded, with these folds stabilized by one or more zinc ions. The physical structure of the folding of the zinc finger DNA binding domain facilitates the protein molecule's ability to attach to deoxyribonucleic acid (DNA), ribonucleic acid (RNA), other proteins or small molecules.

[0003] In the case whereby a zinc finger DNA binding domain facilitates a nuclear binding protein molecule to bind to DNA, the physical structure of the folding of the zinc finger DNA binding domain engages and makes contact with a specific sequence of DNA bases. A particular zinc finger DNA binding domain therefore attaches to a specific sequence of DNA bases. Once a zinc finger DNA binding domain binds to the DNA, this facilitates or represses the possible transcription of a specific segment of the DNA located near the site where the zinc finger DNA binding domain caused the nuclear binding protein molecule to bind to the DNA.

[0004] Nuclear receptors are proteins that sense the presence of ligands such as steroid, thyroid hormones, and certain other proteins. The description of a nuclear receptor is varied in the literature. For purposes of this text, nuclear receptors are commonly comprised of a N-terminal domain, one or more zinc finger DNA binding domains, one or more transactivation domains, a hinge region, a ligand binding domain and a C-terminal domain. In general, nuclear receptors exist in a nonactive form until a ligand binds to the ligand binding domain. Prior to a ligand binding to the nuclear receptor, the nuclear receptor may be prevented from attaching to DNA by the presence of neutralizing proteins. A ligand binding to the ligand binding domain causes: (1) a conformational change in the nuclear receptor which activates the nuclear receptor and (2) removal of the presence of any neutralizing proteins. Separating neutralizing proteins from a nuclear receptor frees the nuclear receptor to traverse to a specific site along the deoxyribonucleic acid. The zinc finger DNA binding domain attaches the nuclear receptor to the DNA at a specific site along the DNA. The transactivation domain interacts with other transcription proteins that ultimately assemble to form a transcription complex. The transcription complex transcribes genetic information in the DNA. The hinge region is thought to facilitate changes in the three-dimensional shape of the nuclear protein.

[0005] Nuclear receptors are subset into at least four categories. The four categories include: (1) Nuclear receptors that originally reside in the cytoplasm and sense the presence of extrinsic ligands, (2) Nuclear receptors that reside in the cytoplasm and sense intrinsic ligands, (3) Nuclear receptors that reside in the nucleus and sense the presence of extrinsic ligands, and (4) Nuclear receptors that reside in the nucleus and sense the presence of intrinsic ligands. Nuclear receptors that sense 'intrinsic' ligands are often referred to as 'orphan' nuclear receptors.

[0006] When an extrinsic ligand or an intrinsic ligand binds to a nuclear receptor that resides in the cytoplasm, the now activated nuclear receptor traverses the cytoplasm, enters the nucleus, traverses the nucleus and attaches to the DNA at a specific binding site as dictated by the zinc finger DNA binding domain present within the nuclear receptor.

[0007] When an extrinsic ligand or an intrinsic ligand binds to a nuclear receptor that resides in nucleus, the now activated nuclear receptor traverses the nucleus and attaches to the DNA at a specific binding site as dictated by the zinc finger DNA binding domain present within the nuclear receptor.

[0008] Examples of extrinsic ligands are steroids and thyroid hormones, which enter the cell from the external environment surrounding the cell. Once an extrinsic ligand enters the cell it attaches to the ligand binding domain of a nuclear receptor residing in the cytoplasm or it attaches to the ligand binding domain of a nuclear receptor residing in the nucleus. Upon an extrinsic ligand binding to the binding domain of a nuclear receptor the result is the nuclear receptor becomes activated, traverses to a specific binding site on the DNA as dictated by the zinc finger DNA binding domain present within the nuclear receptor and binds to that site on the DNA. The binding of the activated nuclear receptor to the DNA at a specific site along the DNA causes coalescing of transcription proteins that results in the assembly of a transcription complex. The transcription complex then transcribes a segment of DNA.

[0009] An intrinsic ligand refers to an activating molecule generated inside the cell that traverses the cytoplasm and binds to the ligand binding domain of a nuclear receptor. Upon an intrinsic ligand binding to the ligand binding domain of a nuclear receptor the result is the nuclear receptor becomes activated, traverses to a specific binding site on the DNA as dictated by the zinc finger DNA binding domain present within the nuclear receptor and binds to that site on the DNA. The binding of the activated nuclear receptor to the DNA at a specific site along the DNA causes coalescing of transcription proteins that results in the assembly of a transcription complex. The transcription complex then transcribes a segment of DNA.

[0010] Nuclear binding proteins (NBP) do not require the binding of a ligand and activation prior to physically binding to the DNA. Nuclear binding proteins are subset into at least two categories, which include: (1) immediately active nuclear binding proteins (iaNBP) and (2) delayed activity nuclear binding proteins (daNBP).

[0011] Immediately active nuclear binding proteins (iaNBP) at a minimum are comprised of a zinc finger DNA binding domain, a transactivation domain, a C-terminal region and a N-terminal region. There may exist more than one transactivation domains. There may exist a hinge domain. There may exist more than one zinc finger DNA binding domain. The zinc finger DNA binding domain attaches the nuclear receptor to the DNA at a specific site along the DNA. The transactivation domain interacts with transcription proteins that ultimately assemble to form a transcription complex. The iaNBP attaches to a specific segment of the DNA as dictated by the zinc finger DNA binding domain present within the iaNBP. Once the iaNBP has bound to the DNA, the iaNBP activates transcription proteins to assemble into a transcription complex. The transcription complex then transcribes a segment of the DNA.

[0012] Delayed activity nuclear binding proteins (daNBP) at a minimum are comprised of a ligand binding domain, a zinc finger DNA binding domain, a transactivation domain, a C-terminal region and a N-terminal region. There may exist more than one transactivation domains. There may exist a hinge domain. There may exist more than one zinc finger DNA binding domain. The zinc finger DNA binding domain attaches the nuclear receptor to the DNA at a specific site along the DNA. The transactivation domain interacts with transcription proteins that ultimately assemble to form a transcription complex. The ligand binding domain acts as a receptor for a ligand to bind to. The daNBP binds to the DNA per attachment of the zinc finger DNA binding domain to the DNA. The daNBP may sit attached to the DNA without activating transcription proteins, until a ligand becomes attached to the daNBP's ligand binding domain. Once a ligand binds to the ligand binding domain of the daNBP, a conformation change occurs in the daNBP molecule. The conformation change in the daNBP activates transcription proteins. Activated transcription proteins assemble into a transcription complex. The transcription complex then transcribes a segment of the DNA.

[0013] Artificial transcription factors (ATF) have been created that utilize zinc finger DNA binding domains to attach to DNA. Artificial transcription factors are comprised of a zinc finger DNA binding domain and either a domain that activates transcription or a domain that represses transcription. Artificial transcription factors attach to the DNA at a specific binding site as dictated by the construction of the zinc finger DNA binding domain. Once an artificial transcription factor binds to the DNA, if the zinc finger DNA binding domain is physically attached to an activating domain, then transcription proteins become activated and a transcription complex is assembled. If an artificial transcription factor binds to the DNA and the zinc finger DNA binding domain is physically attached to a repressor domain, then this form of artificial transcription factor prevents the assembly of a transcription complex, which results in the adjacent DNA not being able to be transcribed. Zinc finger DNA binding domains can be readily designed to attach to specific sequences of the DNA. Artificial transcription factors may be comprised of protein domains exclusively or a combination of one or more protein domains and one or more non-protein elements. Artificial transcription factors may have a ligand binding domain as part of the molecule.

[0014] A 'deoxyribose' is a deoxypentose (C5H10O4) sugar. Deoxyribonucleic acid (DNA) is comprised of three basic elements: a deoxyribose sugar, a phosphate group and nitrogen containing bases. DNA is a macromolecule made up of two chains of repeating deoxyribose sugars linked by phosphodiester bonds between the 3-hydroxyl group of one and the 5-hydroxyl group of the next; the two chains are held antiparallel to each other by weak hydrogen bonds. DNA strands contain a sequence of nucleotides, which include: adenine, cytosine, guanine or thymine. Adenine is always paired with thymine of the opposite strand, and guanine is always paired with cytosine of the opposite strand; one side or strand of a DNA macromolecule is the mirror image of the opposite strand. Nuclear DNA is regarded as the medium for storing the master plan of hereditary information.

[0015] Genes are considered segments of the DNA that represent units of inheritance.

[0016] A chromosome exists in the nucleus of a cell and consists of a DNA double helix bearing a linear sequence of genes, coiled and recoiled around aggregated proteins, termed histones. The number of chromosomes varies from species to species. Most Human cells carries twenty two pairs of chromosomes plus two sex chromosomes; two 'x' chromosomes in women and one 'x' and one 'y' chromosome in men. Chromosomes carry genetic information in the form of units which are referred to as genes.

[0017] Per J. K. Pal, S.S. Ghaskabi, Fundamentals of Molecular Biology, 2009: 'The central dogma of molecular biology . . . states that the genes present in the genome (DNA) are transcribed into mRNAs, which are then translated into polypeptides or proteins, which are phenotypes.' 'Genome, thus, contains the complete set of hereditary information for any organism and is functionally divided into small parts referred to as genes. Each gene is a sequence of nucleotides representing a single protein or RNA. Genome of a living organism may contain as few as 500 genes as in case of Mycoplasma, or as many as 30,000 genes as in case of human beings.' Some references cite as many as 100,000 genes may exist in the human genome.

[0018] The current understanding of the actual biologic structure of a gene is far more elaborate than the historic standard definition of a gene. A gene appears to be comprised of a number of segments loosely strung together along a particular section of DNA. In general there are three segments associated with a gene which include: (1) the Upstream 5' flanking region, (2) the transcriptional unit (often referred to as the open reading frame) and (3) the Downstream 3' flanking region. The Upstream 5' flanking region is comprised of the 'enhancer region', the 'promoter-proximal region', and 'promoter region'. The 'transcriptional unit' or open reading frame starts at a location designated 'transcription start site' (TSS), which is located in a site called the 'initiator region' (inR), which may be described in a general form as Py2CAPy5. The transcription unit is comprised of the combination of segments of DNA nucleotides to be transcribed into RNA and spacing units known as 'introns' that are not transcribed or if transcribed are later removed post transcription, such that they do not appear in the final RNA molecule. In the case of a gene coding for a mRNA molecule, the transcription unit will contain all three elements of the mRNA, which includes: (1) the 5' noncoding region, (2) the translational region and (3) the 3' noncoding region. Interspersed between these regions are introns, which will be either not transcribed or if transcribed removed from the precursor form of mRNA prior to the mRNA reaching its final form. The 'transcriptional unit' is generally considered to be the 'gene'. The Downstream 3' flanking region contains DNA nucleotides that are not transcribed and may contain what has been termed an 'enhancer region'. An enhancer region in the Downstream 3' flanking region is thought to act to promote the gene previously transcribed to be transcribed again.

[0019] On either side of the DNA sequencing comprising a gene and its flanking regions, may be inactive DNA which act as boundaries which have been termed 'insulator elements'. The term 'upstream' refers to DNA sequencing that occurs prior to the TSS if viewed from the 5' end to the 3' end of the DNA; where the term 'downstream' refers to DNA sequencing located after the TSS.

[0020] An 'enhancer region' may or may not be present in the Upstream 5' flanking region. If present, the enhancer region helps facilitate the reading of the gene by encouraging formation of the transcription mechanism. If the enhancer is present, it may exist 200 kb to 17,000 kb upstream from the transcription starting site.

[0021] The 'transcription complex' also referred to as the 'transcription mechanism', in humans, is reported to be comprised of over forty separate proteins that assemble together to ultimately function in a concerted effort to transcribe the nucleotide sequence of the DNA into RNA. The transcription complex (TC) includes elements such as 'general transcription factor Sp1', 'general transcription factor NF1', 'general transcription factor TATA-binding protein', 'TFIID', 'basal transcription complex', and a 'RNA polymerase protein' to name only a few of the forty elements that exist. The elements of the transcription mechanism function as (1) a means to recognize the location of the start of a gene, (2) as proteins to bind the transcription mechanism to the DNA such that transcription may occur or (3) as means of transcribing the DNA nucleotide coding to produce a precursor RNA molecule. There are at least three RNA polymerase proteins which include: RNA polymerase I, RNA polymerase II, and RNA polymerase III. RNA polymerase I tends to be dedicated to transcribing genetic information that will result in the formation of rRNA molecules. RNA polymerase II tends to be dedicated to transcribing genetic information that will result in the formation of mRNA molecules. RNA polymerase III appears to be dedicated to transcribing genetic information that results in the formation of tRNAs, small cellular RNAs and viral RNAs.

[0022] The 'promoter proximal region' is located upstream from the TSS and upstream from the core promoter region. The 'promoter proximal region' includes two sub-regions termed the GC box and the CAAT box. The 'GC box' appears to be a segment rich in guanine-cytosine nucleotide sequences. The GC box binds to the 'general transcription factor Sp1' of the transcription mechanism. The 'CAAT box' is a segment which contains the nucleotide sequence 'GGCCAATCT' located 75 bps upstream from the transcription start site (TSS). The CAAT box binds to the 'general transcription factor NF1' of the transcription mechanism.

[0023] The 'core promoter' region is considered the shortest sequence at which RNA polymerase II can initiate transcription of a gene The core promoter may include the initiator region (inR) and either a TATA box or a DPE. The inR is the region designated Py2CAPy5 that surrounds the transcription start site (TSS). The TATA box is located 25 bps upstream from the TSS. The TATA box acts as a site of attachment of the TFIID, which is a promoter for binding of the RNA polymerase II molecule. The DPE is the 'downstream promoter element' that may appear 28 bps to 32 bps downstream from the TSS. The DPE acts as an alternative site of attachment for the TFIID when the TATA box is not present.

[0024] The transcription mechanism, also referred to as the transcription complex appears to be comprised of different elements depending upon whether rRNA is being transcribed versus mRNA or tRNA or small cellular RNA or viral RNA. The proteins that assemble to assist RNA Polymerase I with transcribing the DNA to produce rRNA appear different than the proteins that assemble to assist RNA polymerase II with transcribing the DNA to produce mRNA or the proteins that assemble to assist RNA polymerase III with transcribing the DNA to produce tRNA, small cellular RNA or viral RNA. A common protein that appears to be present at the initial biding of all three types of RNA polymerase molecules is TATA-binding protein (TBP). TBP appears to be required to attach to the DNA, which then facilitates RNA polymerase to bind to the promoter along the DNA. TBP assembles with TBP-associated factors (TAFs). Together TBF and 11 TAFs comprise the complex referred to as TFIID, which has been previously mentioned in the above text.

[0025] Upstream from the TATA box is the 'initiator element', which may be considered as part of the 'core promoter' region. The initiator element is a segment of the nuclear DNA that binds the basal transcription complex. The basal transcription complex is comprised of a number of proteins that make initial contact with the DNA prior to the RNA polymerase binding to the transcription mechanism. The basal transcription complex is associated with an activator. The activator is a nuclear signaling protein.

[0026] Once the transcription complex is assembled, the transcription complex transcribes the DNA. Transcription of the DNA produces precursor messenger RNA (mRNA), precursor ribosomal RNA (rRNA) or precursor transport RNA (tRNA). In the case of precursor mRNA, the mRNA is further modified, then traverses to the cytoplasm. In the cytoplasm of the cell ribosomes attach to the mRNA. Ribosomes decode mRNA utilizing the process of translation to produce proteins.

[0027] A protein is comprised of a string of amino acids. Proteins can be comprised of only a few amino acids, or a large number of amino acids. Large protein molecules are often referred to as a macromolecule. Proteins can be combined together to form molecules comprised of two or more similar amino acid strands or a protein can be can be comprised of two or more different amino acid strands. When more than one protein are combined into a molecule, this may also be referred as a macromolecule. Proteins can be combined with other molecules such as carbohydrates and lipids. When proteins combine with other molecules this is also often referred to as a macromolecule. Cell surface receptors are considered macromolecules and are often comprised of a protein molecule combined with a carbohydrate molecule to produce a glycoprotein.

[0028] Diabetes mellitus represents an important health issue that affects a significant portion of the world population. In the United

States, about 16 million people suffer from diabetes mellitus. Every year, about 650,000 additional people are diagnosed with this disease. Diabetes mellitus is the seventh leading cause of all deaths.

[0029] Diabetes mellitus represents a state of hyperglycemia, a serum blood sugar that is higher than what is considered the normal range for humans. Glucose, a six-carbon molecule, is a form of sugar. Glucose is absorbed by the cells of the body and converted to energy by the processes of glycolysis, the Krebs cycle and phosporylation. Insulin, a protein, facilitates the transfer of glucose from the blood into cells. Normal range for blood glucose in humans is generally defined as a fasting blood plasma glucose level of between 70 to 110 mg/dl. For descriptive purposes, the term 'plasma' refers to the fluid portion of blood.

[0030] Diabetes mellitus is classified as Type One and Type Two. Type One diabetes mellitus is insulin dependent, which refers to the condition where there is a lack of sufficient insulin circulating in the blood stream and insulin must be provided to the body in order to properly regulate the blood glucose level. When insulin is required to regulate the blood glucose level in the body, this condition is often referred to as insulin dependent diabetes mellitus (IDDM). Type Two diabetes mellitus is noninsulin dependent, often referred to as noninsulin dependent diabetes mellitus (NIDDM), meaning the blood glucose level can be managed without insulin, and instead by means of diet, exercise or intervention with oral medications. Type Two diabetes mellitus is considered a progressive disease, the underlying pathogenic mechanisms including pancreatic Beta cell (also often designated as β-Cell) dysfunction and insulin resistance.

[0031] The pancreas serves as an endocrine gland and an exocrine gland. Functioning as an endocrine gland the pancreas produces and secretes hormones including insulin and glucagon. Insulin acts to reduce levels of glucose circulating in the blood. Beta cells secrete insulin into the blood when a higher than normal level of glucose is detected in the serum. For purposes of this description the terms 'blood', 'blood stream' and 'serum' refer to the same substance.

Glucagon acts to stimulate an increase in glucose circulating in the blood. Beta cells in the pancreas secrete glucagon when a low level of glucose is detected in the serum.

[0032] Glucose enters the body as food and as a result of digestion, glucose enters the blood stream. The Beta cells of the Islets of Langerhans continuously sense the level of glucose in the blood and respond to elevated levels of blood glucose by secreting insulin into the blood. Beta cells produce the protein 'insulin' in their endoplasmic reticulum and store the insulin in vacuoles until it is needed. When Beta cells detect an increase in the glucose level in the blood, Beta cells release insulin into the blood from the described storage vacuoles.

[0033] Insulin is a protein. An insulin protein consists of two chains of amino acids, an alpha chain and a beta chain, linked by two disulfide (S-S) bridges. One chain, the alpha chain consists of 21 amino acids. The second chain the beta chain consists of 30 amino acids.

[0034] Insulin interacts with the cells of the body by means of a cell-surface receptor termed the 'insulin receptor' located on the exterior of a cell's 'outer membrane', otherwise known as the 'plasma membrane'. Insulin interacts with muscle and liver cells by means of the insulin receptor to rapidly remove excess blood sugar when the glucose level in the blood is higher than the upper limit of the normal physiologic range. Recognized functions of insulin include stimulating cells to take up glucose from the blood and convert it to glycogen to facilitate the cells in the body to utilize glucose to generate biochemically usable energy, and to stimulate fat cells to take up glucose and synthesize fat.

[0035] Diabetes Mellitus may be the result of one or more factors. Causes of diabetes mellitus may include: (1) mutation of the insulin gene itself causing miscoding, which results in the production of ineffective insulin molecules; (2) mutations to genes that code for the 'transcription factors' needed for transcription of the insulin gene in the deoxyribonucleic acid (DNA) to create messenger ribonucleic acid (mRNA) molecules, which facilitate the manufacture of the insulin molecule; (3) mutations of the gene encoding for the insulin receptor, which produces inactive or an insufficient number of insulin receptors; (4) mutation to the gene encoding for glucokinase, the enzyme that phosphorylates glucose in the first step of glycolysis; (5) mutations to the genes encoding portions of the potassium channels in the plasma membrane of the Beta cells, preventing proper closure of the channel, thus blocking insulin release; (6) mutations to mitochondrial genes that as a result, decreases the energy available to be used facilitate the release of insulin, therefore reducing insulin secretion; (7) failure of glucose transporters to properly permit the facilitated diffusion of glucose from plasma into the cells of the body.

[0036] The insulin molecule is a protein produced by Beta cells located in the pancreas. A 'pro-insulin messenger RNA' is created in a Beta cell by a transcription complex transcribing the insulin gene from nuclear DNA. The pro-insulin messenger RNA (mRNA) is modified, then travels out of the cytoplasm. Ribosomes, decode the mRNA to produce insulin. Once the biologically active insulin protein is generated it is stored in a vacuole in the Beta cell to await being released into the blood stream.

[0037] Insulin receptors, which appear on the surface of cells, offer binding sites for insulin circulating in the blood. When insulin binds to an insulin receptor, the biologic response inside the cell causes glucose to enter the cell and undergo processing in the cytoplasm. Processed glucose molecules then enter the mitochondria. The mitochondria further process the modified glucose molecules to produce usable energy in the form of adenosine triphosphate molecules (ATP). Thirty-eight ATP molecules may be generated from one molecule of glucose during the process of aerobic respiration. ATP molecules are utilized as an energy source by biologic processes throughout the cell.

[0038] The current medical therapeutic approach to the management of diabetes mellitus has produced limited results. Patients with diabetes generally struggle with an inadequate production of insulin, or an ineffective release of biologically active insulin molecules, or a release of an insufficient number of biologically active insulin molecules, or an insufficient production of cell-surface receptors, or a production of ineffective cell-surface receptors, or a production of ineffective insulin molecules that are unable to interact properly with insulin receptors to produce the required biologic effect. Type One diabetes requires administration of exogenous insulin. The traditional approach to Type Two diabetes has generally first been to adjust the diet to limit the caloric intake the individual consumes. Exercise is used as an initial approach to both Type One and Type Two diabetes as a means of up-regulating the utilization of fats and sugar so as to reduce the amount of circulating plasma glucose. When diet and exercise are inadequate in properly managing Type Two diabetes, oral medications are often introduced. The action of sulfonylureas, a commonly prescribed class of oral medication, is to stimulate the Beta cells to produce additional insulin receptors and enhance the insulin receptors' response to insulin. Biguanides, another form of oral treatment, inhibit gluconeogenesis, the production of glucose in the liver, thereby attempting to reduce plasma glucose levels. Thiazolidinediones (TZDs) lower blood sugar levels by activating peroxisome proliferator-activated receptor gamma (PPAR-γ), a transcription factor, which when activated regulates the activity of various target genes, particularly ones involved in glucose and lipid metabolism. If diet, exercise and oral medications do not produce a satisfactory control of the level of blood glucose in a diabetic patient, exogenous insulin is injected into the body in an effort to normalize the amount of glucose present in the serum. Insulin, a protein, has not successfully been made available as an oral medication to date due to the fact that proteins in general become degraded when they encounter the acid environment present in the stomach.

[0039] Despite strict monitoring of blood glucose and potentially multiple doses of insulin injected throughout the day, many patients with diabetes mellitus still experience devastating adverse effects from elevated blood glucose levels. Microvascular damage and elevated tissue sugar levels contribute to such complications as renal failure, retinopathy involving the eyes, neuropathy, and accelerated heart disease despite aggressive efforts to maintain the blood sugar within the physiologic normal range using exogenous insulin by itself or a combination of exogenous insulin and one or more oral medications. Diabetes remains the number one cause of renal failure in the United States. Especially in diabetic patients whom are dependent upon administering exogenous insulin into their body, though dosing of the insulin may be four or more times a day and even though this may produce adequate control of the blood glucose level to prevent the clinical symptoms of hyperglycemia; this does not unerringly supplement the body's natural capacity to monitor the blood sugar level minute to minute, twenty-four hours a day, and deliver an immediate response to a rise in blood glucose by the release of insulin from Beta cells as required. The deleterious effects of diabetes may still evolve despite strict and persistent control of the glucose level in the blood stream.

[0040] Current treatment approach to managing diabetes may be augmented by the unique approach to utilizing modified viruses as vehicles to transport of nuclear signaling protein molecules into cells in order to increase the production of biologically active insulin. By utilizing modified viruses to transport nuclear signaling protein molecules to facilitate the production of mRNAs, which would then facilitate the assembly of the necessary proteins. A diabetic would require the necessary proteins to adequately control the blood glucose level by utilizing inherent regulatory mechanisms rather than exogenous therapies.

[0041] Present medical care is attempting to utilize viruses to deliver genetic information into cells. Research in the field of gene therapy has involved certain naturally occurring viruses. Some of the common viral vectors that have been investigated include: Adeno-associated virus, Adenovirus, Alphavirus, Epstein-Barr virus, Gammaretrovirus, Herpes simplex virus, Letivirus, Poliovirus, Rhabdovirus, Vaccinia virus. Naturally occurring virus vectors are limited to the naturally occurring external probes that are affixed to the outer wall of the virus. The external probes fixed to the outside wall of a virus virion dictate which type of cell the virus can engage and infect. Therefore, as an example, the function of the adenovirus, a respiratory virus, is strictly limited to engaging and infecting specific lung cells. Used as a medical treatment device, the adenovirus can only deliver gene therapy to specific lung cells, which severely limits this vector's usefulness as a deliver device. The therapeutic function of all naturally occurring viral vectors is limited to delivering a DNA or RNA payload to the cell type the viral vector naturally targets as its host cell.

[0042] Naturally occurring viruses also have the disadvantage of being susceptible to detection and elimination by a body's immune system. Viruses have been infecting humans for hundreds of thousands of years. A human's innate immune system is very efficient at detecting the presence of most naturally occurring viruses when such a virus is inside the body. The human immune system is quite capable of generating a vigorous response to most intruding viruses, attacking and neutralizing virus virions whenever a virus virion physically exists are outside the exterior wall of the virus's host cell. If gene therapy in its current state were to become a clinical therapeutic tool, the naturally occurring viruses selected for gene therapy research will have limited effectiveness due the fact that once the viral vector is introduced into the body, the body's the immune system will quickly engage and eliminate the viral vectors, possibly before the vector is able to deliver its payload to its host cell or target cell.

[0043] Cichutek, K., 2001 (US Patent No. 6,323,031 B1) teaches preparation and use of novel lentiviral SiVagm-derived vectors for gene transfer into selected cell types, specifically into proliferatively active and resting human cells.

[0044] Cichutek teaches that it is indeed plausible to re-configure an existing virus and use it as a transport vehicle, though Cichutek's specification and claims are too limited to describe a method that will work for all cell types, if indeed if it will work for any cell type.

[0045] Cichutek describes vectors for 'gene transfer'; in the claims the language that is used is 'genetic information'. Cichutek's Claim 1 of the cited patent states 'A propagation-incompetent SIVagm vector comprising a viral core and a viral envelope, wherein the viral core comprises a simian immunodeficiency virus (SIVagm) viral core of the African vervet monkey Chlorocebus.' Cichutek's does not describe in his claims any further details of the intended payload other than the stating 'SIVagm viral core' in claim 1; in claims 5 & 6 Cichutek describes only 'genetic information'. Transfer of 'genetic information' dramatically limits the useful application of Cichutek's patent in the treatment of medical diseases.

[0046] Cichutek does not claim the use of specific glycogen probes to target specific types of cells. Cichutek's approach is dependent upon the probes naturally present on the viral vectors reported in the patent, which will direct the viral vectors to only those cells the viruses naturally use as their host cell. Cichutek's approach is very restrictive, limited to gene transfer to only cells the viruses use as their natural host cell.

[0047] It is questionable that Cichutek's approach as described in the specification and claims is feasible. Cichutek's claim 4, states 'The SIVagm vector of claim 1, wherein the viral envelope further comprises a single chain antibody (scFv) or a ligand of a cell surface molecule.' By use of the words 'a' and 'or' in the claim, the claim is limited in the singular, meaning Cichutek claims a single chain antibody or a singular ligand. Singular type antibodies or ligands can be used for cell to cell communication, but to open an access portal into a cell and insert a payload into the cell requires two different types antibodies or ligands. As an example human immunodeficiency virus requires the use of both the gp120 and gp41 probes to open a portal into a T-Helper cell and insert its genome into the T-Helper cell. The gp120 probe engages the CD4+ cell-surface receptor on the T-cell. Once the gp120 probe has successfully engaged a CD4+ cell-surface receptor on the target T-Helper cell, then the HIV virion's gp41 probe can engage either a CXCR4 or a CCR5 cell-surface receptor on the T-Helper cell in order to open up an access portal for HIV to insert its genome into a T-Helper cell. It is well documented in the medical literature that a genetic defect leading to an abnormality in the CXCR4 cell-surface receptor prevents HIV virions from opening an access portal and inserting its genetic payload into such T-Helper cells. This genetic defect offers the subset of people carrying the genetic defect resistance to HIV infection. This example demonstrates the need for at least two types of glycoprotein probes to be present on the surface of a viral vector in order for a viral vector to be capable of opening an access portal and delivering the payload the vector carries into its host cell or target cell.

[0048] A delivery system that offered a defined means of targeting specific types of cells, would invoke minimal or no response by the innate immune system when present in the body, and a delivery system that would be capable of inserting into cells a wide variety of nuclear signaling proteins would significantly improve the current medical treatment options available to clinicians treating patients.

[0049] The solution to arriving at a versatile, workable delivery system that will meet the needs of a number of medical treatments involves three important elements. These elements include:

  (1) configurable glycoprotein probes whereby more than one type of glycoprotein probe is to be used to engage and access specific target cell types in order to successfully deliver a payload into a specific cell type,
  (2) an external envelope comprised of a protein shell or lipid layer expressing the least number of cell-surface markers, such as the use of a stem cell to act as the host cell to manufacture the delivery devices,
  (3) configuring the core of the vector to enable it to carry and deliver nuclear signaling proteins.

[0050] Viruses are obligate parasites. Viruses simply represent a carrier of genetic material and by themselves viruses are unable to replicate or carry out any form of biologic function outside their host cell. A 'virion' refers to the physical structure of a single complete virus as it exists outside of the host cell. Viruses are generally comprised of one or more nested shells constructed of one or more layers of protein, some with a lipid outer envelope, a genetic payload that represents the instruction code necessary to replicate the virus, and protein enzymes to help facilitate the genetic payload in the function of replicating copies of the virus once the genetic payload has been delivered to a host cell. Located on the outer shell or envelope of a virus are probes. The function of a virus's probes is to locate and engage a host cell's receptors. The virus's surface probes are designed to detect, make contact with and functionally engage one or more receptors located on the exterior of a cell type that will offer the virus the proper environment in which to construct copies of itself. A host cell provides the virus the proper biologic machinery for the virus to successfully replicate itself. Once the virus's genome is inside the host cell, the viral genome takes command of the cell's production machinery and causes the host cell to generate copies of the virus. As the viral copies exit the host cell, these virions set off in search of other host cells to infect.

[0051] Naturally occurring viruses exist in a number of differing shapes. The shape of a virus may be rod or filament like, icosahedral, or complex structures combining filament and polygonal shapes. Viruses generally have their outer wall comprised of a protein coat or an envelope comprised of lipids.

[0052] An outer envelope comprised of lipids may be in the form of one or two phospholipid layers. When the outer envelope is comprised of two phospholipid layers this is termed a lipid bilayer. A phospholipid is a composite molecule comprised of a polar or hydrophilic region on one end and a nonpolar or hydrophobic region on the opposite end. A lipid bilayer covering a virus, like the membrane of a cell, is constructed with the hydrophilic region of one of the phospholipid layers pointed toward the exterior of the virion and the hydrophilic region of the second phospholipid layer pointed inward toward the center of the virus virion; with the hydrophobic regions of each of the two lipid layers pointed toward each other. The outer envelope of some forms of virus may be comprised of an outer lipid layer or lipid bilayer affixed to a protein matrix for support, the protein matrix being located closer to the center of the virus virion than the lipid layer or lipid bilayer.

[0053] Spherical viruses are generally spherical in shape and may be comprised of an outer envelope and one inner shell or an outer envelope and multiple inner shells. Inner shells are approximately spherical in shape; this is because the proteins comprising the protein matrix shell have an irregular shape to their structure. In the case of a spherical virus with an outer envelope and one inner shell, the inner shell is often referred to as a nucleocapsid shell comprised of numerous capsid proteins attached to each other. In the case of a spherical virus being comprised of an outer envelope and multiple inner shells, the outermost inner viral shells may be referred to as comprised of a quantity of matrix proteins, where the innermost shell is referred to as a nucleocapsid and is comprised of a quantity of capsid proteins. The inner protein shells are nested inside each other.

[0054] Viruses carry genetic material in the form of deoxyribonucleic acid (DNA) or ribonucleic acid (RNA) in their nucleocapsid often referred to as the core. A virus is therefore generally considered to be a DNA virus if its genome is comprised of DNA or the virus is considered a RNA virus if its genome is comprised of RNA. Viruses may also carry enzymes as part of their payload. An enzyme such as 'reverse transcriptase' transforms a RNA viral genome into DNA. Protease enzymes modify the viral genome once it has entered a host cell. An integrase enzyme assists a DNA viral genome with insertion into the host cell's nuclear DNA. The payload is carried inside the virus's nucleocapsid shell.

[0055] The probes attached to the exterior of a virus are constructed to engage specific cell-surface receptors on specific cell types in the body. Only a cell that expresses cell-surface receptors that are capable of being engaged by the probes of a specific virus can act as a host for the virus. Viruses often use two probes to access a host cell. The first probe makes an initial attachment to the host cell, while the action of the virus's second probe often in conjunction with the action of the first probe cause an access portal to be created in the host cell's exterior plasma membrane. Once an access portal is formed, the virus inserts the contents of its payload into the host cell. Once the virus's genome is inside the cytoplasm of the host cell, any enzymes that accompanied the viral genome into the cell, may begin to modify or assist the virus's genome with infecting and taking control of the host cell's biologic functions.

439

[0056] Probes are attached to the external envelope of a virus virion. Probes may be in the form of a protein structure or may be in the form of a glycoprotein molecule. For viruses constructed with a protein matrix as its outer envelope, the probes tend to be protein structures. A portion of the protein structure probe is fixed or anchored in the protein matrix, while a portion of the protein structure probe extends out and away from the protein matrix. The portion of the protein structure probe extending out away from the virus virion is referred to as the 'exterior domain', the portion anchored in the protein matrix is the 'transcending domain'. Some protein probes have a third segment that extends through the envelope and exists inside the virus virion, which is referred to as the 'interior domain'. The exterior domain of a protein structure probe is intended to engage a specific cell-surface receptor on a biologically active cell the virus is targeting as its host cell.

[0057] Viruses that utilize a lipid layer as the outer envelope, are constructed with probes that tend to be glycoproteins. A glycoprotein is comprised of a protein segment and a carbohydrate segment. The carbohydrate segment of the glycoprotein molecule is fixed or anchored in the lipid layer of the outer envelope, while the protein segment extends outward and away from the outer envelope. The protein portion of a glycoprotein probe that extends outward and away from the outer envelope of a virus virion is intended to engage a cell-surface receptor on a biologically active cell the virus is targeting as its host cell.

[0058] Some forms of viruses that utilize a lipid layer as its envelope use protein structure probes. In this case, the portion of the protein structure probe that extends outward and away from the outer envelope is the 'exterior domain', the portion that is anchored in the lipid layer is the 'transcending domain' and again some protein structure probes have an 'interior domain' that exist inside the virion, which may also help anchor the protein structure probe to the virion. The exterior domain of a protein structure probe that extends outward and away from the outer envelope of a virus virion is intended to engage a cell-surface receptor on a biologically active cell the virus is targeting as its host cell.

[0059] When a virus carries a DNA payload and the viral DNA is inserted into the host cell, the virus's DNA travels to the host cell's nucleus and is known to become inserted into the host cell's own native DNA. In the case where a virus is carrying its genetic payload as RNA, the virus inserts the RNA payload into the host cell and may also insert one or more enzymes to facilitate the RNA being utilized properly to replicate copies of the virus. Once inside the host cell, some species of virus facilitate use of the viral RNA by having the RNA converted to DNA. Once the viral RNA has been converted to DNA, the virus's DNA travels to the host cell's nucleus and is known to become inserted into the host cell's native DNA. Once a virus's genetic material has been inserted into the host cell's native DNA, the virus's genetic material takes command of certain cell functions and redirects the resources of the host cell to generate copies of the virus. Other forms of RNA viruses bypass the need to use the nuclear DNA and simply utilize portions of the viral genome to act as messenger RNA. RNA viruses that bypass the host cell's DNA, cause the cell in general to generate copies of the necessary parts of the virus directly from the virus's RNA genome.

[0060] The human immunodeficiency virus (HIV) has an outer envelope comprised of a lipid bilayer. The lipid bilayer covers a protein matrix consisting of p17^{gag} proteins. Inside the p17^{gag} protein is nested a nucleocapsid comprised of p24^{gag} proteins. Inside the nucleocapsid HIV carries its payload. HIV's genetic payload consists of two single strands of RNA. In addition to the two strands of HIV RNA, there are proteins that are carried in the core of the nucleocapsid along with the two RNA strands. These proteins include 'reverse transcriptase', 'integrase' and 'protease' molecules.

[0061] The T-Helper cell acts as HIV's host cell. HIV locates its host by utilizing at least two different types of probes located on its envelope. The HIV virion utilizes two types of glycoprotein probes affixed to the outer surface of its external envelope to engage a T-Helper cell. HIV utilizes a glycoprotein probe 120 to locate a CD4 cell-surface receptor on a T-Helper cell. Once an HIV glycoprotein 120 probe has successfully engaged a CD4 cell surface-receptor on a T-Helper cell a conformational change occurs in the probe and a glycoprotein 41 probe is exposed. The glycoprotein 41 probe's intent is to engage a CXCR4 or CCR5 cell-surface receptor on the same T-Helper cell. Once a glycoprotein 41 probe on the HIV virion successfully engages a CXCR4 or CCR5 cell-surface receptor, the HIV virion opens an access portal through the T-Helper cell's outer membrane.

[0062] Once the HIV virion has opened an access portal through the T-Helper cell's outer plasma membrane, the HIV virion inserts two positive strand RNA molecules it carries into the T-Helper cell. Each RNA strand is approximately 9500 nucleotides in length. Inserted along with the RNA strands are the enzymes reverse transcriptase, protease and integrase. Once the virus's genome gains access to the interior of the T-Helper cell, in the cytoplasm the pair of RNA molecules are transformed to deoxyribonucleic acid by the reverse transcriptase enzyme. Following modification of the virus's genome to DNA, the virus's genetic information migrates to the host cell's nucleus. In the nucleus, with the assistance of the integrase protein, the HIV's DNA becomes inserted into the T-Helper cell's native DNA. When the timing is appropriate, the now integrated viral DNA is decoded by the host cell's polymerase molecules and the virus's genetic information commands certain cell functions to carry out the replication process to construct copies of the human deficiency virus.

[0063] The outer layer of the HIV virion is comprised of a portion of the T-Helper cell's outer cell membrane. In the final stage of the replication process, as a copy of the HIV capsid, carrying the HIV genome, buds through the host cell's cell membrane the capsid acquires as its external envelope, a wrapping of lipid bilayer from the host cell's cell membrane. In the case of HIV, since the surface of the pathogen is covered by an envelope comprised of lipid bilayer taken from the host T-Helper cells, this feature allows the HIV virion the capacity to eluded the immune systems, since the cells comprising the immune system may find it difficult to tell the difference between the surface of an infectious HIV virion and the surface characteristics of a noninfected T-Helper cell.

[0064] The Hepatitis C virus (HCV) is a positive sense RNA virus, meaning a type of RNA that is capable of bypassing the need for involving the host cell's nucleus by having its RNA genome function as messenger RNA. Hepatitis C infects liver cells. The Hepatitis C viral genome becomes divided once it gains access to the interior of a liver host cell. Portions of the subdivisions of the Hepatitis C genome directly interact with ribosomes to produce proteins necessary to construct copies of the virus.

[0065] HCV belongs to the Flaviviridae family and is the only member of the Hepacivirus genus. There are considered to be at least 100 different strains of Hepatitis C virus based on genome sequencing variability.

[0066] HCV is comprised of an outer lipoprotein envelope and an internal nucleocapsid. The genetic payload is carried within the nucleocapsid. In its natural state, present on the surface of the outer envelope of the Hepatitis C virus are probes that detect receptors present on the surface of liver cells. The glycoprotein E1 probe and the glycoprotein E2 probe have been identified to be affixed to the surface of HCV. The E2 probe binds with high affinity to the large external loop of a CD81 cell-surface receptor. CD81 is found on the surface of many cell types including liver cells. Once the E2 probe has engaged the CD81 cell-surface receptor, cofactors on the surface of HCV's external envelope engage either or both the low density lipoprotein receptor (LDLR) or the scavenger receptor class B type I (SR-BI) present on the liver cell in order to effect the mechanism to facilitate HCV breaching the cell membrane and inserting its RNA genome payload through the plasma cell membrane of the liver cell into the liver cell. Upon successful engagement of the HCV surface probes with a liver cell's cell-surface receptors, HCV inserts the single strand of RNA and other payload elements it carries into the liver cell targeted to be a host cell. The HCV RNA genome then interacts with enzymes and ribosomes inside the liver cell in a translational process to produce the proteins required to construct copies of the protein components of HCV. The HCV genome undergoes a method of transcription to replicate copies of the virus's RNA genome. Inside the host, pieces of the HCV virus are assembled together and ultimately loaded with a copy of the HCV genome. Replicas of the original HCV then escape the host cell and migrate the environment in search of additional host liver cells to infect and continue the replication process.

[0067] The HCV's naturally occurring genetic payload consists of a single molecule of linear positive sense, single stranded RNA approximately 9600 nucleotides in length. By means of a translational process a polyprotein of approximately 3000 amino acids is generated. This polyprotein is cleaved post translation by host and viral proteases into individual viral proteins which include: the structural proteins of C, E1, E2, the nonstructural proteins NS1, NS2, NS3, NS4A, NS4B, NS5A, NS5B, p7 and ARFP/F protein. Hepatitis C virus's proteins direct the host liver cell to construction copies of the Hepatitis C virus. A membrane associated replicase complex consisting of the virus's nonstructural proteins NS3 and NS5B facilitate the replication of the viral genome. The membrane of the endoplasmic reticulum appears to be the site of protein maturation and viral assembly. Once copies of the Hepatitis C Virus are generated, they exit the host cell and each copy of HCV migrates in search of another appropriate liver cell that will act as a host to continue the replication process.

[0068] Hepatitis C virus life-cycle demonstrates that copies of a virus virion can be generated by inserting RNA into a host cell that functions as messenger RNA in the host cell. The Hepatitis C viral RNA genome functions as messenger RNA, acting as the template in conjunction with the biologic machinery of a host cell to produce the components that comprise copies of the Hepatitis C virion and the Hepatitis C viral RNA provides the biologic instructions to assemble the components into complete copies of the Hepatitis C virions. The Hepatitis C virus life-cycle clearly demonstrates that viral virions can be manufactured by a host cell without involving the nucleus of the cell.

[0069] Deciphering the existence, replication and behavior of viruses provides clear examples of several fundamental concepts, which include: (1) Viruses target specific cells in the body by means of identifying and engaging such target cells utilizing the probes projecting outward from the virus's exterior shell to make contact with cell-surface receptors located on the surface of the target cells, and (2) Viruses are capable of carrying various types of payloads including DNA, RNA and a variety of proteins.

[0070] Current gene therapy approach to attempting to deliver a payload to cells in the body use modified forms of existing viruses to act as transport devices to deliver genetic information. This approach is severely limited by restricting the virus virion to the target only cells the viral vector naturally seeks out and infects. Current gene therapy approach is further limited by using the pre-existing size of naturally occurring viruses, rather than being able to modify the size of the structure to be able to tailor the volumetric carrying capacity of the payload portion of the modified virus. Further gene therapy is restricted to utilizing naturally occurring viruses to deliver only genetic information; it has not previously been appreciated by those skilled in the art that virus-like transport devices might deliver to a variety of specific cell types a wide variety of differing payloads such as signaling proteins.

[0071] A dramatic, not previously recognized by those expert in the art is the need to develop a transport vehicle that can be fashioned to seek out specific types of cells and deliver to these cells nuclear signals. The external envelope of a transport should be constructed so as not to alert the immune system of its presence to prevent rejection of the vehicles. Transport vehicles should be capable of being configured to target any specific cell type and engage and deliver their payload only to that specific cell type. To this point, no such device has been conceived.

BRIEF SUMMARY OF THE INVENTION

[0072] Utilization of configurable microscopic medical payload delivery devices to deliver nuclear signaling proteins to specific cell types facilitates a dramatic new approach to medical care. By selecting the type of probes that are present on the surface of the configurable microscopic medical payload delivery devices, specific types of cells can be targeted. By delivering nuclear signaling proteins to specific cell types, genes can be activated or inactivated in those specific cell types. A wide variety of medical conditions are treatable by utilizing this new and unique approach.

DETAILED DESCRIPTION

[0073] The future of medical treatment will be the widespread utilization of configurable microscopic medical payload delivery devices (CMMPDD) to deliver nuclear signaling proteins directly to targeted cell types in the body.

[0074] For purposes of this text an 'external envelope' refers to the outermost covering of a virus or a virus-like transport device or a configurable microscopic medical payload delivery device. The external envelope may be comprised of a lipid layer, a lipid bilayer, the combination of a lipid layer affixed to a protein matrix or the combination of a lipid bilayer affixed to a protein matrix.

[0075] For purposes of this text an 'internal shell' refers to a protein matrix shell nested inside the external envelope. The inner most protein matrix shell is termed the nucleocapsid. The proteins that comprise the nucleocapsid are termed capsid proteins. In the center or core of the nucleocapsid is where the payload is carried.

[0076] For purposes of this text 'external probes' are molecular structures that are utilized to locate and engage cell-surface receptors on biologically active cells. External probes are generally comprised of a portion which is anchored or fixed in the external envelope and a second portion that extends out and away from the external envelope. External probes may be comprised solely of a protein structure or an external probe may be a glycoprotein molecule.

[0077] For purposes of this text 'glycoprotein molecule' refers to a molecule comprised of a carbohydrate region and a protein region. Glycoprotein molecules that act as probes are generally anchored or fixed to a lipid layer utilizing the carbohydrate portion of the molecule as an anchor. The protein portion of the glycoprotein molecule which extends outward and away from the external envelope the glycoprotein has been affixed such that the protein region may function as a probe to locate and attach to the cell-surface receptor it was created to engage.

[0078] The concept of configurable microscopic medical payload delivery devices is modeled after naturally existing viruses. Configurable microscopic medical payload delivery devices in general are spherical in shape; though other shapes may be used as function might warrant the use of a particular shape. The spherical configurable microscopic medical payload delivery devices are comprised of an external envelope and one or more inner nested protein shells. A quantity of exterior protein structure probes and/ or glycoprotein probes are anchored in the exterior lipid envelope and extend out and away from the exterior lipid envelope. Nesting of protein shells refers to progressively smaller diameter shells fitting snugly inside protein shells of a larger diameter. Inside the inner most protein shell, referred to as the nucleocapsid, is a cavity referred to as the core of the device. The core of the device is the space where the medically therapeutic payload the device carries is located.

[0079] Configurable microscopic medical payload delivery devices are generated to target certain specific cell types in the body. Configurable microscopic medical payload delivery devices target specific cell types by the configuration of probes affixed to the external envelope of the CMMPDD. By affixing specific probes to the external envelope of the CMMPDD, these probes intended to engage and attach only to specific cell-surface receptors located on certain cell types in the body, the CMMPDD will deliver its payload only to those cell types that express compatible and engagable specific cell-surface receptors. In a similar fashion where the exterior probes of a naturally occurring virus engage specific cell-surface receptors present on the surface of the virus's host cell and only the designated host cell, the CMMPDD's exterior probes are configured to engage cell-surface receptors on a specific type of target cell. In this manner, the payload of medication or biologic tools carried by CMMPDD will be delivered only to specific types of cells in the body. The exterior probes on the surface of a CMMPDD will vary as needed so as to effect the CMMPDD delivery of payloads to cell types as needed to effect a medical treatment.

[0080] The size of configurable microscopic medical payload delivery devices is to depend upon the volume size of the payload the CMMPDD is required to carry and deliver to a target cell. The size of a CMMPDD is dependent upon the diameter of the inner protein matrix shells. The diameter of each inner protein matrix shell is governed by the number of protein molecules utilized to construct the protein matrix shell at the time the protein matrix shell is generated. Increasing the number of proteins that comprise a protein matrix shell, increases the diameter of the protein matrix shell. The external lipid envelope wraps around and covers the outermost protein matrix shell. The larger the volume of the core of the CMMPDD, the greater the physical size payload the CMMPDD is able to carry. The size of the configurable microscopic medical payload delivery device is to be the size of cell (approximately 10^{-4} m in diameter) or less, generally detectable by a light microscope or, as needed, an electron microscope. The size of the CMMPDD is not to be too large such that it would generate a burden to the body by damaging organ tissues through clogging blood vessels, and the maintaining a small enough size that the CMMPDD can be properly disposed of by the body once the CMMPDD has delivered its payload to its target cell. The dimensions of each type of CMMPDD are to be tailored to the mission of the CMMPDD, which takes into account the type of target cell, the size of the payload that is to be delivered to the target cells and the length of time the CMMPDD may engage the target cell.

[0081] Being enveloped in an external lipid layer, configurable microscopic medical payload delivery devices possess the advantage of having their exterior appear similar to the plasma membrane that acts as an outside covering for the cells that comprise the body. By appearing similar to existing plasma membranes, the CMMPDDs appear similar to naturally occurring structures found in the body, affording the CMMPDD the capability to avoid detection by a body's immune system because the exterior of the CMMPDD mimics the cells comprising the body and the surveillance cells of the immune system find it difficult to discern between the CMMPDD and naturally occurring cells comprising the body.

[0082] To carry out the process of manufacturing a configurable microscopic medical payload delivery device, a primitive cell such as a stem cell is selected. The reason for utilizing primitive cells such as stems cells as the host cell, is that the CMMPDD acquires its outer envelope from the host cell and the more primitive the host cell, the fewer in number the identifying protein markers are present on the surface of the CMMPDD. The fewer the identifying surface proteins present on the outer envelope of the CMMPDD, the less likely a body's immune system will identify the CMMPDD as an invader and therefore less likely the body's immune system will react to the presence of the CMMPDD and reject the CMMPDD by attacking and neutralizing the CMMPDD.

[0083] Stem cells used as host cells to manufacture quantities of CMMPDD product are selected per histocompatibility markers present on their surface. Certain histocompatibility markers present on the surface of the final CMMPDD product will be less likely to cause a reaction in a specific patient based on the genetic profile of the patient's histocompatibility markers. A similar histocompatibility match is done when donor organs are selected to be given to recipients to avoid rejection of the donor organ by the recipient's immune system.

[0084] The selected stem cell used to manufacture configurable microscopic medical payload delivery devices goes through several steps of maturation before it is capable of generating therapeutic CMMPDD product. Messenger RNA would be inserted into the host stem cell that would code for the general physical outer structures of the CMMPDD. Messenger RNA would be inserted into the host that would generate surface probes that would target the surface receptors on specifically target cells. Messenger RNA would be inserted into the host that would be used to generate the payload of nuclear signaling proteins. Similar to how copies of a naturally occurring virus, such as the Hepatitis C virus or HIV, are produced, assembled and released from a host cell, copies of the CMMPDD would be produced, assembled and released from a host cell. Once released from the host cell, the copies of the CMMPDD would be collected, then pooled together to produce a therapeutic dose that would result in a medically beneficial effect.

[0085] The construction of the configurable microscopic medical payload delivery devices is performed by taking stem cells and inserting modified viral genetic programming into the stem cells. Stem cells are chosen as the host cell due to the low number of surface markers, which leads to less antigenicity in configurable microscopic medical payload delivery devices when the configurable microscopic medical payload delivery devices are released by the host cells and wrapped in an outer envelope comprised of the host cells' plasma membrane.

[0086] The stem cells used as host cells are suspended in a broth of nutrients and are kept at an optimum temperature to govern the rate of production of the CMMPDD product. Similar to the natural production of the Hepatitis C virus, the configurable microscopic medical payload delivery devices 'production genome' is introduced into the host stem cells. The configurable microscopic medical payload delivery devices production genome carries genetic instructions to cause the host cells to manufacture the configurable microscopic medical payload delivery devices' outer protein wall, the inner protein matrixes, the surface probes the configurable microscopic medical payload delivery device is to have affixed to its outer envelope and the nuclear signaling proteins the configurable microscopic medical payload delivery devices are to carry; and the instructions to assemble the various pieces into the final form of the configurable microscopic medical payload delivery devices and the instructions to activate the budding process. The resultant configurable microscopic medical payload delivery devices are collected from the nutrient broth surrounding the host cells and placed together into doses to be used as a treatment for a medical disease.

[0087] The 'production genome' are an array of messenger RNAs that are directly translated by the host cell's internal enzymes. The production genome dictates the characteristics of the final version of the CMMPDD that buds from the host stem cell and is released and is to be utilized as a medical treatment. The production genome is specifically tailored to code for the surface probes that will seek and engage a specific type of target cell. The production genome also carries the instructions to code for the production of the type of nuclear signaling proteins to be delivered to the specific type of target cell. The 'production genome' varies depending upon the configuration of the CMMPDD and the type of nuclear signaling proteins the CMMPDD will transport to effect a specific medical treatment on a specific type of cell.

[0088] The configurable microscopic medical payload delivery device transporting nuclear signaling proteins represents a very versatile medical treatment delivery device. There are an estimated 30,000 to 100,000 genes located in the human genome. CMMPDD could be used to deliver nuclear signaling proteins to activate or inactivate any of the chromosomal genes in any specific cell type in the body.

[0089] As an example of this method, to treat diabetes mellitus utilizing configurable microscopic medical payload delivery devices to deliver to Beta cells messenger RNA coded to produce insulin, the following production process is followed in the lab: (1) human stem cells are selected. (2) Into the selected stem cells is placed the production genome constructed, in this case, specifically as a means to treat diabetes mellitus. The RNA production genome contains genetic instructions to cause the host stem cells to manufacture the configurable microscopic medical payload delivery devices' outer protein wall, the inner protein matrix, surface probes to include glycoprotein probes that engage the GPR40 cell-surface receptor present on the surface of Beta cells located in the Islets of Langerhans in the pancreas, and the payload of nuclear signaling proteins, in this case the nuclear signaling proteins to activate the production of the insulin molecules in Beta cells; and the biologic instructions to assemble the components into the final form of the configurable microscopic medical payload delivery devices; and the biologic instructions to activate the budding process. (3) Upon insertion of the RNA production genome dedicated to producing a nuclear signaling proteins configured to activate the genes to generate messenger RNA that will result in the production of insulin, into the host stem cells, host stem cells respond by (i) simultaneously translating the different segments of the RNA production genome to produce the proteins that comprise the exterior protein wall, the inner protein matrix molecules, the surface probes to seek out and engage Beta cells, the nuclear signaling protein payload to produce insulin, and (ii) decoding the RNA instructions to assemble the components into the configurable microscopic medical payload delivery devices. (4) Upon assembly, the configurable microscopic medical payload delivery devices bud through the cell membrane of the host stem cell. (5) At the time of the budding process, the configurable microscopic medical payload delivery devices acquire an outside envelope wrapped over the outer protein shell, this outer envelope comprised of a portion of the plasma membrane from the host stem cell as the configurable microscopic medical payload delivery devices exit the host cell. (6) The resultant configurable microscopic medical payload delivery devices are collected from the nutrient broth surrounding the host stem cells. (7) The configurable microscopic medical payload delivery devices are washed in sterile solvent to remove contaminants. (8) The configurable microscopic medical payload delivery devices are removed from the sterile solvent and suspended in a hypoallergenic liquid medium. (9) The configurable microscopic medical payload delivery devices are separated into individual quantities to facilitate storage and delivery to physicians and patients. (10) The configurable microscopic medical payload delivery devices transported in the hypoallergenic liquid medium is administered to a diabetic patient per injection in a dose that is tailored to receiving patient's requirement to produce sufficient amount of insulin to control the blood sugar. (11) Upon being injected into the body, the configurable microscopic medical payload delivery devices migrate to the Beta cells located in the Islets of Langerhans by means of the patient's blood stream. (12) Upon the configurable microscopic medical payload delivery devices reaching the Beta cells, the configurable microscopic medical payload delivery devices engage the cell-surface receptors located on the Beta cells and insert the payload they carry into the Beta cells. The payload, in this case being nuclear signaling proteins to activated the genes responsible for the Beta cell's production of insulin molecules. The increase in insulin production by Beta cells successfully manages diabetes mellitus.

Conclusions, Ramification, and Scope

[0090] Accordingly, the reader will see that the configurable microscopic medical payload delivery device to deliver nuclear signaling proteins to specific targeted cell types provides advantages over existing art by (1) being a delivery device that seeks out specific types of cells, (2) by being a delivery device that is versatile enough to deliver a variety of potential nuclear signaling proteins to accomplish various medical treatments and (3) by being a delivery device constructed with a surface envelope that will avoid detection by the innate immune system so as not to activate the immune system to its presence; for these reasons this represents a new and unique medical delivery device that has never before been recognized nor appreciated by those skilled in the art.

[0091] Although the description above contains specificities, these should not be construed as limiting the scope of the invention but as merely providing illustrations of some of the presently preferred embodiments of the invention.

[0092] Thus the scope of the invention should be determined by the appended claims and their legal equivalents, rather than by the examples given.

CLAIMS: Reserved.

PATENT APPLICATION
SPECIFICATION NUMBER 4

TITLE OF THE INVENTION:

CONFIGURABLE MICROSCOPIC MEDICAL PAYLOAD DELIVERY DEVICE TO DELIVER CONTROL RNAS TO SPECIFIC CELLS TO MANAGE DIABETES MELLITUS AND GENETIC DEFICIENCY DISORDERS

BACKGROUND OF THE INVENTION

Field of the Invention

This invention relates to any medical device intended to correct a protein deficiency or genetic deficiency in the body by utilizing a configurable microscopic medical payload delivery device to insert one or more control RNAs into one or more specific cell types in the body to improve cell function.

Description of Background Art

[0001] For purposes of this text a 'control RNA' molecule (conRNA) is an RNA molecule intended to attach to nuclear deoxyribonucleic

454

acid for the purpose of initiating or inhibiting the process of transcription of a segment of the deoxyribonucleic acid.

[0002] A 'deoxyribose' is a deoxypentose (C5H10O4) sugar. Deoxyribonucleic acid (DNA) is comprised of three basic elements: a deoxyribose sugar, a phosphate group and nitrogen containing bases. DNA is a macromolecule made up of two chains of repeating deoxyribose sugars linked by phosphodiester bonds between the 3-hydroxyl group of one and the 5-hydroxyl group of the next; the two chains are held antiparallel to each other by weak hydrogen bonds. DNA strands contain a sequence of nucleotides, which include: adenine, cytosine, guanine or thymine. Adenine is always paired with thymine of the opposite strand, and guanine is always paired with cytosine of the opposite strand; one side or strand of a DNA macromolecule is the mirror image of the opposite strand. Nuclear DNA is regarded as the medium for storing the master plan of hereditary information.

[0003] Genes are considered segments of the DNA that represent units of inheritance.

[0004] A chromosome exists in the nucleus of a cell and consists of a DNA double helix bearing a linear sequence of genes, coiled and recoiled around aggregated proteins, termed histones. The number of chromosomes varies from species to species. Most Human cells carries twenty two pairs of chromosomes plus two sex chromosomes; two 'x' chromosomes in women and one 'x' and one 'y' chromosome in men. Chromosomes carry genetic information in the form of units which are referred to as genes.

[0005] Per J. K. Pal, S.S. Ghaskabi, Fundamentals of Molecular Biology, 2009: 'The central dogma of molecular biology . . . states that the genes present in the genome (DNA) are transcribed into mRNAs, which are then translated into polypeptides or proteins, which are phenotypes.' 'Genome, thus, contains the complete set of hereditary information for any organism and is functionally divided into small parts referred to as genes. Each gene is a sequence of nucleotides representing a single protein or RNA. Genome of a living organism may contain as few as 500 genes as in case of Mycoplasma, or as many as 30,000 genes as in case of human beings.' Some references cite as many as 100,000 genes may exist in the human genome.

[0006] The current understanding of the actual biologic structure of a gene is far more elaborate than the historic standard definition of a gene. A gene appears to be comprised of a number of segments loosely strung together along a particular section of DNA. In general there are three segments associated with a gene which include: (1) the Upstream 5' flanking region, (2) the transcriptional unit (often referred to as the open reading frame) and (3) the Downstream 3' flanking region. The Upstream 5' flanking region is comprised of the 'enhancer region', the 'promoter-proximal region', and 'promoter region'. The 'transcriptional unit' or open reading frame starts at a location designated 'transcription start site' (TSS), which is located in a site called the 'initiator region' (inR), which may be described in a general form as Py2CAPy5. The transcription unit is comprised of the combination of segments of DNA nucleotides to be transcribed into RNA and spacing units known as 'introns' that are not transcribed or if transcribed are later removed post transcription, such that they do not appear in the final RNA molecule. In the case of a gene coding for a mRNA molecule, the transcription unit will contain all three elements of the mRNA, which includes: (1) the 5' noncoding region, (2) the translational region and (3) the 3' noncoding region. Interspersed between these regions are introns, which will be either not transcribed or if transcribed removed from the precursor form of mRNA prior to the mRNA reaching its final form. The 'transcriptional unit' is generally considered to be the 'gene'. The Downstream 3' flanking region contains DNA nucleotides that are not transcribed and may contain what has been termed an 'enhancer region'. An enhancer region in the Downstream 3' flanking region is thought to act to promote the gene previously transcribed to be transcribed again.

[0007] On either side of the DNA sequencing comprising a gene and its flanking regions, may be inactive DNA which act as boundaries which have been termed 'insulator elements'. The term 'upstream' refers to DNA sequencing that occurs prior to the TSS if viewed from the 5' end to the 3' end of the DNA; where the term 'downstream' refers to DNA sequencing located after the TSS.

[0008] An 'enhancer region' may or may not be present in the Upstream 5' flanking region. If present, the enhancer region helps facilitate the reading of the gene by encouraging formation of the transcription mechanism. If the enhancer is present, it may exist 200 kb to 17,000 kb upstream from the transcription starting site.

[0009] The 'transcription complex' also referred to as the 'transcription mechanism', in humans, is reported to be comprised of over forty separate proteins that assemble together to ultimately function in a concerted effort to transcribe the nucleotide sequence of the DNA into RNA. The transcription complex (TC) includes elements such as 'general transcription factor Sp1', 'general transcription factor NF1', 'general transcription factor TATA-binding protein', 'TFIID', 'basal transcription complex', and a 'RNA polymerase protein' to name only a few of the forty elements that exist. The elements of the transcription mechanism function as (1) a means to recognize the location of the start of a gene, (2) as proteins to bind the transcription mechanism to the DNA such that transcription may occur or (3) as means of transcribing the DNA nucleotide coding to produce a precursor RNA molecule. There are at least three RNA polymerase proteins which include: RNA polymerase I, RNA polymerase II, and RNA polymerase III. RNA polymerase I tends to be dedicated to transcribing genetic information that will result in the formation of rRNA molecules. RNA polymerase II tends to be dedicated to transcribing genetic information that will result in the formation of mRNA molecules. RNA polymerase III appears to be dedicated to transcribing genetic information that results in the formation of tRNAs, small cellular RNAs and viral RNAs.

[0010] The 'promoter proximal region' is located upstream from the TSS and upstream from the core promoter region. The 'promoter proximal region' includes two sub-regions termed the GC box and the CAAT box. The 'GC box' appears to be a segment rich in guanine-cytosine nucleotide sequences. The GC box binds to the 'general transcription factor Sp1' of the transcription mechanism. The

'CAAT box' is a segment which contains the nucleotide sequence 'GGCCAATCT' located 75 bps upstream from the transcription start site (TSS). The CAAT box binds to the 'general transcription factor NF1' of the transcription mechanism.

[0011] The 'core promoter' region is considered the shortest sequence at which RNA polymerase II can initiate transcription of a gene The core promoter may include the initiator region (inR) and either a TATA box or a DPE. The inR is the region designated Py2CAPy5 that surrounds the transcription start site (TSS). The TATA box is located 25 bps upstream from the TSS. The TATA box acts as a site of attachment of the TFIID, which is a promoter for binding of the RNA polymerase II molecule. The DPE is the 'downstream promoter element' that may appear 28 bps to 32 bps downstream from the TSS. The DPE acts as an alternative site of attachment for the TFIID when the TATA box is not present.

[0012] The transcription mechanism, also referred to as the transcription complex appears to be comprised of different elements depending upon whether rRNA is being transcribed versus mRNA or tRNA or small cellular RNA or viral RNA. The proteins that assemble to assist RNA Polymerase I with transcribing the DNA to produce rRNA appear different than the proteins that assemble to assist RNA polymerase II with transcribing the DNA to produce mRNA or the proteins that assemble to assist RNA polymerase III with transcribing the DNA to produce tRNA, small cellular RNA or viral RNA. A common protein that appears to be present at the initial biding of all three types of RNA polymerase molecules is TATA-binding protein (TBP). TBP appears to be required to attach to the DNA, which then facilitates RNA polymerase to bind to the promoter along the DNA. TBP assembles with TBP-associated factors (TAFs). Together TBF and 11 TAFs comprise the complex referred to as TFIID, which has been previously mentioned in the above text.

[0013] Upstream from the TATA box is the 'initiator element', which may be considered as part of the 'core promoter' region. The initiator element is a segment of the nuclear DNA that binds the basal transcription complex. The basal transcription complex is comprised of a number of proteins that make initial contact with the DNA prior to the RNA polymerase binding to the transcription mechanism. The basal transcription complex is associated with an activator. The activator is a control RNA.

[0014] Once the transcription complex is assembled, the transcription complex transcribes the DNA. Transcription of the DNA produces precursor messenger RNA (mRNA), precursor ribosomal RNA (rRNA), precursor transport RNA (tRNA) or control RNA (conRNA), or other RNAs. In the case of precursor mRNA, the mRNA is further modified, then traverses to the cytoplasm. In the cytoplasm of the cell ribosomes attach to the mRNA. Ribosomes decode mRNA utilizing the process of translation to produce proteins.

[0015] A protein is comprised of a string of amino acids. Proteins can be comprised of only a few amino acids, or a large number of amino acids. Large protein molecules are often referred to as a macromolecule. Proteins can be combined together to form molecules comprised of two or more similar amino acid strands or a protein can be can be comprised of two or more different amino acid strands. When more than one protein are combined into a molecule, this may also be referred as a macromolecule. Proteins can be combined with other molecules such as carbohydrates and lipids. When proteins combine with other molecules this is also often referred to as a macromolecule. Cell surface receptors are considered macromolecules and are often comprised of a protein molecule combined with a carbohydrate molecule to produce a glycoprotein.

[0016] Diabetes mellitus represents an important health issue that affects a significant portion of the world population. In the United States, about 16 million people suffer from diabetes mellitus. Every year, about 650,000 additional people are diagnosed with this disease. Diabetes mellitus is the seventh leading cause of all deaths.

[0017] Diabetes mellitus represents a state of hyperglycemia, a serum blood sugar that is higher than what is considered the normal range for humans. Glucose, a six-carbon molecule, is a form of sugar. Glucose is absorbed by the cells of the body and converted to energy by the processes of glycolysis, the Krebs cycle and phosporylation. Insulin, a protein, facilitates the transfer of glucose from the blood into cells. Normal range for blood glucose in humans is generally defined as a fasting blood plasma glucose level of between 70 to 110 mg/dl. For descriptive purposes, the term 'plasma' refers to the fluid portion of blood.

[0018] Diabetes mellitus is classified as Type One and Type Two. Type One diabetes mellitus is insulin dependent, which refers to the condition where there is a lack of sufficient insulin circulating in the blood stream and insulin must be provided to the body in order to properly regulate the blood glucose level. When insulin is required to regulate the blood glucose level in the body, this condition is often referred to as insulin dependent diabetes mellitus (IDDM). Type Two diabetes mellitus is noninsulin dependent, often referred to as noninsulin dependent diabetes mellitus (NIDDM), meaning the blood glucose level can be managed without insulin, and instead by means of diet, exercise or intervention with oral medications. Type Two diabetes mellitus is considered a progressive disease, the underlying pathogenic mechanisms including pancreatic Beta cell (also often designated as β-Cell) dysfunction and insulin resistance.

[0019] The pancreas serves as an endocrine gland and an exocrine gland. Functioning as an endocrine gland the pancreas produces and secretes hormones including insulin and glucagon. Insulin acts to reduce levels of glucose circulating in the blood. Beta cells secrete insulin into the blood when a higher than normal level of glucose is detected in the serum. For purposes of this description the terms 'blood', 'blood stream' and 'serum' refer to the same substance. Glucagon acts to stimulate an increase in glucose circulating in the blood. Beta cells in the pancreas secrete glucagon when a low level of glucose is detected in the serum.

[0020] Glucose enters the body as food and as a result of digestion, glucose enters the blood stream. The Beta cells of the Islets of

Langerhans continuously sense the level of glucose in the blood and respond to elevated levels of blood glucose by secreting insulin into the blood. Beta cells produce the protein 'insulin' in their endoplasmic reticulum and store the insulin in vacuoles until it is needed. When Beta cells detect an increase in the glucose level in the blood, Beta cells release insulin into the blood from the described storage vacuoles.

[0021] Insulin is a protein. An insulin protein consists of two chains of amino acids, an alpha chain and a beta chain, linked by two disulfide (S-S) bridges. One chain, the alpha chain consists of 21 amino acids. The second chain the beta chain consists of 30 amino acids.

[0022] Insulin interacts with the cells of the body by means of a cell-surface receptor termed the 'insulin receptor' located on the exterior of a cell's 'outer membrane', otherwise known as the 'plasma membrane'. Insulin interacts with muscle and liver cells by means of the insulin receptor to rapidly remove excess blood sugar when the glucose level in the blood is higher than the upper limit of the normal physiologic range. Recognized functions of insulin include stimulating cells to take up glucose from the blood and convert it to glycogen to facilitate the cells in the body to utilize glucose to generate biochemically usable energy, and to stimulate fat cells to take up glucose and synthesize fat.

[0023] Diabetes Mellitus may be the result of one or more factors. Causes of diabetes mellitus may include: (1) mutation of the insulin gene itself causing miscoding, which results in the production of ineffective insulin molecules; (2) mutations to genes that code for the 'transcription factors' needed for transcription of the insulin gene in the deoxyribonucleic acid (DNA) to create messenger ribonucleic acid (mRNA) molecules, which facilitate the manufacture of the insulin molecule; (3) mutations of the gene encoding for the insulin receptor, which produces inactive or an insufficient number of insulin receptors; (4) mutation to the gene encoding for glucokinase, the enzyme that phosphorylates glucose in the first step of glycolysis; (5) mutations to the genes encoding portions of the potassium channels in the plasma membrane of the Beta cells, preventing proper closure of the channel, thus blocking insulin release; (6) mutations to mitochondrial genes that as a result, decreases the energy available to be used facilitate the release of insulin, therefore reducing insulin secretion; (7) failure of glucose transporters to properly permit the facilitated diffusion of glucose from plasma into the cells of the body.

[0024] The insulin molecule is a protein produced by Beta cells located in the pancreas. A 'pro-insulin messenger RNA' is created in a Beta cell by a transcription complex transcribing the insulin gene from nuclear DNA. The pro-insulin messenger RNA (mRNA) is modified, then travels out of the cytoplasm. Ribosomes, decode the mRNA to produce insulin. Once the biologically active insulin protein is generated it is stored in a vacuole in the Beta cell to await being released into the blood stream.

[0025] Insulin receptors, which appear on the surface of cells, offer binding sites for insulin circulating in the blood. When insulin binds to an insulin receptor, the biologic response inside the cell causes glucose to enter the cell and undergo processing in the cytoplasm. Processed glucose molecules then enter the mitochondria. The mitochondria further process the modified glucose molecules to produce usable energy in the form of adenosine triphosphate molecules (ATP). Thirty-eight ATP molecules may be generated from one molecule of glucose during the process of aerobic respiration. ATP molecules are utilized as an energy source by biologic processes throughout the cell.

[0026] The current medical therapeutic approach to the management of diabetes mellitus has produced limited results. Patients with diabetes generally struggle with an inadequate production of insulin, or an ineffective release of biologically active insulin molecules, or a release of an insufficient number of biologically active insulin molecules, or an insufficient production of cell-surface receptors, or a production of ineffective cell-surface receptors, or a production of ineffective insulin molecules that are unable to interact properly with insulin receptors to produce the required biologic effect. Type One diabetes requires administration of exogenous insulin. The traditional approach to Type Two diabetes has generally first been to adjust the diet to limit the caloric intake the individual consumes. Exercise is used as an initial approach to both Type One and Type Two diabetes as a means of up-regulating the utilization of fats and sugar so as to reduce the amount of circulating plasma glucose. When diet and exercise are inadequate in properly managing Type Two diabetes, oral medications are often introduced. The action of sulfonylureas, a commonly prescribed class of oral medication, is to stimulate the Beta cells to produce additional insulin receptors and enhance the insulin receptors' response to insulin. Biguanides, another form of oral treatment, inhibit gluconeogenesis, the production of glucose in the liver, thereby attempting to reduce plasma glucose levels. Thiazolidinediones (TZDs) lower blood sugar levels by activating peroxisome proliferator-activated receptor gamma (PPAR-γ), a transcription factor, which when activated regulates the activity of various target genes, particularly ones involved in glucose and lipid metabolism. If diet, exercise and oral medications do not produce a satisfactory control of the level of blood glucose in a diabetic patient, exogenous insulin is injected into the body in an effort to normalize the amount of glucose present in the serum. Insulin, a protein, has not successfully been made available as an oral medication to date due to the fact that proteins in general become degraded when they encounter the acid environment present in the stomach.

[0027] Despite strict monitoring of blood glucose and potentially multiple doses of insulin injected throughout the day, many patients with diabetes mellitus still experience devastating adverse effects from elevated blood glucose levels. Microvascular damage and elevated tissue sugar levels contribute to such complications as renal failure, retinopathy involving the eyes, neuropathy, and accelerated heart disease despite aggressive efforts to maintain the blood sugar within the physiologic normal range using exogenous insulin by itself or a combination of exogenous insulin and one or more oral medications. Diabetes remains the number one cause of renal failure in the United States. Especially in diabetic patients whom are dependent upon administering exogenous insulin into their body, though dosing of the insulin may be four or more times a day and even though this may produce adequate control of the blood glucose level to prevent the clinical symptoms of hyperglycemia; this does not unerringly supplement the body's natural capacity to monitor the blood sugar level minute to minute, twenty-four hours a day, and deliver an immediate response to a rise in blood glucose by the release of insulin from Beta cells as required. The deleterious effects of diabetes may still evolve despite strict and persistent control of the glucose level in the blood stream.

[0028] Current treatment approach to managing diabetes may be augmented by the unique approach to utilizing modified viruses as vehicles to transport of control RNA molecules into cells in order to increase the production of biologically active insulin. By utilizing modified viruses to transport control RNA molecules to facilitate the production of mRNAs, which would then facilitate the assembly of the necessary proteins. A diabetic would require the necessary proteins to adequately control the blood glucose level by utilizing inherent regulatory mechanisms rather than exogenous therapies.

[0029] Present medical care is attempting to utilize viruses to deliver genetic information into cells. Research in the field of gene therapy has involved certain naturally occurring viruses. Some of the common viral vectors that have been investigated include: Adeno-associated virus, Adenovirus, Alphavirus, Epstein-Barr virus, Gammaretrovirus, Herpes simplex virus, Letivirus, Poliovirus, Rhabdovirus, Vaccinia virus. Naturally occurring virus vectors are limited to the naturally occurring external probes that are affixed to the outer wall of the virus. The external probes fixed to the outside wall of a virus virion dictate which type of cell the virus can engage and infect. Therefore, as an example, the function of the adenovirus, a respiratory virus, is strictly limited to engaging and infecting specific lung cells. Used as a medical treatment device, the adenovirus can only deliver gene therapy to specific lung cells, which severely limits this vector's usefulness as a deliver device. The therapeutic function of all naturally occurring viral vectors is limited to delivering a DNA or RNA payload to the cell type the viral vector naturally targets as its host cell.

[0030] Naturally occurring viruses also have the disadvantage of being susceptible to detection and elimination by a body's immune system. Viruses have been infecting humans for hundreds of thousands of years. A human's innate immune system is very efficient at detecting the presence of most naturally occurring viruses when such a virus is inside the body. The human immune system is quite capable of generating a vigorous response to most intruding viruses, attacking and neutralizing virus virions whenever a virus virion physically exists are outside the exterior wall of the virus's host cell. If gene therapy in its current state were to become a clinical therapeutic tool, the naturally occurring viruses selected for gene therapy research will have limited effectiveness due the fact that once the viral vector is introduced into the body, the body's the immune system will quickly engage and eliminate the viral vectors, possibly before the vector is able to deliver its payload to its host cell or target cell.

[0031] Cichutek, K., 2001 (US Patent No. 6,323,031 B1) teaches preparation and use of novel lentiviral SiVagm-derived vectors for gene transfer into selected cell types, specifically into proliferatively active and resting human cells.

[0032] Cichutek teaches that it is indeed plausible to re-configure an existing virus and use it as a transport vehicle, though Cichutek's specification and claims are too limited to describe a method that will work for all cell types, if indeed if it will work for any cell type.

[0033] Cichutek describes vectors for 'gene transfer'; in the claims the language that is used is 'genetic information'. Cichutek's Claim 1 of the cited patent states 'A propagation-incompetent SIVagm vector comprising a viral core and a viral envelope, wherein the viral core comprises a simian immunodeficiency virus (SIVagm) viral core of the African vervet monkey Chlorocebus.' Cichutek's does not describe in his claims any further details of the intended payload other than the stating 'SIVagm viral core' in claim 1; in claims 5 & 6 Cichutek describes only 'genetic information'. Transfer of 'genetic information' dramatically limits the useful application of Cichutek's patent in the treatment of medical diseases.

[0034] Cichutek does not claim the use of specific glycogen probes to target specific types of cells. Cichutek's approach is dependent upon the probes naturally present on the viral vectors reported in the patent, which will direct the viral vectors to only those cells the viruses naturally use as their host cell. Cichutek's approach is very restrictive, limited to gene transfer to only cells the viruses use as their natural host cell.

[0035] It is questionable that Cichutek's approach as described in the specification and claims is feasible. Cichutek's claim 4, states 'The SIVagm vector of claim 1, wherein the viral envelope further comprises a single chain antibody (scFv) or a ligand of a cell surface molecule.' By use of the words 'a' and 'or' in the claim, the claim is limited in the singular, meaning Cichutek claims a single chain antibody or a singular ligand. Singular type antibodies or ligands can be used for cell to cell communication, but to open an access portal into a cell and insert a payload into the cell requires two different types antibodies or ligands. As an example human immunodeficiency virus requires the use of both the gp120 and gp41 probes to open a portal into a T-Helper cell and insert its genome into the T-Helper cell. The gp120 probe engages the CD4+ cell-surface receptor on the T-cell. Once the gp120 probe has successfully engaged a CD4+ cell-surface receptor on the target T-Helper cell, then the HIV virion's gp41 probe can engage either a CXCR4 or a CCR5 cell-surface receptor on the T-Helper cell in order to open up an access portal for HIV to insert its genome into a T-Helper cell. It is well documented in the medical literature that a genetic defect leading to an abnormality in the CXCR4 cell-surface receptor prevents HIV virions from opening an access portal and inserting its genetic payload into such T-Helper cells. This genetic defect offers the subset of people carrying the genetic defect resistance to HIV infection. This example demonstrates the need for at least two types of glycoprotein probes to be present on the surface of a viral vector in order for a viral vector to be capable of opening an access portal and delivering the payload the vector carries into its host cell or target cell.

[0036] A delivery system that offered a defined means of targeting specific types of cells, would invoke minimal or no response by the innate immune system when present in the body, and a delivery system that would be capable of inserting into cells a wide variety of control RNAs would significantly improve the current medical treatment options available to clinicians treating patients.

[0037] The solution to arriving at a versatile, workable delivery system that will meet the needs of a number of medical treatments involves three important elements. These elements include:

1) configurable glycoprotein probes whereby more than one type of glycoprotein probe is to be used to engage and access specific target cell types in order to successfully deliver a payload into a specific cell type,
2) an external envelope comprised of a protein shell or lipid layer expressing the least number of cell-surface markers, such as the use of a stem cell to act as the host cell to manufacture the delivery devices,
3) configuring the core of the vector to enable it to carry and deliver control RNAs.

[0038] Viruses are obligate parasites. Viruses simply represent a carrier of genetic material and by themselves viruses are unable to replicate or carry out any form of biologic function outside their host cell. A 'virion' refers to the physical structure of a single complete virus as it exists outside of the host cell. Viruses are generally comprised of one or more nested shells constructed of one or more layers of protein, some with a lipid outer envelope, a genetic payload that represents the instruction code necessary to replicate the virus, and protein enzymes to help facilitate the genetic payload in the function of replicating copies of the virus once the genetic payload has been delivered to a host cell. Located on the outer shell or envelope of a virus are probes. The function of a virus's probes is to locate and engage a host cell's receptors. The virus's surface probes are designed to detect, make contact with and functionally engage one or more receptors located on the exterior of a cell type that will offer the virus the proper environment in which to construct copies of itself. A host cell provides the virus the proper biologic machinery for the virus to successfully replicate itself. Once the virus's genome is inside the host cell, the viral genome takes command of the cell's production machinery and causes the host cell to generate copies of the virus. As the viral copies exit the host cell, these virions set off in search of other host cells to infect.

[0039] Naturally occurring viruses exist in a number of differing shapes. The shape of a virus may be rod or filament like, icosahedral, or complex structures combining filament and polygonal shapes. Viruses generally have their outer wall comprised of a protein coat or an envelope comprised of lipids.

[0040] An outer envelope comprised of lipids may be in the form of one or two phospholipid layers. When the outer envelope is comprised of two phospholipid layers this is termed a lipid bilayer. A phospholipid is a composite molecule comprised of a polar or hydrophilic region on one end and a nonpolar or hydrophobic region on the opposite end. A lipid bilayer covering a virus, like the membrane of a cell, is constructed with the hydrophilic region of one of the phospholipid layers pointed toward the exterior of the virion and the hydrophilic region of the second phospholipid layer pointed inward toward the center of the virus virion; with the hydrophobic regions of each of the two lipid layers pointed toward each other. The outer envelope of some forms of virus may be comprised of an outer lipid layer or lipid bilayer affixed to a protein matrix for support, the protein matrix being located closer to the center of the virus virion than the lipid layer or lipid bilayer.

[0041] Spherical viruses are generally spherical in shape and may be comprised of an outer envelope and one inner shell or an outer envelope and multiple inner shells. Inner shells are approximately spherical in shape; this is because the proteins comprising the protein matrix shell have an irregular shape to their structure. In the case of a spherical virus with an outer envelope and one inner shell, the inner shell is often referred to as a nucleocapsid shell comprised of numerous capsid proteins attached to each other. In the case of a spherical virus being comprised of an outer envelope and multiple inner shells, the outermost inner viral shells may be referred to as comprised of a quantity of matrix proteins, where the innermost shell is referred to as a nucleocapsid and is comprised of a quantity of capsid proteins. The inner protein shells are nested inside each other.

[0042] Viruses carry genetic material in the form of deoxyribonucleic acid (DNA) or ribonucleic acid (RNA) in their nucleocapsid often referred to as the core. A virus is therefore generally considered to be a DNA virus if its genome is comprised of DNA or the virus is considered a RNA virus if its genome is comprised of RNA. Viruses may also carry enzymes as part of their payload. An enzyme such as 'reverse transcriptase' transforms a RNA viral genome into DNA. Protease enzymes modify the viral genome once it has entered a host cell. An integrase enzyme assists a DNA viral genome with insertion into the host cell's nuclear DNA. The payload is carried inside the virus's nucleocapsid shell.

[0043] The probes attached to the exterior of a virus are constructed to engage specific cell-surface receptors on specific cell types in the body. Only a cell that expresses cell-surface receptors that are capable of being engaged by the probes of a specific virus can act as a host for the virus. Viruses often use two probes to access a host cell. The first probe makes an initial attachment to the host cell, while the action of the virus's second probe often in conjunction with the action of the first probe cause an access portal to be created in the host cell's exterior plasma membrane. Once an access portal is formed, the virus inserts the contents of its payload into the host cell. Once the virus's genome is inside the cytoplasm of the host cell, any enzymes that accompanied the viral genome into the cell, may begin to modify or assist the virus's genome with infecting and taking control of the host cell's biologic functions.

[0044] Probes are attached to the external envelope of a virus virion. Probes may be in the form of a protein structure or may be in the form of a glycoprotein molecule. For viruses constructed with a protein matrix as its outer envelope, the probes tend to be protein structures. A portion of the protein structure probe is fixed or anchored in the protein matrix, while a portion of the protein structure probe extends out and away from the protein matrix. The portion of the protein structure probe extending out away from the virus virion is referred to as the 'exterior domain', the portion anchored in the protein matrix is the 'transcending domain'. Some protein probes have a third segment that extends through the envelope and exists inside the virus virion, which is referred to as the 'interior domain'. The exterior domain of a protein structure probe is intended to engage a specific cell-surface receptor on a biologically active cell the virus is targeting as its host cell.

[0045] Viruses that utilize a lipid layer as the outer envelope, are constructed with probes that tend to be glycoproteins. A glycoprotein is comprised of a protein segment and a carbohydrate segment. The carbohydrate segment of the glycoprotein molecule is fixed or anchored in the lipid layer of the outer envelope, while the protein segment extends outward and away from the outer envelope. The protein portion of a glycoprotein probe that extends outward and away from the outer envelope of a virus virion is intended to engage a cell-surface receptor on a biologically active cell the virus is targeting as its host cell.

[0046] Some forms of viruses that utilize a lipid layer as its envelope use protein structure probes. In this case, the portion of the protein structure probe that extends outward and away from the outer envelope is the 'exterior domain', the portion that is anchored in the lipid layer is the 'transcending domain' and again some protein structure probes have an 'interior domain' that exist inside the virion, which may also help anchor the protein structure probe to the virion. The exterior domain of a protein structure probe that extends outward and away from the outer envelope of a virus virion is intended to engage a cell-surface receptor on a biologically active cell the virus is targeting as its host cell.

[0047] When a virus carries a DNA payload and the viral DNA is inserted into the host cell, the virus's DNA travels to the host cell's nucleus and is known to become inserted into the host cell's own native DNA. In the case where a virus is carrying its genetic payload as RNA, the virus inserts the RNA payload into the host cell and may also insert one or more enzymes to facilitate the RNA being utilized properly to replicate copies of the virus. Once inside the host cell, some species of virus facilitate use of the viral RNA by having the RNA converted to DNA. Once the viral RNA has been converted to DNA, the virus's DNA travels to the host cell's nucleus and is known to become inserted into the host cell's native DNA. Once a virus's genetic material has been inserted into the host cell's native DNA, the virus's genetic material takes command of certain cell functions and redirects the resources of the host cell to generate copies of the virus. Other forms of RNA viruses bypass the need to use the nuclear DNA and simply utilize portions of the viral genome to act as messenger RNA. RNA viruses that bypass the host cell's DNA, cause the cell in general to generate copies of the necessary parts of the virus directly from the virus's RNA genome.

[0048] The human immunodeficiency virus (HIV) has an outer envelope comprised of a lipid bilayer. The lipid bilayer covers a protein matrix consisting of p17^{gag} proteins. Inside the p17^{gag} protein is nested a nucleocapsid comprised of p24^{gag} proteins. Inside the nucleocapsid HIV carries its payload. HIV's genetic payload consists of two single strands of RNA. In addition to the two strands of HIV RNA, there are proteins that are carried in the core of the nucleocapsid along with the two RNA strands. These proteins include 'reverse transcriptase', 'integrase' and 'protease' molecules.

[0049] The T-Helper cell acts as HIV's host cell. HIV locates its host by utilizing at least two different types of probes located on its envelope. The HIV virion utilizes two types of glycoprotein probes affixed to the outer surface of its external envelope to engage a T-Helper cell. HIV utilizes a glycoprotein probe 120 to locate a CD4 cell-surface receptor on a T-Helper cell. Once an HIV glycoprotein 120 probe has successfully engaged a CD4 cell surface-receptor on a T-Helper cell a conformational change occurs in the probe and a glycoprotein 41 probe is exposed. The glycoprotein 41 probe's intent is to engage a CXCR4 or CCR5 cell-surface receptor on the same T-Helper cell. Once a glycoprotein 41 probe on the HIV virion successfully engages a CXCR4 or CCR5 cell-surface receptor, the HIV virion opens an access portal through the T-Helper cell's outer membrane.

[0050] Once the HIV virion has opened an access portal through the T-Helper cell's outer plasma membrane, the HIV virion inserts two positive strand RNA molecules it carries into the T-Helper cell. Each RNA strand is approximately 9500 nucleotides in length. Inserted along with the RNA strands are the enzymes reverse transcriptase, protease and integrase. Once the virus's genome gains access to the interior of the T-Helper cell, in the cytoplasm the pair of RNA molecules are transformed to deoxyribonucleic acid by the reverse transcriptase enzyme. Following modification of the virus's genome to DNA, the virus's genetic information migrates to the host cell's nucleus. In the nucleus, with the assistance of the integrase protein, the HIV's DNA becomes inserted into the T-Helper cell's native DNA. When the timing is appropriate, the now integrated viral DNA is decoded by the host cell's polymerase molecules and the virus's genetic information commands certain cell functions to carry out the replication process to construct copies of the human deficiency virus.

[0051] The outer layer of the HIV virion is comprised of a portion of the T-Helper cell's outer cell membrane. In the final stage of the replication process, as a copy of the HIV capsid, carrying the HIV genome, buds through the host cell's cell membrane the capsid acquires as its external envelope, a wrapping of lipid bilayer from the host cell's cell membrane. In the case of HIV, since the surface of the pathogen is covered by an envelope comprised of lipid bilayer taken from the host T-Helper cells, this feature allows the HIV virion the capacity to eluded the immune systems, since the cells comprising the immune system may find it difficult to tell the difference between the surface of an infectious HIV virion and the surface characteristics of a noninfected T-Helper cell.

[0052] The Hepatitis C virus (HCV) is a positive sense RNA virus, meaning a type of RNA that is capable of bypassing the need for involving the host cell's nucleus by having its RNA genome function as messenger RNA. Hepatitis C infects liver cells. The Hepatitis C viral genome becomes divided once it gains access to the interior of a liver host cell. Portions of the subdivisions of the Hepatitis C genome directly interact with ribosomes to produce proteins necessary to construct copies of the virus.

[0053] HCV belongs to the Flaviviridae family and is the only member of the Hepacivirus genus. There are considered to be at least 100 different strains of Hepatitis C virus based on genome sequencing variability.

[0054] HCV is comprised of an outer lipoprotein envelope and an internal nucleocapsid. The genetic payload is carried within the nucleocapsid. In its natural state, present on the surface of the outer envelope of the Hepatitis C virus are probes that detect receptors present on the surface of liver cells. The glycoprotein E1 probe and the glycoprotein E2 probe have been identified to be affixed to the surface of HCV. The E2 probe binds with high affinity to the large external loop of a CD81 cell-surface receptor. CD81 is found on the surface of many cell types including liver cells. Once the E2 probe has engaged the CD81 cell-surface receptor, cofactors on the surface of HCV's external envelope engage either or both the low density lipoprotein receptor (LDLR) or the scavenger receptor class B type I (SR-BI) present on the liver cell in order to effect the mechanism to facilitate HCV breaching the cell membrane and inserting its RNA genome payload through the plasma cell membrane of the liver cell into the liver cell. Upon successful engagement of the HCV surface probes with a liver cell's cell-surface receptors, HCV inserts the single strand of RNA and other payload elements it carries into the liver cell targeted to be a host cell. The HCV RNA genome then interacts with enzymes and ribosomes inside the liver cell in a translational process to produce the proteins required to construct copies of the protein components of HCV. The HCV genome undergoes a method of transcription to replicate copies of the virus's RNA genome. Inside the host, pieces of the HCV virus are assembled together and ultimately loaded with a copy of the HCV genome. Replicas of the original HCV then escape the host cell and migrate the environment in search of additional host liver cells to infect and continue the replication process.

[0055] The HCV's naturally occurring genetic payload consists of a single molecule of linear positive sense, single stranded RNA approximately 9600 nucleotides in length. By means of a translational process a polyprotein of approximately 3000 amino

473

acids is generated. This polyprotein is cleaved post translation by host and viral proteases into individual viral proteins which include: the structural proteins of C, E1, E2, the nonstructural proteins NS1, NS2, NS3, NS4A, NS4B, NS5A, NS5B, p7 and ARFP/F protein. Hepatitis C virus's proteins direct the host liver cell to construction copies of the Hepatitis C virus. A membrane associated replicase complex consisting of the virus's nonstructural proteins NS3 and NS5B facilitate the replication of the viral genome. The membrane of the endoplasmic reticulum appears to be the site of protein maturation and viral assembly. Once copies of the Hepatitis C Virus are generated, they exit the host cell and each copy of HCV migrates in search of another appropriate liver cell that will act as a host to continue the replication process.

[0056] Hepatitis C virus life-cycle demonstrates that copies of a virus virion can be generated by inserting RNA into a host cell that functions as messenger RNA in the host cell. The Hepatitis C viral RNA genome functions as messenger RNA, acting as the template in conjunction with the biologic machinery of a host cell to produce the components that comprise copies of the Hepatitis C virion and the Hepatitis C viral RNA provides the biologic instructions to assemble the components into complete copies of the Hepatitis C virions. The Hepatitis C virus life-cycle clearly demonstrates that viral virions can be manufactured by a host cell without involving the nucleus of the cell.

[0057] Deciphering the existence, replication and behavior of viruses provides clear examples of several fundamental concepts, which include: (1) Viruses target specific cells in the body by means of identifying and engaging such target cells utilizing the probes projecting outward from the virus's exterior shell to make contact with cell-surface receptors located on the surface of the target cells, and (2) Viruses are capable of carrying various types of payloads including DNA, RNA and a variety of proteins.

[0058] Current gene therapy approach to attempting to deliver a payload to cells in the body use modified forms of existing viruses to act as transport devices to deliver genetic information. This approach is severely limited by restricting the virus virion to the target only cells the viral vector naturally seeks out and infects. Current gene therapy approach is further limited by using the pre-existing size of naturally occurring viruses, rather than being able to modify the size of the structure to be able to tailor the volumetric carrying capacity of the payload portion of the modified virus. Further gene therapy is restricted to utilizing naturally occurring viruses to deliver only genetic information; it has not previously been appreciated by those skilled in the art that virus-like transport devices might deliver to a variety of specific cell types a wide variety of differing payloads such as signaling proteins.

[0059] A dramatic, not previously recognized by those expert in the art is the need to develop a transport vehicle that can be fashioned to seek out specific types of cells and deliver to these cells nuclear signals. The external envelope of a transport should be constructed so as not to alert the immune system of its presence to prevent rejection of the vehicles. Transport vehicles should be capable of being configured to target any specific cell type and engage and deliver their payload only to that specific cell type. To this point, no such device has been conceived.

BRIEF SUMMARY OF THE INVENTION

[0060] Utilization of configurable microscopic medical payload delivery devices to deliver control RNAs to specific cell types facilitates a dramatic new approach to medical care. By selecting the type of probes that are present on the surface of the configurable microscopic medical payload delivery devices, specific types of cells can be targeted. By delivering control RNAs to specific cell types, genes can be activated or inactivated in those specific cell types. A wide variety of medical conditions are treatable by utilizing this new and unique approach.

DETAILED DESCRIPTION

[0061] The future of medical treatment will be the widespread utilization of configurable microscopic medical payload delivery devices (CMMPDD) to deliver control RNAs directly to targeted cell types in the body.

[0062] For purposes of this text an 'external envelope' refers to the outermost covering of a virus or a virus-like transport device or a configurable microscopic medical payload delivery device. The external envelope may be comprised of a lipid layer, a lipid bilayer, the combination of a lipid layer affixed to a protein matrix or the combination of a lipid bilayer affixed to a protein matrix.

[0063] For purposes of this text an 'internal shell' refers to a protein matrix shell nested inside the external envelope. The inner most protein matrix shell is termed the nucleocapsid. The proteins that comprise the nucleocapsid are termed capsid proteins. In the center or core of the nucleocapsid is where the payload is carried.

[0064] For purposes of this text 'external probes' are molecular structures that are utilized to locate and engage cell-surface receptors on biologically active cells. External probes are generally comprised of a portion which is anchored or fixed in the external envelope and a second portion that extends out and away from the external envelope. External probes may be comprised solely of a protein structure or an external probe may be a glycoprotein molecule.

[0065] For purposes of this text 'glycoprotein molecule' refers to a molecule comprised of a carbohydrate region and a protein region. Glycoprotein molecules that act as probes are generally anchored or fixed to a lipid layer utilizing the carbohydrate portion of the molecule as an anchor. The protein portion of the glycoprotein molecule which extends outward and away from the external envelope the glycoprotein has been affixed such that the protein region may function as a probe to locate and attach to the cell-surface receptor it was created to engage.

[0066] The concept of configurable microscopic medical payload delivery devices is modeled after naturally existing viruses. Configurable microscopic medical payload delivery devices in general are spherical in shape; though other shapes may be used as function might warrant the use of a particular shape. The spherical configurable microscopic medical payload delivery devices are comprised of an external envelope and one or more inner nested protein shells. A quantity of exterior protein structure probes and/ or glycoprotein probes are anchored in the exterior lipid envelope and extend out and away from the exterior lipid envelope. Nesting of protein shells refers to progressively smaller diameter shells fitting snugly inside protein shells of a larger diameter. Inside the inner most protein shell, referred to as the nucleocapsid, is a cavity referred to as the core of the device. The core of the device is the space where the medically therapeutic payload the device carries is located.

[0067] Configurable microscopic medical payload delivery devices are generated to target certain specific cell types in the body. Configurable microscopic medical payload delivery devices target specific cell types by the configuration of probes affixed to the external envelope of the CMMPDD. By affixing specific probes to the external envelope of the CMMPDD, these probes intended to engage and attach only to specific cell-surface receptors located on certain cell types in the body, the CMMPDD will deliver its payload only to those cell types that express compatible and engagable specific cell-surface receptors. In a similar fashion where the exterior probes of a naturally occurring virus engage specific cell-surface receptors present on the surface of the virus's host cell and only the designated host cell, the CMMPDD's exterior probes are configured to engage cell-surface receptors on a specific type of target cell. In this manner, the payload of medication or biologic tools carried by CMMPDD will be delivered only to specific types of cells in the body. The exterior probes on the surface of a CMMPDD will vary as needed so as to effect the CMMPDD delivery of payloads to cell types as needed to effect a medical treatment.

[0068] The size of configurable microscopic medical payload delivery devices is to depend upon the volume size of the payload the CMMPDD is required to carry and deliver to a target cell. The size of a CMMPDD is dependent upon the diameter of the inner protein matrix shells. The diameter of each inner protein matrix shell is governed by the number of protein molecules utilized to construct the protein matrix shell at the time the protein matrix shell is generated. Increasing the number of proteins that comprise a protein matrix shell, increases the diameter of the protein matrix shell. The external lipid envelope wraps around and covers the outermost protein matrix shell. The larger the volume of the core of the CMMPDD, the greater the physical size payload the CMMPDD is able to carry. The size of the configurable microscopic medical payload delivery device is to be the size of cell (approximately 10^{-4} m in diameter) or less, generally detectable by a light microscope or, as needed, an electron microscope. The size of the CMMPDD is not to be too large such that it would generate a burden to the body by damaging organ tissues through clogging blood vessels, and the maintaining a small enough size that the CMMPDD can be properly disposed of by the body once the CMMPDD has delivered its payload to its target cell. The dimensions of each type of CMMPDD are to be tailored to the mission of the CMMPDD, which takes into account the type of target cell, the size of the payload that is to be delivered to the target cells and the length of time the CMMPDD may engage the target cell.

[0069] Being enveloped in an external lipid layer, configurable microscopic medical payload delivery devices possess the advantage of having their exterior appear similar to the plasma membrane that acts as an outside covering for the cells that comprise the body. By appearing similar to existing plasma membranes, the CMMPDDs appear similar to naturally occurring structures found in the body, affording the CMMPDD the capability to avoid detection by a body's immune system because the exterior of the CMMPDD mimics the cells comprising the body and the surveillance cells of the immune system find it difficult to discern between the CMMPDD and naturally occurring cells comprising the body.

[0070] To carry out the process of manufacturing a configurable microscopic medical payload delivery device, a primitive cell such as a stem cell is selected. The reason for utilizing primitive cells such as stems cells as the host cell, is that the CMMPDD acquires its outer envelope from the host cell and the more primitive the host cell, the fewer in number the identifying protein markers are present on the surface of the CMMPDD. The fewer the identifying surface proteins present on the outer envelope of the CMMPDD, the less likely a body's immune system will identify the CMMPDD as an invader and therefore less likely the body's immune system will react to the presence of the CMMPDD and reject the CMMPDD by attacking and neutralizing the CMMPDD.

[0071] Stem cells used as host cells to manufacture quantities of CMMPDD product are selected per histocompatibility markers present on their surface. Certain histocompatibility markers present on the surface of the final CMMPDD product will be less likely to cause a reaction in a specific patient based on the genetic profile of the patient's histocompatibility markers. A similar histocompatibility match is done when donor organs are selected to be given to recipients to avoid rejection of the donor organ by the recipient's immune system.

[0072] The selected stem cell used to manufacture configurable microscopic medical payload delivery devices goes through several steps of maturation before it is capable of generating therapeutic CMMPDD product. Messenger RNA is inserted into the host stem cell that would code for the general physical outer structures of the CMMPDD. Messenger RNA is inserted into the host that would generate surface probes that would target the surface receptors on specifically target cells. Messenger RNA is inserted into the host that would be used to generate the payload of control RNAs. Similar to how copies of a naturally occurring virus, such as the Hepatitis C virus or HIV, are produced, assembled and released from a host cell, copies of the CMMPDD are produced, assembled and released from a host cell. Once released from the host cell, the copies of the CMMPDD would be collected, then pooled together to produce a therapeutic dose to result in a medically beneficial effect.

[0073] The construction of the configurable microscopic medical payload delivery devices is performed by taking stem cells and inserting modified viral genetic programming into the stem cells.

Stem cells are chosen as the host cell due to the low number of surface markers, which leads to less antigenicity in configurable microscopic medical payload delivery devices when the configurable microscopic medical payload delivery devices are released by the host cells and wrapped in an outer envelope comprised of the host cells' plasma membrane.

[0074] The stem cells used as host cells are suspended in a broth of nutrients and are kept at an optimum temperature to govern the rate of production of the CMMPDD product. Similar to the natural production of the Hepatitis C virus, the configurable microscopic medical payload delivery devices 'production genome' is introduced into the host stem cells. The configurable microscopic medical payload delivery devices production genome carries genetic instructions to cause the host cells to manufacture the configurable microscopic medical payload delivery devices' outer protein wall, the inner protein matrixes, the surface probes the configurable microscopic medical payload delivery device is to have affixed to its outer envelope and the control RNAs the configurable microscopic medical payload delivery devices are to carry; and the instructions to assemble the various pieces into the final form of the configurable microscopic medical payload delivery devices and the instructions to activate the budding process. The resultant configurable microscopic medical payload delivery devices are collected from the nutrient broth surrounding the host cells and placed together into doses to be used as a treatment for a medical disease.

[0075] The 'production genome' are an array of messenger RNAs that are directly translated by the host cell's internal enzymes. The production genome dictates the characteristics of the final version of the CMMPDD that buds from the host stem cell and is released and is to be utilized as a medical treatment. The production genome is specifically tailored to code for the surface probes that will seek and engage a specific type of target cell. The production genome also carries the instructions to code for the production of the type of control RNAs to be delivered to the specific type of target cell. The 'production genome' varies depending upon the configuration of the CMMPDD and the type of control RNAs the

CMMPDD is to transport to effect a specific medical treatment on a specific type of cell.

[0076] The configurable microscopic medical payload delivery device transporting control RNAs represents a very versatile medical treatment delivery device. There are an estimated 30,000 to 100,000 genes located in the human genome. CMMPDD could be used to deliver control RNAs to activate or inactivate any of the chromosomal genes in any specific cell type in the body.

[0077] As an example of this method, to treat diabetes mellitus utilizing configurable microscopic medical payload delivery devices to deliver to Beta cells messenger RNA coded to produce insulin, the following production process is followed in the lab: (1) human stem cells are selected. (2) Into the selected stem cells is placed the production genome constructed, in this case, specifically as a means to treat diabetes mellitus. The RNA production genome contains genetic instructions to cause the host stem cells to manufacture the configurable microscopic medical payload delivery devices' outer protein wall, the inner protein matrix, surface probes to include glycoprotein probes that engage the GPR40 cell-surface receptor present on the surface of Beta cells located in the Islets of Langerhans in the pancreas, and the payload of control RNAs, in this case the control RNAs to activate the production of the insulin molecules in Beta cells; and the biologic instructions to assemble the components into the final form of the configurable microscopic medical payload delivery devices; and the biologic instructions to activate the budding process. (3) Upon insertion of the RNA production genome dedicated to producing a control RNAs configured to activate the genes to generate messenger RNA that will result in the production of insulin, into the host stem cells, host stem cells respond by (i) simultaneously translating the different segments of the RNA production genome to produce the proteins that comprise the exterior protein wall, the inner protein matrix molecules, the surface probes to seek out and engage Beta cells, the control RNA payload to produce insulin, and (ii) decoding the RNA instructions to assemble the components into the configurable microscopic medical payload delivery devices. (4) Upon assembly, the configurable microscopic medical payload delivery devices bud through the cell membrane of the host stem cell. (5) At the time of the budding process, the configurable microscopic medical payload delivery devices acquire an outside envelope wrapped over the outer protein shell, this outer envelope comprised of a portion of the plasma membrane from the host stem cell as the configurable microscopic medical payload delivery devices exit the host cell. (6) The resultant configurable microscopic medical payload delivery devices are collected from the nutrient broth surrounding the host stem cells. (7) The configurable microscopic medical payload delivery devices are washed in sterile solvent to remove contaminants. (8) The configurable microscopic medical payload delivery devices are removed from the sterile solvent and suspended in a hypoallergenic liquid medium. (9) The configurable microscopic medical payload delivery devices are separated into individual quantities to facilitate storage and delivery to physicians and patients. (10) The configurable microscopic medical payload delivery devices transported in the hypoallergenic liquid medium is administered to a diabetic patient per injection in a dose that is tailored to receiving patient's requirement to produce sufficient amount of insulin to control the blood sugar. (11) Upon being injected into the body, the configurable microscopic medical payload delivery devices migrate to the Beta cells located in the Islets of Langerhans by means of the patient's blood stream. (12) Upon the configurable microscopic medical payload delivery devices reaching the Beta cells, the configurable microscopic medical payload delivery devices engage the cell-surface receptors located on the Beta cells and insert the payload they carry into the Beta cells. The payload, in this case being control RNAs to activated the genes responsible for the Beta cell's production of insulin molecules. The increase in insulin production by Beta cells successfully manages diabetes mellitus.

Conclusions, Ramification, and Scope

[0078] Accordingly, the reader will see that the configurable microscopic medical payload delivery device to deliver control RNAs to specific targeted cell types provides advantages over existing art by (1) being a delivery device that seeks out specific types of cells,

(2) by being a delivery device that is versatile enough to deliver a variety of potential control RNAs to accomplish various medical treatments and (3) by being a delivery device constructed with a surface envelope that will avoid detection by the innate immune system so as not to activate the immune system to its presence; for these reasons this represents a new and unique medical delivery device that has never before been recognized nor appreciated by those skilled in the art.

[0079] Although the description above contains specificities, these should not be construed as limiting the scope of the invention but as merely providing illustrations of some of the presently preferred embodiments of the invention.

[0080] Thus the scope of the invention should be determined by the appended claims and their legal equivalents, rather than by the examples given.

CLAIMS: Reserved.

PATENT APPLICATION
SPECIFICATION NUMBER 5

TITLE OF THE INVENTION:

CONFIGURABLE MICROSCOPIC MEDICAL PAYLOAD DELIVERY DEVICE TO DELIVER COMMAND RNAS TO SPECIFIC CELLS TO MANAGE DIABETES MELLITUS AND GENETIC DEFICIENCY DISORDERS

BACKGROUND OF THE INVENTION

Field of the Invention

This invention relates to any medical device intended to correct a protein deficiency or genetic deficiency in the body by utilizing a configurable microscopic medical payload delivery device to insert one or more command RNAs into one or more specific cell types in the body to improve cell function.

Description of Background Art

[0001] For purposes of this text a 'command RNA' molecule (comRNA) is an RNA molecule that functions like a messenger RNA, but where an messenger RNA is translated in the cytoplasm of a cell to produce single chain proteins, the command RNA provides instructions deciphered and/or translated in the smooth endoplasmic retinaculum organelle as to how to build complex multi-chained proteins, phospholipids and cholesterol.

[0002] A 'deoxyribose' is a deoxypentose (C5H10O4) sugar. Deoxyribonucleic acid (DNA) is comprised of three basic elements: a deoxyribose sugar, a phosphate group and nitrogen containing bases. DNA is a macromolecule made up of two chains of repeating deoxyribose sugars linked by phosphodiester bonds between the 3-hydroxyl group of one and the 5-hydroxyl group of the next; the two chains are held antiparallel to each other by weak hydrogen bonds. DNA strands contain a sequence of nucleotides, which include: adenine, cytosine, guanine or thymine. Adenine is always paired with thymine of the opposite strand, and guanine is always paired with cytosine of the opposite strand; one side or strand of a DNA macromolecule is the mirror image of the opposite strand. Nuclear DNA is regarded as the medium for storing the master plan of hereditary information.

[0003] Genes are considered segments of the DNA that represent units of inheritance.

[0004] A chromosome exists in the nucleus of a cell and consists of a DNA double helix bearing a linear sequence of genes, coiled and recoiled around aggregated proteins, termed histones. The number of chromosomes varies from species to species. Most Human cells carries twenty two pairs of chromosomes plus two sex chromosomes; two 'x' chromosomes in women and one 'x' and one 'y' chromosome in men. Chromosomes carry genetic information in the form of units which are referred to as genes.

[0005] Per J. K. Pal, S.S. Ghaskabi, Fundamentals of Molecular Biology, 2009: 'The central dogma of molecular biology . . . states that the genes present in the genome (DNA) are transcribed into mRNAs, which are then translated into polypeptides or proteins, which are phenotypes.' 'Genome, thus, contains the complete set of hereditary information for any organism and is functionally divided into small parts referred to as genes. Each gene is a sequence of nucleotides representing a single protein or RNA. Genome of a living organism may contain as few as 500 genes as in case of Mycoplasma, or as many as 30,000 genes as in case of human beings.' Some references cite as many as 100,000 genes may exist in the human genome.

[0006] The current understanding of the actual biologic structure of a gene is far more elaborate than the historic standard definition of a gene. A gene appears to be comprised of a number of segments loosely strung together along a particular section of DNA. In general there are three segments associated with a gene which include: (1) the Upstream 5' flanking region, (2) the transcriptional unit (often referred to as the open reading frame) and (3) the Downstream 3' flanking region. The Upstream 5' flanking region is comprised of the 'enhancer region', the 'promoter-proximal region', and 'promoter region'. The 'transcriptional unit' or open reading frame starts at a location designated 'transcription start site' (TSS), which is located in a site called the 'initiator region' (inR), which may be described in a general form as Py2CAPy5. The transcription unit is comprised of the combination of segments of DNA nucleotides to be transcribed into RNA and spacing units known as 'introns' that are not transcribed or if transcribed are later removed post transcription, such that they do not appear in the final RNA molecule. In the case of a gene coding for a mRNA molecule, the transcription unit will contain all three elements of the mRNA, which includes: (1) the 5' noncoding region, (2) the translational region and (3) the 3' noncoding region. Interspersed between these regions are introns, which will be either not transcribed or if transcribed removed from the precursor form of mRNA prior to the mRNA reaching its final form. The 'transcriptional unit' is generally considered to be the 'gene'. The Downstream 3' flanking region contains DNA nucleotides that are not transcribed and may contain what has been termed an 'enhancer region'. An enhancer region in the Downstream 3' flanking region is thought to act to promote the gene previously transcribed to be transcribed again.

[0007] On either side of the DNA sequencing comprising a gene and its flanking regions, may be inactive DNA which act as boundaries which have been termed 'insulator elements'. The term 'upstream' refers to DNA sequencing that occurs prior to the TSS if viewed from the 5' end to the 3' end of the DNA; where the term 'downstream' refers to DNA sequencing located after the TSS.

[0008] An 'enhancer region' may or may not be present in the Upstream 5' flanking region. If present, the enhancer region helps facilitate the reading of the gene by encouraging formation of the transcription mechanism. If the enhancer is present, it may exist 200 kb to 17,000 kb upstream from the transcription starting site.

[0009] The 'transcription complex' also referred to as the 'transcription mechanism', in humans, is reported to be comprised of over forty separate proteins that assemble together to ultimately function in a concerted effort to transcribe the nucleotide sequence of the DNA into RNA. The transcription complex (TC) includes elements such as 'general transcription factor Sp1', 'general transcription factor NF1', 'general transcription factor TATA-binding protein', 'TFIID', 'basal transcription complex', and a 'RNA polymerase protein' to name only a few of the forty elements that exist. The elements of the transcription mechanism function as (1) a means to recognize the location of the start of a gene, (2) as proteins to bind the transcription mechanism to the DNA such that transcription may occur or (3) as means of transcribing the DNA nucleotide coding to produce a precursor RNA molecule. There are at least three RNA polymerase proteins which include: RNA polymerase I, RNA polymerase II, and RNA polymerase III. RNA polymerase I tends to be dedicated to transcribing genetic information that will result in the formation of rRNA molecules. RNA polymerase II tends to be dedicated to transcribing genetic information that will result in the formation of mRNA molecules. RNA polymerase III appears to be dedicated to transcribing genetic information that results in the formation of tRNAs, small cellular RNAs and viral RNAs.

[0010] The 'promoter proximal region' is located upstream from the TSS and upstream from the core promoter region. The 'promoter proximal region' includes two sub-regions termed the GC box and the CAAT box. The 'GC box' appears to be a segment rich in guanine-cytosine nucleotide sequences. The GC box binds to the 'general transcription factor Sp1' of the transcription mechanism. The 'CAAT box' is a segment which contains the nucleotide sequence 'GGCCAATCT' located 75 bps upstream from the transcription start site (TSS). The CAAT box binds to the 'general transcription factor NF1' of the transcription mechanism.

[0011] The 'core promoter' region is considered the shortest sequence at which RNA polymerase II can initiate transcription of a gene The core promoter may include the initiator region (inR) and either a TATA box or a DPE. The inR is the region designated Py2CAPy5 that surrounds the transcription start site (TSS). The TATA box is located 25 bps upstream from the TSS. The TATA box acts as a site of attachment of the TFIID, which is a promoter for binding of the RNA polymerase II molecule. The DPE is the 'downstream promoter element' that may appear 28 bps to 32 bps downstream from the TSS. The DPE acts as an alternative site of attachment for the TFIID when the TATA box is not present.

[0012] The transcription mechanism, also referred to as the transcription complex appears to be comprised of different elements depending upon whether rRNA is being transcribed versus mRNA or tRNA or small cellular RNA or viral RNA. The proteins that assemble to assist RNA Polymerase I with transcribing the DNA to produce rRNA appear different than the proteins that assemble to assist RNA polymerase II with transcribing the DNA to produce mRNA or the proteins that assemble to assist RNA polymerase III with transcribing the DNA to produce tRNA, small cellular RNA or viral RNA. A common protein that appears to be present at the initial biding of all three types of RNA polymerase molecules is TATA-binding protein (TBP). TBP appears to be required to attach to the DNA, which then facilitates RNA polymerase to bind to the promoter along the DNA. TBP assembles with TBP-associated factors (TAFs). Together TBF and 11 TAFs comprise the complex referred to as TFIID, which has been previously mentioned in the above text.

[0013] Upstream from the TATA box is the 'initiator element', which may be considered as part of the 'core promoter' region. The initiator element is a segment of the nuclear DNA that binds the basal transcription complex. The basal transcription complex is comprised of a number of proteins that make initial contact with the DNA prior to the RNA polymerase binding to the transcription mechanism. The basal transcription complex is associated with an activator. The activator is a command RNA.

[0014] Once the transcription complex is assembled, the transcription complex transcribes the DNA. Transcription of the DNA produces precursor messenger RNA (mRNA), precursor ribosomal RNA (rRNA) or precursor transport RNA (tRNA) or command RNA (comRNA) or other RNAs. In the case of precursor mRNA, the mRNA is further modified, then traverses to the cytoplasm. In the cytoplasm of the cell ribosomes attach to the mRNA. Ribosomes decode mRNA utilizing the process of translation to produce proteins.

[0015] A protein is comprised of a string of amino acids. Proteins can be comprised of only a few amino acids, or a large number of amino acids. Large protein molecules are often referred to as a macromolecule. Proteins can be combined together to form molecules comprised of two or more similar amino acid strands or a protein can be can be comprised of two or more different amino acid strands. When more than one protein are combined into a molecule, this may also be referred as a macromolecule. Proteins can be combined with other molecules such as carbohydrates and lipids. When proteins combine with other molecules this is also often referred to as a macromolecule. Cell surface receptors are considered macromolecules and are often comprised of a protein molecule combined with a carbohydrate molecule to produce a glycoprotein.

[0016] A phospholipid is a molecule comprised of a phosphate group, two alcohols and one or two fatty acid chains. Cholesterol is an organic compound of the steroid family with the chemical formula $C_{27}H_{46}O$. Cholesterol is essential to life, it is a primary constituent of the membrane. Both molecules are constructed in the smooth endoplasmic reticulum.

[0017] Diabetes mellitus represents an important health issue that affects a significant portion of the world population. In the United States, about 16 million people suffer from diabetes mellitus. Every year, about 650,000 additional people are diagnosed with this disease. Diabetes mellitus is the seventh leading cause of all deaths.

[0018] Diabetes mellitus represents a state of hyperglycemia, a serum blood sugar that is higher than what is considered the normal range for humans. Glucose, a six-carbon molecule, is a form of sugar. Glucose is absorbed by the cells of the body and converted to energy by the processes of glycolysis, the Krebs cycle and phosporylation. Insulin, a protein, facilitates the transfer of glucose from the blood into cells. Normal range for blood glucose in humans is generally defined as a fasting blood plasma glucose level of between 70 to 110 mg/dl. For descriptive purposes, the term 'plasma' refers to the fluid portion of blood.

[0019] Diabetes mellitus is classified as Type One and Type Two. Type One diabetes mellitus is insulin dependent, which refers to the condition where there is a lack of sufficient insulin circulating in the blood stream and insulin must be provided to the body in order to properly regulate the blood glucose level. When insulin is required to regulate the blood glucose level in the body, this condition is often referred to as insulin dependent diabetes mellitus (IDDM). Type Two diabetes mellitus is noninsulin dependent, often referred to as noninsulin dependent diabetes mellitus (NIDDM), meaning the blood glucose level can be managed without insulin, and instead by means of diet, exercise or intervention with oral medications. Type Two diabetes mellitus is considered a progressive disease, the underlying pathogenic mechanisms including pancreatic Beta cell (also often designated as β-Cell) dysfunction and insulin resistance.

[0020] The pancreas serves as an endocrine gland and an exocrine gland. Functioning as an endocrine gland the pancreas produces and secretes hormones including insulin and glucagon. Insulin acts to reduce levels of glucose circulating in the blood. Beta cells secrete insulin into the blood when a higher than normal level of glucose is detected in the serum. For purposes of this description the terms 'blood', 'blood stream' and 'serum' refer to the same substance. Glucagon acts to stimulate an increase in glucose circulating in the blood. Beta cells in the pancreas secrete glucagon when a low level of glucose is detected in the serum.

[0021] Glucose enters the body as food and as a result of digestion, glucose enters the blood stream. The Beta cells of the Islets of Langerhans continuously sense the level of glucose in the blood and respond to elevated levels of blood glucose by secreting insulin into the blood. Beta cells produce the protein 'insulin' in their endoplasmic reticulum and store the insulin in vacuoles until it is needed. When Beta cells detect an increase in the glucose level in the blood, Beta cells release insulin into the blood from the described storage vacuoles.

[0022] Insulin is a protein. An insulin protein consists of two chains of amino acids, an alpha chain and a beta chain, linked by two disulfide (S-S) bridges. One chain, the alpha chain consists of 21 amino acids. The second chain the beta chain consists of 30 amino acids.

[0023] Insulin interacts with the cells of the body by means of a cell-surface receptor termed the 'insulin receptor' located on the exterior of a cell's 'outer membrane', otherwise known as the 'plasma membrane'. Insulin interacts with muscle and liver cells by means of the insulin receptor to rapidly remove excess blood sugar when the glucose level in the blood is higher than the upper limit of the normal physiologic range. Recognized functions of insulin include stimulating cells to take up glucose from the blood and convert it to glycogen to facilitate the cells in the body to utilize glucose to generate biochemically usable energy, and to stimulate fat cells to take up glucose and synthesize fat.

[0024] Diabetes Mellitus may be the result of one or more factors. Causes of diabetes mellitus may include: (1) mutation of the insulin gene itself causing miscoding, which results in the production of ineffective insulin molecules; (2) mutations to genes that code for the 'transcription factors' needed for transcription of the insulin gene in the deoxyribonucleic acid (DNA) to create messenger ribonucleic acid (mRNA) molecules, which facilitate the manufacture of the insulin molecule; (3) mutations of the gene encoding for the insulin receptor, which produces inactive or an insufficient number of insulin receptors; (4) mutation to the gene encoding for glucokinase, the enzyme that phosphorylates glucose in the first step of glycolysis; (5) mutations to the genes encoding portions of the potassium channels in the plasma membrane of the Beta cells, preventing proper closure of the channel, thus blocking insulin release; (6) mutations to mitochondrial genes that as a result, decreases the energy available to be used facilitate the release of insulin, therefore reducing insulin secretion; (7) failure of glucose transporters to properly permit the facilitated diffusion of glucose from plasma into the cells of the body.

[0025] The insulin molecule, comprised of two polypeptide chains, is produced by Beta cells located in the pancreas. Command RNAs provide the instructions necessary to produce complex molecules such as insulin. Command RNAs act as the templates for transcription of the polypeptide chains and the instructions necessary to properly join the two polypeptide chains with disulfide linkages to create the insulin molecule. Once the biologically active insulin protein is generated it is stored in a vacuole in the Beta cell to await being released into the blood stream.

[0026] Insulin receptors, which appear on the surface of cells, offer binding sites for insulin circulating in the blood. When insulin binds to an insulin receptor, the biologic response inside the cell causes glucose to enter the cell and undergo processing in the cytoplasm. Processed glucose molecules then enter the mitochondria. The mitochondria further process the modified glucose molecules to produce usable energy in the form of adenosine triphosphate molecules (ATP). Thirty-eight ATP molecules may be generated from one molecule of glucose during the process of aerobic respiration. ATP molecules are utilized as an energy source by biologic processes throughout the cell.

[0027] The current medical therapeutic approach to the management of diabetes mellitus has produced limited results. Patients with diabetes generally struggle with an inadequate production of insulin, or an ineffective release of biologically active insulin molecules, or a release of an insufficient number of biologically active insulin molecules, or an insufficient production of cell-surface receptors, or a production of ineffective cell-surface receptors, or a production of ineffective insulin molecules that are unable to interact properly with insulin receptors to produce the required biologic effect. Type One diabetes requires administration of exogenous insulin. The traditional approach to Type Two diabetes has generally first been to adjust the diet to limit the caloric intake the individual consumes. Exercise is used as an initial approach to both Type One and Type Two diabetes as a means of up-regulating the utilization of fats and sugar so as to reduce the amount of circulating plasma glucose. When diet and exercise are inadequate in properly managing Type Two diabetes, oral medications are often introduced. The action of sulfonylureas, a commonly prescribed class of oral medication, is to stimulate the Beta cells to produce additional insulin receptors and enhance the insulin receptors' response to insulin. Biguanides, another form of oral treatment, inhibit gluconeogenesis, the production of glucose in the liver, thereby attempting to reduce plasma glucose levels. Thiazolidinediones (TZDs) lower blood sugar levels by activating peroxisome proliferator-activated receptor gamma (PPAR-γ), a transcription factor, which when activated regulates the activity of various target genes, particularly ones involved in glucose and lipid metabolism. If diet, exercise and oral medications do not produce a satisfactory control of the level of blood glucose in a diabetic patient, exogenous insulin is injected into the body in an effort to normalize the amount of glucose present in the serum. Insulin, a protein, has not successfully been made available as an oral medication to date due to the fact that proteins in general become degraded when they encounter the acid environment present in the stomach.

[0028] Despite strict monitoring of blood glucose and potentially multiple doses of insulin injected throughout the day, many patients with diabetes mellitus still experience devastating adverse effects from elevated blood glucose levels. Microvascular damage and elevated tissue sugar levels contribute to such complications as renal failure, retinopathy involving the eyes, neuropathy, and accelerated heart disease despite aggressive efforts to maintain the blood sugar within the physiologic normal range using exogenous insulin by itself or a combination of exogenous insulin and one or more oral medications. Diabetes remains the number one cause of renal failure in the United States. Especially in diabetic patients whom are dependent upon administering exogenous insulin into their body, though dosing of the insulin may be four or more times a day and even though this may produce adequate control of the blood glucose level to prevent the clinical symptoms of hyperglycemia; this does not unerringly supplement the body's natural capacity to monitor the blood sugar level minute to minute, twenty-four hours a day, and deliver an immediate response to a rise in blood glucose by the release of insulin from Beta cells as required. The deleterious effects of diabetes may still evolve despite strict and persistent control of the glucose level in the blood stream.

[0029] Current treatment approach to managing diabetes may be augmented by the unique approach to utilizing modified viruses as vehicles to transport of command RNA molecules into cells in order to increase the production of biologically active insulin. By utilizing modified viruses to transport command RNA molecules to facilitate the production and assembly of the necessary proteins. A diabetic would require the necessary proteins to adequately control the blood glucose level by utilizing inherent regulatory mechanisms rather than exogenous therapies.

[0030] Present medical care is attempting to utilize viruses to deliver genetic information into cells. Research in the field of gene therapy has involved certain naturally occurring viruses. Some of the common viral vectors that have been investigated include: Adeno-associated virus, Adenovirus, Alphavirus, Epstein-Barr virus, Gammaretrovirus, Herpes simplex virus, Letivirus, Poliovirus,

Rhabdovirus, Vaccinia virus. Naturally occurring virus vectors are limited to the naturally occurring external probes that are affixed to the outer wall of the virus. The external probes fixed to the outside wall of a virus virion dictate which type of cell the virus can engage and infect. Therefore, as an example, the function of the adenovirus, a respiratory virus, is strictly limited to engaging and infecting specific lung cells. Used as a medical treatment device, the adenovirus can only deliver gene therapy to specific lung cells, which severely limits this vector's usefulness as a deliver device. The therapeutic function of all naturally occurring viral vectors is limited to delivering a DNA or RNA payload to the cell type the viral vector naturally targets as its host cell.

[0031] Naturally occurring viruses also have the disadvantage of being susceptible to detection and elimination by a body's immune system. Viruses have been infecting humans for hundreds of thousands of years. A human's innate immune system is very efficient at detecting the presence of most naturally occurring viruses when such a virus is inside the body. The human immune system is quite capable of generating a vigorous response to most intruding viruses, attacking and neutralizing virus virions whenever a virus virion physically exists are outside the exterior wall of the virus's host cell. If gene therapy in its current state were to become a clinical therapeutic tool, the naturally occurring viruses selected for gene therapy research will have limited effectiveness due the fact that once the viral vector is introduced into the body, the body's the immune system will quickly engage and eliminate the viral vectors, possibly before the vector is able to deliver its payload to its host cell or target cell.

[0032] Cichutek, K., 2001 (US Patent No. 6,323,031 B1) teaches preparation and use of novel lentiviral SiVagm-derived vectors for gene transfer into selected cell types, specifically into proliferatively active and resting human cells.

[0033] Cichutek teaches that it is indeed plausible to re-configure an existing virus and use it as a transport vehicle, though Cichutek's specification and claims are too limited to describe a method that will work for all cell types, if indeed if it will work for any cell type.

[0034] Cichutek describes vectors for 'gene transfer'; in the claims the language that is used is 'genetic information'. Cichutek's Claim 1 of the cited patent states 'A propagation-incompetent SIVagm vector comprising a viral core and a viral envelope, wherein the viral core comprises a simian immunodeficiency virus (SIVagm) viral core of the African vervet monkey Chlorocebus.' Cichutek's does not describe in his claims any further details of the intended payload other than the stating 'SIVagm viral core' in claim 1; in claims 5 & 6 Cichutek describes only 'genetic information'. Transfer of 'genetic information' dramatically limits the useful application of Cichutek's patent in the treatment of medical diseases.

[0035] Cichutek does not claim the use of specific glycogen probes to target specific types of cells. Cichutek's approach is dependent upon the probes naturally present on the viral vectors reported in the patent, which will direct the viral vectors to only those cells the viruses naturally use as their host cell. Cichutek's approach is very restrictive, limited to gene transfer to only cells the viruses use as their natural host cell.

[0036] It is questionable that Cichutek's approach as described in the specification and claims is feasible. Cichutek's claim 4, states 'The SIVagm vector of claim 1, wherein the viral envelope further comprises a single chain antibody (scFv) or a ligand of a cell surface molecule.' By use of the words 'a' and 'or' in the claim, the claim is limited in the singular, meaning Cichutek claims a single chain antibody or a singular ligand. Singular type antibodies or ligands can be used for cell to cell communication, but to open an access portal into a cell and insert a payload into the cell requires two different types antibodies or ligands. As an example human immunodeficiency virus requires the use of both the gp120 and gp41 probes to open a portal into a T-Helper cell and insert its genome into the T-Helper cell. The gp120 probe engages the CD4+ cell-surface receptor on the T-cell. Once the gp120 probe has successfully engaged a CD4+ cell-surface receptor on the target T-Helper cell, then the HIV virion's gp41 probe can engage either a CXCR4 or a CCR5 cell-surface receptor on the T-Helper cell in order to open up an access portal for HIV to insert its genome into a T-Helper cell. It is well documented in the medical literature that a genetic defect leading to an abnormality in the CXCR4 cell-surface receptor prevents HIV virions from opening an access portal and inserting its genetic payload into such T-Helper cells. This genetic defect offers the subset of people carrying the genetic defect resistance to HIV infection. This example demonstrates the need for at least two types of glycoprotein probes to be present on the surface of a viral vector in order for a viral vector to be capable of opening an access portal and delivering the payload the vector carries into its host cell or target cell.

[0037] A delivery system that offered a defined means of targeting specific types of cells, would invoke minimal or no response by the innate immune system when present in the body, and a delivery system that would be capable of inserting into cells a wide variety of command RNAs would significantly improve the current medical treatment options available to clinicians treating patients.

[0038] The solution to arriving at a versatile, workable delivery system that will meet the needs of a number of medical treatments involves three important elements. These elements include:

1) configurable glycoprotein probes whereby more than one type of glycoprotein probe is to be used to engage and access specific target cell types in order to successfully deliver a payload into a specific cell type,
2) an external envelope comprised of a protein shell or lipid layer expressing the least number of cell-surface markers, such as the use of a stem cell to act as the host cell to manufacture the delivery devices,
3) configuring the core of the vector to enable it to carry and deliver command RNAs.

[0039] Viruses are obligate parasites. Viruses simply represent a carrier of genetic material and by themselves viruses are unable to replicate or carry out any form of biologic function outside their host cell. A 'virion' refers to the physical structure of a single complete virus as it exists outside of the host cell. Viruses are generally comprised of one or more nested shells constructed of one or more layers of protein, some with a lipid outer envelope, a genetic payload that represents the instruction code necessary to replicate the virus, and protein enzymes to help facilitate the genetic payload in the function of replicating copies of the virus once the genetic payload has been delivered to a host cell. Located on the outer shell or envelope of a virus are probes. The function of a virus's probes is to locate and engage a host cell's receptors. The virus's surface probes are designed to detect, make contact with and functionally engage one or more receptors located on the exterior of a cell type that will offer the virus the proper environment in which to construct copies of itself. A host cell provides the virus the proper biologic machinery for the virus to successfully replicate itself. Once the virus's genome is inside the host cell, the viral genome takes command of the cell's production machinery and causes the host cell to generate copies of the virus. As the viral copies exit the host cell, these virions set off in search of other host cells to infect.

[0040] Naturally occurring viruses exist in a number of differing shapes. The shape of a virus may be rod or filament like, icosahedral, or complex structures combining filament and polygonal shapes. Viruses generally have their outer wall comprised of a protein coat or an envelope comprised of lipids.

[0041] An outer envelope comprised of lipids may be in the form of one or two phospholipid layers. When the outer envelope is comprised of two phospholipid layers this is termed a lipid bilayer. A phospholipid is a composite molecule comprised of a polar or hydrophilic region on one end and a nonpolar or hydrophobic region on the opposite end. A lipid bilayer covering a virus, like the membrane of a cell, is constructed with the hydrophilic region of one of the phospholipid layers pointed toward the exterior of the virion and the hydrophilic region of the second phospholipid layer pointed inward toward the center of the virus virion; with the hydrophobic regions of each of the two lipid layers pointed toward each other. The outer envelope of some forms of virus may be comprised of an outer lipid layer or lipid bilayer affixed to a protein matrix for support, the protein matrix being located closer to the center of the virus virion than the lipid layer or lipid bilayer.

[0042] Spherical viruses are generally spherical in shape and may be comprised of an outer envelope and one inner shell or an outer envelope and multiple inner shells. Inner shells are approximately spherical in shape; this is because the proteins comprising the protein matrix shell have an irregular shape to their structure. In the case of a spherical virus with an outer envelope and one inner shell, the inner shell is often referred to as a nucleocapsid shell comprised of numerous capsid proteins attached to each other. In the case of a spherical virus being comprised of an outer envelope and multiple inner shells, the outermost inner viral shells may be referred to as comprised of a quantity of matrix proteins, where the innermost shell is referred to as a nucleocapsid and is comprised of a quantity of capsid proteins. The inner protein shells are nested inside each other.

[0043] Viruses carry genetic material in the form of deoxyribonucleic acid (DNA) or ribonucleic acid (RNA) in their nucleocapsid often referred to as the core. A virus is therefore generally considered to be a DNA virus if its genome is comprised of DNA or the virus is considered a RNA virus if its genome is comprised of RNA. Viruses may also carry enzymes as part of their payload. An enzyme such as 'reverse transcriptase' transforms a RNA viral genome into DNA. Protease enzymes modify the viral genome once it has entered a host cell. An integrase enzyme assists a DNA viral genome with insertion into the host cell's nuclear DNA. The payload is carried inside the virus's nucleocapsid shell.

[0044] The probes attached to the exterior of a virus are constructed to engage specific cell-surface receptors on specific cell types in the body. Only a cell that expresses cell-surface receptors that are capable of being engaged by the probes of a specific virus can act as a host for the virus. Viruses often use two probes to access a host cell. The first probe makes an initial attachment to the host cell, while the action of the virus's second probe often in conjunction with the action of the first probe cause an access portal to be created in the host cell's exterior plasma membrane. Once an access portal is formed, the virus inserts the contents of its payload into the host cell. Once the virus's genome is inside the cytoplasm of the host cell, any enzymes that accompanied the viral genome into the cell, may begin to modify or assist the virus's genome with infecting and taking control of the host cell's biologic functions.

[0045] Probes are attached to the external envelope of a virus virion. Probes may be in the form of a protein structure or may be in the form of a glycoprotein molecule. For viruses constructed with a protein matrix as its outer envelope, the probes tend to be protein structures. A portion of the protein structure probe is fixed or anchored in the protein matrix, while a portion of the protein structure probe extends out and away from the protein matrix. The portion of the protein structure probe extending out away from the virus virion is referred to as the 'exterior domain', the portion anchored in the protein matrix is the 'transcending domain'. Some protein probes have a third segment that extends through the envelope and exists inside the virus virion, which is referred to as the 'interior domain'. The exterior domain of a protein structure probe is intended to engage a specific cell-surface receptor on a biologically active cell the virus is targeting as its host cell.

[0046] Viruses that utilize a lipid layer as the outer envelope, are constructed with probes that tend to be glycoproteins. A glycoprotein is comprised of a protein segment and a carbohydrate segment. The carbohydrate segment of the glycoprotein molecule is fixed or anchored in the lipid layer of the outer envelope, while the protein segment extends outward and away from the outer envelope. The protein portion of a glycoprotein probe that extends outward and away from the outer envelope of a virus virion is intended to engage a cell-surface receptor on a biologically active cell the virus is targeting as its host cell.

[0047] Some forms of viruses that utilize a lipid layer as its envelope use protein structure probes. In this case, the portion of the protein structure probe that extends outward and away from the outer envelope is the 'exterior domain', the portion that is anchored in the lipid layer is the 'transcending domain' and again some protein structure probes have an 'interior domain' that exist inside the virion, which may also help anchor the protein structure probe to the virion. The exterior domain of a protein structure probe that extends outward and away from the outer envelope of a virus virion is intended to engage a cell-surface receptor on a biologically active cell the virus is targeting as its host cell.

[0048] When a virus carries a DNA payload and the viral DNA is inserted into the host cell, the virus's DNA travels to the host cell's nucleus and is known to become inserted into the host cell's own native DNA. In the case where a virus is carrying its genetic payload as RNA, the virus inserts the RNA payload into the host cell and may also insert one or more enzymes to facilitate the RNA being utilized properly to replicate copies of the virus. Once inside the host cell, some species of virus facilitate use of the viral RNA by having the RNA converted to DNA. Once the viral RNA has been converted to DNA, the virus's DNA travels to the host cell's nucleus and is known to become inserted into the host cell's native DNA. Once a virus's genetic material has been inserted into the host cell's native DNA, the virus's genetic material takes command of certain cell functions and redirects the resources of the host cell to generate copies of the virus. Other forms of RNA viruses bypass the need to use the nuclear DNA and simply utilize portions of the viral genome to act as messenger RNA. RNA viruses that bypass the host cell's DNA, cause the cell in general to generate copies of the necessary parts of the virus directly from the virus's RNA genome.

[0049] The human immunodeficiency virus (HIV) has an outer envelope comprised of a lipid bilayer. The lipid bilayer covers a protein matrix consisting of $p17^{gag}$ proteins. Inside the $p17^{gag}$ protein is nested a nucleocapsid comprised of $p24^{gag}$ proteins. Inside the nucleocapsid HIV carries its payload. HIV's genetic payload consists of two single strands of RNA. In addition to the two strands of HIV RNA, there are proteins that are carried in the core of the nucleocapsid along with the two RNA strands. These proteins include 'reverse transcriptase', 'integrase' and 'protease' molecules.

[0050] The T-Helper cell acts as HIV's host cell. HIV locates its host by utilizing at least two different types of probes located on its envelope. The HIV virion utilizes two types of glycoprotein probes affixed to the outer surface of its external envelope to engage a T-Helper cell. HIV utilizes a glycoprotein probe 120 to locate a CD4 cell-surface receptor on a T-Helper cell. Once an HIV glycoprotein 120 probe has successfully engaged a CD4 cell surface-receptor on a T-Helper cell a conformational change occurs in the probe and a glycoprotein 41 probe is exposed. The glycoprotein 41 probe's intent is to engage a CXCR4 or CCR5 cell-surface receptor on the same T-Helper cell. Once a glycoprotein 41 probe on the HIV virion successfully engages a CXCR4 or CCR5 cell-surface receptor, the HIV virion opens an access portal through the T-Helper cell's outer membrane.

[0051] Once the HIV virion has opened an access portal through the T-Helper cell's outer plasma membrane, the HIV virion inserts two positive strand RNA molecules it carries into the T-Helper cell. Each RNA strand is approximately 9500 nucleotides in length. Inserted along with the RNA strands are the enzymes reverse transcriptase, protease and integrase. Once the virus's genome gains access to the interior of the T-Helper cell, in the cytoplasm the pair of RNA molecules are transformed to deoxyribonucleic acid by the reverse transcriptase enzyme. Following modification of the virus's genome to DNA, the virus's genetic information migrates to the host cell's nucleus. In the nucleus, with the assistance of the integrase protein, the HIV's DNA becomes inserted into the T-Helper cell's native DNA. When the timing is appropriate, the now integrated viral DNA is decoded by the host cell's polymerase molecules and the virus's genetic information commands certain cell functions to carry out the replication process to construct copies of the human deficiency virus.

[0052] The outer layer of the HIV virion is comprised of a portion of the T-Helper cell's outer cell membrane. In the final stage of the replication process, as a copy of the HIV capsid, carrying the HIV genome, buds through the host cell's cell membrane the capsid acquires as its external envelope, a wrapping of lipid bilayer from the host cell's cell membrane. In the case of HIV, since the surface of the pathogen is covered by an envelope comprised of lipid bilayer taken from the host T-Helper cells, this feature allows the HIV virion the capacity to eluded the immune systems, since the cells comprising the immune system may find it difficult to tell the difference between the surface of an infectious HIV virion and the surface characteristics of a noninfected T-Helper cell.

[0053] The Hepatitis C virus (HCV) is a positive sense RNA virus, meaning a type of RNA that is capable of bypassing the need for involving the host cell's nucleus by having its RNA genome function as messenger RNA. Hepatitis C infects liver cells. The Hepatitis C viral genome becomes divided once it gains access to the interior of a liver host cell. Portions of the subdivisions of the Hepatitis C genome directly interact with ribosomes to produce proteins necessary to construct copies of the virus.

[0054] HCV belongs to the Flaviviridae family and is the only member of the Hepacivirus genus. There are considered to be at least 100 different strains of Hepatitis C virus based on genome sequencing variability.

[0055] HCV is comprised of an outer lipoprotein envelope and an internal nucleocapsid. The genetic payload is carried within the nucleocapsid. In its natural state, present on the surface of the outer envelope of the Hepatitis C virus are probes that detect receptors present on the surface of liver cells. The glycoprotein E1 probe and the glycoprotein E2 probe have been identified to be affixed to the surface of HCV. The E2 probe binds with high affinity to the large external loop of a CD81 cell-surface receptor. CD81 is found on the surface of many cell types including liver cells. Once the E2 probe has engaged the CD81 cell-surface receptor, cofactors on the surface of HCV's external envelope engage either or both the low density lipoprotein receptor (LDLR) or the scavenger receptor class B type I (SR-BI) present on the liver cell in order to effect the mechanism to facilitate HCV breaching the cell membrane and inserting its RNA genome payload through the plasma cell membrane of the liver cell into the liver cell. Upon successful engagement of the HCV surface probes with a liver cell's cell-surface receptors,

HCV inserts the single strand of RNA and other payload elements it carries into the liver cell targeted to be a host cell. The HCV RNA genome then interacts with enzymes and ribosomes inside the liver cell in a translational process to produce the proteins required to construct copies of the protein components of HCV. The HCV genome undergoes a method of transcription to replicate copies of the virus's RNA genome. Inside the host, pieces of the HCV virus are assembled together and ultimately loaded with a copy of the HCV genome. Replicas of the original HCV then escape the host cell and migrate the environment in search of additional host liver cells to infect and continue the replication process.

[0056] The HCV's naturally occurring genetic payload consists of a single molecule of linear positive sense, single stranded RNA approximately 9600 nucleotides in length. By means of a translational process a polyprotein of approximately 3000 amino acids is generated. This polyprotein is cleaved post translation by host and viral proteases into individual viral proteins which include: the structural proteins of C, E1, E2, the nonstructural proteins NS1, NS2, NS3, NS4A, NS4B, NS5A, NS5B, p7 and ARFP/F protein. Hepatitis C virus's proteins direct the host liver cell to construction copies of the Hepatitis C virus. A membrane associated replicase complex consisting of the virus's nonstructural proteins NS3 and NS5B facilitate the replication of the viral genome. The membrane of the endoplasmic reticulum appears to be the site of protein maturation and viral assembly. Once copies of the Hepatitis C Virus are generated, they exit the host cell and each copy of HCV migrates in search of another appropriate liver cell that will act as a host to continue the replication process.

[0057] Hepatitis C virus life-cycle demonstrates that copies of a virus virion can be generated by inserting RNA into a host cell that functions as messenger RNA in the host cell. The Hepatitis C viral RNA genome functions as messenger RNA, acting as the template in conjunction with the biologic machinery of a host cell to produce the components that comprise copies of the Hepatitis C virion and the Hepatitis C viral RNA provides the biologic instructions to assemble the components into complete copies of the Hepatitis C virions. The Hepatitis C virus life-cycle clearly demonstrates that viral virions can be manufactured by a host cell without involving the nucleus of the cell.

[0058] Deciphering the existence, replication and behavior of viruses provides clear examples of several fundamental concepts, which include: (1) Viruses target specific cells in the body by means of identifying and engaging such target cells utilizing the probes projecting outward from the virus's exterior shell to make contact with cell-surface receptors located on the surface of the target cells, and (2) Viruses are capable of carrying various types of payloads including DNA, RNA and a variety of proteins.

[0059] Current gene therapy approach to attempting to deliver a payload to cells in the body use modified forms of existing viruses to act as transport devices to deliver genetic information. This approach is severely limited by restricting the virus virion to the target only cells the viral vector naturally seeks out and infects. Current gene therapy approach is further limited by using the pre-existing size of naturally occurring viruses, rather than being able to modify the size of the structure to be able to tailor the volumetric carrying capacity of the payload portion of the modified virus. Further gene therapy is restricted to utilizing naturally occurring viruses to deliver only genetic information; it has not previously been appreciated by those skilled in the art that virus-like transport devices might deliver to a variety of specific cell types a wide variety of differing payloads such as signaling proteins.

[0060] A dramatic, not previously recognized by those expert in the art is the need to develop a transport vehicle that can be fashioned to seek out specific types of cells and deliver to these cells nuclear signals. The external envelope of a transport should be constructed so as not to alert the immune system of its presence to prevent rejection of the vehicles. Transport vehicles should be capable of being configured to target any specific cell type and engage and deliver their payload only to that specific cell type. To this point, no such device has been conceived.

BRIEF SUMMARY OF THE INVENTION

[0061] Utilization of configurable microscopic medical payload delivery devices to deliver command RNAs to specific cell types facilitates a dramatic new approach to medical care. By selecting the type of probes that are present on the surface of the configurable microscopic medical payload delivery devices, specific types of cells can be targeted. By delivering command RNAs to specific cell types a wide variety of complex proteins and molecules can be generated in those specific cell types to produce medically beneficial results. A wide variety of medical conditions are treatable by utilizing this new and unique approach.

DETAILED DESCRIPTION

[0062] The future of medical treatment will be the widespread utilization of configurable microscopic medical payload delivery devices (CMMPDD) to deliver command RNAs directly to targeted cell types in the body.

[0063] For purposes of this text an 'external envelope' refers to the outermost covering of a virus or a virus-like transport device or a configurable microscopic medical payload delivery device. The external envelope may be comprised of a lipid layer, a lipid bilayer, the combination of a lipid layer affixed to a protein matrix or the combination of a lipid bilayer affixed to a protein matrix.

[0064] For purposes of this text an 'internal shell' refers to a protein matrix shell nested inside the external envelope. The inner most protein matrix shell is termed the nucleocapsid. The proteins that comprise the nucleocapsid are termed capsid proteins. In the center or core of the nucleocapsid is where the payload is carried.

[0065] For purposes of this text 'external probes' are molecular structures that are utilized to locate and engage cell-surface receptors on biologically active cells. External probes are generally comprised of a portion which is anchored or fixed in the external envelope and a second portion that extends out and away from the external envelope. External probes may be comprised solely of a protein structure or an external probe may be a glycoprotein molecule.

[0066] For purposes of this text 'glycoprotein molecule' refers to a molecule comprised of a carbohydrate region and a protein region. Glycoprotein molecules that act as probes are generally anchored or fixed to a lipid layer utilizing the carbohydrate portion of the molecule as an anchor. The protein portion of the glycoprotein molecule which extends outward and away from the external envelope the glycoprotein has been affixed such that the protein region may function as a probe to locate and attach to the cell-surface receptor it was created to engage.

[0067] The concept of configurable microscopic medical payload delivery devices is modeled after naturally existing viruses. Configurable microscopic medical payload delivery devices in general are spherical in shape; though other shapes may be used as function might warrant the use of a particular shape. The spherical configurable microscopic medical payload delivery devices are comprised of an external envelope and one or more inner nested protein shells. A quantity of exterior protein structure probes and/ or glycoprotein probes are anchored in the exterior lipid envelope and extend out and away from the exterior lipid envelope. Nesting of protein shells refers to progressively smaller diameter shells fitting snugly inside protein shells of a larger diameter. Inside the inner most protein shell, referred to as the nucleocapsid, is a cavity referred to as the core of the device. The core of the device is the space where the medically therapeutic payload the device carries is located.

[0068] Configurable microscopic medical payload delivery devices are generated to target certain specific cell types in the body. Configurable microscopic medical payload delivery devices target specific cell types by the configuration of probes affixed to the external envelope of the CMMPDD. By affixing specific probes to the external envelope of the CMMPDD, these probes intended to engage and attach only to specific cell-surface receptors located on certain cell types in the body, the CMMPDD will deliver its payload only to those cell types that express compatible and engagable specific cell-surface receptors. In a similar fashion where the exterior probes of a naturally occurring virus engage specific cell-surface receptors present on the surface of the virus's host cell and only the designated host cell, the CMMPDD's exterior probes are configured to engage cell-surface receptors on a specific type of target cell. In this manner, the payload of medication or biologic tools carried by CMMPDD will be delivered only to specific types of cells in the body. The exterior probes on the surface of a CMMPDD will vary as needed so as to effect the CMMPDD delivery of payloads to cell types as needed to effect a medical treatment.

[0069] The size of configurable microscopic medical payload delivery devices is to depend upon the volume size of the payload the CMMPDD is required to carry and deliver to a target cell. The size of a CMMPDD is dependent upon the diameter of the inner protein matrix shells. The diameter of each inner protein matrix shell is governed by the number of protein molecules utilized to construct the protein matrix shell at the time the protein matrix shell is generated. Increasing the number of proteins that comprise a protein matrix shell, increases the diameter of the protein matrix shell. The external lipid envelope wraps around and covers the outermost protein matrix shell. The larger the volume of the core of the CMMPDD, the greater the physical size payload the CMMPDD is able to carry. The size of the configurable microscopic medical payload delivery device is to be the size of cell (approximately 10^{-4} m in diameter) or less, generally detectable by a light microscope or, as needed, an electron microscope. The size of the CMMPDD is not to be too large such that it would generate a burden to the body by damaging organ tissues through clogging blood vessels, and the maintaining a small enough size that the CMMPDD can be properly disposed of by the body once the CMMPDD has delivered its payload to its target cell. The dimensions of each type of CMMPDD are to be tailored to the mission of the CMMPDD, which takes into account the type of target cell, the size of the payload that is to be delivered to the target cells and the length of time the CMMPDD may engage the target cell.

[0070] Being enveloped in an external lipid layer, configurable microscopic medical payload delivery devices possess the advantage of having their exterior appear similar to the plasma membrane that acts as an outside covering for the cells that comprise the body. By appearing similar to existing plasma membranes, the CMMPDDs appear similar to naturally occurring structures found in the body, affording the CMMPDD the capability to avoid detection by a body's immune system because the exterior of the CMMPDD mimics the cells comprising the body and the surveillance cells of the immune system find it difficult to discern between the CMMPDD and naturally occurring cells comprising the body.

[0071] To carry out the process of manufacturing a configurable microscopic medical payload delivery device, a primitive cell such as a stem cell is selected. The reason for utilizing primitive cells such as stems cells as the host cell, is that the CMMPDD acquires its outer envelope from the host cell and the more primitive the host cell, the fewer in number the identifying protein markers are present on the surface of the CMMPDD. The fewer the identifying surface proteins present on the outer envelope of the CMMPDD, the less likely a body's immune system will identify the CMMPDD as an invader and therefore less likely the body's immune system will react to the presence of the CMMPDD and reject the CMMPDD by attacking and neutralizing the CMMPDD.

[0072] Stem cells used as host cells to manufacture quantities of CMMPDD product are selected per histocompatibility markers present on their surface. Certain histocompatibility markers present on the surface of the final CMMPDD product will be less likely to cause a reaction in a specific patient based on the genetic profile of the patient's histocompatibility markers. A similar histocompatibility match is done when donor organs are selected to be given to recipients to avoid rejection of the donor organ by the recipient's immune system.

[0073] The selected stem cell used to manufacture configurable microscopic medical payload delivery devices goes through several steps of maturation before it is capable of generating therapeutic CMMPDD product. Messenger RNA is inserted into the host stem cell that would code for the general physical outer structures of the CMMPDD. Messenger RNA is inserted into the host that would generate surface probes that would target the surface receptors on specifically target cells. Messenger RNA is inserted into the host that would be used to generate the payload of command RNAs. Similar to how copies of a naturally occurring virus, such as the Hepatitis C virus or HIV, are produced, assembled and released from a host cell, copies of the CMMPDD are produced, assembled and released from a host cell. Once released from the host cell, the copies of the CMMPDD would be collected, then pooled together to produce a therapeutic dose to result in a medically beneficial effect.

[0074] The construction of the configurable microscopic medical payload delivery devices is performed by taking stem cells and inserting modified viral genetic programming into the stem cells. Stem cells are chosen as the host cell due to the low number of surface markers, which leads to less antigenicity in configurable microscopic medical payload delivery devices when the configurable microscopic medical payload delivery devices are released by the host cells and wrapped in an outer envelope comprised of the host cells' plasma membrane.

[0075] The stem cells used as host cells are suspended in a broth of nutrients and are kept at an optimum temperature to govern the rate of production of the CMMPDD product. Similar to the natural production of the Hepatitis C virus, the configurable microscopic medical payload delivery devices 'production genome' is introduced into the host stem cells. The configurable microscopic medical payload delivery devices production genome carries genetic instructions to cause the host cells to manufacture the configurable microscopic medical payload delivery devices' outer protein wall, the inner protein matrixes, the surface probes the configurable microscopic medical payload delivery device is to have affixed to its outer envelope and the command RNAs the configurable microscopic medical payload delivery devices are to carry; and the instructions to assemble the various pieces into the final form of the configurable microscopic medical payload delivery devices and the instructions to activate the budding process. The resultant configurable microscopic medical payload delivery devices are collected from the nutrient broth surrounding the host cells and placed together into doses to be used as a treatment for a medical disease.

[0076] The 'production genome' are an array of messenger RNAs that are directly translated by the host cell's internal enzymes. The production genome dictates the characteristics of the final version of the CMMPDD that buds from the host stem cell and is released and is to be utilized as a medical treatment. The production genome is specifically tailored to code for the surface probes that will seek and engage a specific type of target cell. The production genome also carries the instructions to code for the production of the type of command RNAs to be delivered to the specific type of target cell. The 'production genome' varies depending upon the configuration of the CMMPDD and the type of command RNAs the CMMPDD is to transport to effect a specific medical treatment on a specific type of cell.

[0077] The configurable microscopic medical payload delivery device transporting command RNAs represents a very versatile medical treatment delivery device. There are an estimated 30,000 differing proteins generated by human cells; many of these proteins being complex molecules with (1) either more than one polypeptide chain or (2) a combination of a protein chain combined with another type of molecule other than a molecule. CMMPDD could be used to deliver command RNAs to generate any complex protein in any specific cell type in the body.

[0078] As an example of this method, to treat diabetes mellitus utilizing configurable microscopic medical payload delivery devices to deliver to Beta cells messenger RNA coded to produce insulin, the following production process is followed in the lab: (1) human stem cells are selected. (2) Into the selected stem cells is placed the production genome constructed, in this case, specifically as a means to treat diabetes mellitus. The RNA production genome contains genetic instructions to cause the host stem cells to manufacture the configurable microscopic medical payload delivery devices' outer protein wall, the inner protein matrix, surface probes to include glycoprotein probes that engage the GPR40 cell-surface receptor present on the surface of Beta cells located in the Islets of Langerhans in the pancreas, and the payload of command RNAs coded to generate insulin molecules; and the biologic instructions to assemble the components into the final form of the configurable microscopic medical payload delivery devices; and the biologic instructions to activate the budding process. (3) Upon insertion of the RNA production genome dedicated to producing a command RNAs configured to activate the genes to generate messenger RNA that will result in the production of insulin, into the host stem cells, host stem cells respond by (i) simultaneously translating the different segments of the RNA production genome to produce the proteins that comprise the exterior protein wall, the inner protein matrix molecules, the surface probes to seek out and engage Beta cells, the command RNA payload to produce insulin, and (ii) decoding the RNA instructions to assemble the components into the configurable microscopic medical payload delivery devices. (4) Upon assembly, the configurable microscopic medical payload delivery devices bud through the cell membrane of the host stem cell. (5) At the time of the budding process, the configurable microscopic medical payload delivery devices acquire an outside envelope wrapped over the outer protein shell, this outer envelope comprised of a portion of the plasma membrane from the host stem cell as the configurable microscopic medical payload delivery devices exit the host cell. (6) The resultant configurable microscopic medical payload delivery devices are collected from the nutrient broth surrounding the host stem cells. (7) The configurable microscopic medical payload delivery devices are washed in sterile solvent to remove contaminants. (8) The configurable microscopic medical payload delivery devices are removed from the sterile solvent and suspended in a hypoallergenic liquid medium. (9) The configurable microscopic medical payload delivery devices are separated into individual quantities to facilitate storage and delivery to physicians and patients. (10) The configurable microscopic medical payload delivery devices transported in the hypoallergenic liquid medium is administered to a diabetic patient per injection in a dose that is tailored to receiving patient's requirement to produce sufficient amount of insulin to control the blood sugar. (11) Upon being injected into the body, the configurable microscopic medical payload delivery devices migrate to the Beta cells located in the Islets of Langerhans by means of the patient's blood stream. (12) Upon the configurable microscopic medical payload delivery devices reaching the Beta cells, the configurable microscopic medical payload delivery devices engage the cell-surface receptors located on the Beta cells and insert the payload they carry into the Beta cells. The payload being command RNAs configured to produce insulin molecules. The increase in insulin production by Beta cells successfully manages diabetes mellitus.

Conclusions, Ramification, and Scope

[0079] Accordingly, the reader will see that the configurable microscopic medical payload delivery device to deliver command RNAs to specific targeted cell types provides advantages over existing art by (1) being a delivery device that seeks out specific types of cells, (2) by being a delivery device that is versatile enough to deliver a variety of potential command RNAs to accomplish various medical treatments and (3) by being a delivery device constructed with a surface envelope that will avoid detection by the innate immune system so as not to activate the immune system to its presence; for these reasons this represents a new and unique medical delivery device that has never before been recognized nor appreciated by those skilled in the art.

[0080] Although the description above contains specificities, these should not be construed as limiting the scope of the invention but as merely providing illustrations of some of the presently preferred embodiments of the invention.

[0081] Thus the scope of the invention should be determined by the appended claims and their legal equivalents, rather than by the examples given.

CLAIMS: Reserved.